Library of
Davidson College

PSYCHOPHYSIOLOGY OF THE GASTROINTESTINAL TRACT

Experimental and Clinical Applications

PSYCHOPHYSIOLOGY OF THE GASTROINTESTINAL TRACT
Experimental and Clinical Applications

Edited by
Rupert Hölzl
Max Planck Institute of Psychiatry
Munich, Federal Republic of Germany

and
William E. Whitehead
Johns Hopkins School of Medicine
Baltimore, Maryland

PLENUM PRESS • NEW YORK AND LONDON

Library of Congress Cataloging in Publication Data

Main entry under title:

Psychophysiology of the gastrointestinal tract.

Includes bibliographies and index.
1. Gastrointestinal system—Diseases—Psychosomatic aspects. I. Hölzl, Rupert. II. Whitehead, William E. [DNLM: 1. Gastrointestinal diseases—Psychology—Congresses. 2. Gastrointestinal diseases—Physiopathology—Congresses. 3. Psychosomatic medicine—Congresses. 4. Gastrointestinal system—Physiology—Congresses. WI 100 P974 1980]
RC802.P76 1983   616.3′08   83-4033
ISBN 0-306-41089-3

© 1983 Plenum Press, New York
A Division of Plenum Publishing Corporation
233 Spring Street, New York, N.Y. 10013

All rights reserved

No part of this book may be reproduced, stored in a retrieval system, or transmitted in any form or by any means, electronic, mechanical, photocopying, microfilming, recording, or otherwise, without written permission from the Publisher

Printed in the United States of America

To
the Max-Planck-Gesellschaft
and the
Deutsche Forschungsgemeinschaft,
who generously supported the conference
out of which this book grew.

To
Helga, Phebe, and our parents,
who were so patient.

CONTRIBUTORS

GYÖRGY ÁDÁM Department of Comparative Physiology, Eötvös University of Budapest, Budapest, Hungary

HEINRICH A. BRÜCHLE Department of Psychology, Max Planck Institute of Psychiatry, Munich, The Federal Republic of Germany

HERBERT LIVINGSTON DUTHIE Welsh National School of Medicine, Cardiff, Wales

BERNARD T. ENGEL Gerontology Research Center (Baltimore), National Institute on Aging, National Institutes of Health, P.H.S., U.S. Department of Health and Human Services, Bethesda, and the Baltimore City Hospital, Baltimore, Maryland

RUPERT HÖLZL Department of Psychology, Max Planck Institute of Psychiatry, Munich, The Federal Republic of Germany

PAUL R. LATIMER Behavior Therapy and Research Unit, Temple University Medical School, Philadelphia, Pennsylvania

GERHARD M. MÜLLER Department of Psychology, Max Planck Institute of Psychiatry, Munich, The Federal Republic of Germany

WILLIAM C. ORR Department of Clinical Physiology, Presbyterian Hospital, Oklahoma City, Oklahoma

ROBERT PAZULINEK Department of Human Development Counseling, George Peabody College of Vanderbilt University, Nashville, Tennessee

THOMAS SAJWAJ Behavioral Medicine Program, Lamar Medical Center, Vernon, Alabama

MARVIN M. SCHUSTER The Johns Hopkins School of Medicine and the Division of Digestive Diseases, Baltimore City Hospital, Baltimore, Maryland

GEORG STACHER Psychophysiology Unit at the Psychiatric and at the First Surgical Clinic, University of Vienna, Vienna, Austria

ROBERT M. STERN Department of Psychology, The Pennsylvania State University, University Park, Pennsylvania

BARBARA B. WALKER Ann Arbor Veterans Administration Medical Center and University of Michigan, Ann Arbor, Michigan

WILLIAM E. WHITEHEAD Department of Psychiatry, the Johns Hopkins School of Medicine, and Department of Medicine, Baltimore City Hospital, Baltimore, Maryland

PETER R. WELGAN Department of Psychiatry and Human Behavior, University of California at Irvine and 1001 Dove Street, Suite 280, Newport Beach, California

FOREWORD

Over a quarter century ago, Flanders Dunbar, in her 1954 compendium on "Emotion and Bodily Changes," surveyed over 5,000 references on psychosomatic interrelationships, including a literature on psychic factors in gastrointestinal disorders dating back to 1845. The title of the present volume suggests a line of descent from these early initiatives, but important changes are in the making. Indeed, the form and substance of long overdue reformulations are clearly reflected in the scholarly contributions which enhance this report of the 1980 Munich symposium proceedings.

Traditional psychosomatic approaches to understanding the gastrointestinal system and its functional disorders have been based in large part on two virtually unchallenged assumptions. In the first instance, unobserved (indeed unobservable) "psychological processes" have been considered causally related to disease onset and/or to fluctuations in the course of the disease. And secondly, it has been assumed that "psychotherapeutic" interventions for disease management should be designed to alter these hypothesized "psychic" antecedents. More recently, however, a new paradigm for analyzing the relationships involving disordered physiological functions and behavioral interactions has been developed within the framework of what has been termed *behavioral medicine*. The conceptual boundaries of this relatively new approach to behavioral physiology have not yet been firmly established, but the major differences between the new "behavioral" model and the traditional "psychosomatic" model are brought into sharp relief by the experimental and clinical contributions to the present volume.

In contrast to conventional psychosomatic formulations, more contemporary behavioral models focus upon operationally definable constructs. Most importantly, the behavioral medicine approach illustrated in these proceedings depends upon a thorough analysis of changes in physiology and behavior to identify relevant interactions as a basis for intervention—either direct behavioral manipulation of physiology or alteration of other behaviors related to the disorder or its treatment. Demonstration of a causal relationship between "psychological" processes and either the etiology or course of the disease is not a necessary precondition for behavioral intervention. And since a behavioral approach which takes physiology as its starting point is clearly relevant to virtually all medical disorders, applications are not constrained by the need to define such disorders as "psychosomatic" in nature.

It is clearly within this operational framework that the present volume is presented as perhaps the first substantive bridge between the traditional psychosomatic approach and the contemporary behavioral medicine approach to gastrointestinal disease. The obvious emphasis upon physiological measurement and objective behavioral analysis reflected in the ensuing chapters satisfies the operational requirements of a sound behavioral physiology. By the same token, the broad scope of environmental interactions to which more "psychosocially" oriented approaches have called attention have not been neglected. To the extent that such formulations have proven less than fruitful in the past, difficulty in specifying the physiological rationale for hypothesized relationships may well have been at the core of the problem. A clear formulation of how such environmental and behavioral variables interact with gastrointestinal function is obviously essential to asking the correct experimental questions and interpreting clinical observations. The strengths of the present volume reside in just such an analysis of the pathophysiology of gastrointestinal disorders and its relationship to the processes which mediate contact with behavior–environment interactions.

In this latter regard, the varied contributions represented in these proceedings are importantly linked to another *experimental* tradition which has been somewhat neglected over the past several decades. In 1956, Sawrey and Weisz first reported the production of gastric ulcers in rats under conditions which they described as behavioral "conflict." Although a range of confounding environmental conditions complicated the interpretation of these findings, several subsequent experiments with both laboratory primates and humans confirmed the demonstratively powerful influence of behavioral interactions upon the gastrointestinal system and its functional disorders. Despite extensive experimental work stimulated by these early findings, "laboratory stress" models for peptic ulcer disease were considered of questionable relevance to human clinical problems. But the stage had been set for an experimental analytic approach to the behavioral physiology of the gastrointestinal system, and renewed research interest in the esophagus and colon served to broaden the scope of investigative emphasis. A timely, comprehensive, and authoritative coverage of the most recent progress in experimental and clinical applications as they relate to the psychophysiology of the gastrointestinal tract is provided by the impressive and well-organized collection of contributions presented in the ensuing pages of this volume.

Joseph V. Brady

Professor of Behavioral Biology
The Johns Hopkins School of Medicine

PREFACE

This book contains a collection of papers based on contributions to the First International Symposium on "The Psychophysiology of the Gut: Clinical and Experimental Applications," which was held at Schloss Ringberg/Tegernsee in Bavaria, June 30–July 4, 1980. The conference was sponsored by the Deutsche Forschungsgemeinschaft and the Max-Planck-Gesellschaft. The purpose of both the conference and the resulting book are to stimulate more psychophysiologists to engage in research on the gastrointestinal tract. It was our feeling that the understanding and treatment of gastrointestinal diseases could be advanced greatly if psychophysiologists and behavioral psychologists could be enticed to collaborate with gastroenterologists on these problems.

The need for such collaborative research is great, and it is apparent to gastroenterologists. An estimated 40%–70% of consultations to gastroenterology clinics are for functional disorders which most physicians feel they cannot treat adequately. Moreover, the contributions of biofeedback and behavioral approaches to the successful treatment of fecal incontinence and ruminative vomiting syndrome are known to most gastroenterologists and have made them receptive to collaboration. Within the last few years the American Gastroenterological Association has created a task force to stimulate research along these lines, and the National Institute on Arthritis, Diabetes, and Digestive and Kidney Diseases sponsored a workshop in 1979 for a similar purpose. Clearly the time is right.

The goal of stimulating more psychophysiologists to undertake this research has determined the format of the conference and the book. We wanted first to describe the physiological measurement techniques in sufficient detail so that people outside the area would know how to begin. Second, we attempted to summarize the basic psychophysiology of each part of the gastrointestinal tract; that is, the evidence that the organ is responsive to environmental events. Lastly, we sought to describe applications of psychophysiological methods to treatment and to identify directions for future research.

We brought together at a Bavarian castle a small group of people whom we regarded as the most outstanding scientists in the area of gastrointestinal psychophysiology and asked them to discuss these topics for a week. Each participant presented one or more formal papers on methodology, responsiveness to environmental events, or application, but more than half the meeting was devoted to informal discussion. The participants were then requested to revise their papers after they returned home so as to incorporate the discussion. The result, we hope, is a rather comprehensive statement on the state of the art in those areas of gastrointestinal psychophysiology we chose to emphasize.

The reader will notice that some topics have been omitted. We did not deal with the small intestine or the gall bladder because these organs are relatively inaccessible to psychophysiological measurement. (Psychophysiological studies require continuous measurement, preferably in real time.) There is consequently no significant literature on the responsiveness of these organs to environmental events, and we do not anticipate that there will be. The experimental literature on salivation was omitted because, from the perspective of understanding and treating gastrointestinal disorders, salivation is trivial; collaboration between gastroenterologists and psychophysiologists on the study of salivation is unlikely. We have also omitted any specific discussion of the extensive literature on the respondent conditioning of gastrointestinal responses, although Pavlovian conditioning is alluded to by several authors. This occurred because little work on Pavlovian conditioning in humans is currently being done, with the exception of the conditioned taste aversion work of Garcia and his colleagues (cf. Chapter 17).

The book is divided into major anatomical divisions—esophagus, stomach, colon, and rectum—plus a section on visceral perception at the end. Each section begins with an introduction by one of the editors which provides the background necessary to understand the papers which follow.

The editors would like to acknowledge some of the people who helped us to organize the symposium and to prepare the manuscripts. Foremost among these was Silvia Pattay, who managed the detailed arrangements for the conference with such competence and who spent long hours transcribing the taped discussions and editing manuscripts. Neither the conference nor the book could have happened without her. Particular thanks are also due to Suzi Chntek, Henry Brüchle, and Gerhard Müller from the Psychology Department of the Max Planck Institute of Psychiatry, who also worked to make the conference a success. Henry Brüchle's and Gerhard Müller's pleasant and stimulating collaboration with one of us (Rupert Hölzl) may certainly be called one of the roots out of which the conference and, finally, the book have grown. E. Darcie Morrill also helped with the editing of manuscripts, and the John F. Kennedy Institute for Handicapped Children in Baltimore helped with the typing. Finally, we would like to thank Professor E. Ploog and Professor J. Brengelman of the Max Planck Institute for their valuable support in our efforts to organize the symposium. We hope that this book and the further research it may stimulate will justify their efforts.

Rupert Hölzl
William E. Whitehead

CONTENTS

Part I
Esophagus.................................... 1
RUPERT HÖLZL

Chapter 1
Studies of Esophageal Function during Waking and Sleep
WILLIAM C. ORR

1. Introduction................................... 5
2. Tests of Esophageal Function 6
   2.1. Esophageal Motility........................ 6
   2.2. Clinical Tests of Acid Clearance............. 12
   2.3. Esophageal pH Monitoring 12
3. Esophageal Function during Sleep.................. 14
4. Implications and Future Studies................... 19
5. References..................................... 20

Chapter 2
The Responsiveness of the Esophagus to Environmental Stimuli
GEORG STACHER

1. Introduction................................... 21
2. Types of Esophageal Motility 21
3. Relation of Tertiary Contractions to Psychological Stress 22
4. Experimental Studies of Acoustically Induced Esophageal Contractions................................... 24
   4.1. Intensity of Stimuli Required to Produce Contractions 24
   4.2. Orienting versus Defense Reactions 25

5. Implications for Understanding and Treatment of Esophageal Motor Disorders ... 28
6. References ... 30

Chapter 3
Disorders of the Esophagus: Applications of Psychophysiological Methods to Treatment
MARVIN M. SCHUSTER

1. Introduction ... 33
2. Disorders of the Esophagus ... 33
   2.1. Globus Hystericus ... 34
   2.2. Diffuse Esophageal Spasm ... 34
   2.3. Reflux Esophagitis ... 34
   2.4. Achalasia ... 35
3. Physiology of the Lower Esophageal Sphincter ... 36
   3.1. Reflex Motor Responses ... 36
   3.2. Pharmacology of the LES ... 36
4. Biofeedback Training to Raise Lower Esophageal Sphincter Pressure ... 37
5. References ... 42

Chapter 4
Psychological Treatment Approaches to Psychogenic Vomiting and Rumination
ROBERT PAZULINEC AND THOMAS SAJWAJ

1. Introduction ... 43
2. Clinical Syndrome ... 44
   2.1. Topography ... 44
   2.2. Etiology ... 46
   2.3. Clinical Consequences ... 48
3. Treatment Approaches ... 49
   3.1. Medical Interventions ... 49
   3.2. Massive Attention ... 50
   3.3. Psychotherapy ... 51
   3.4. Peripheral Electric Shock Therapy ... 52
   3.5. Taste Aversion Methods ... 54
   3.6. Differential Reinforcement and Other Behavioral Techniques ... 56
4. Comparison of Treatment Approaches ... 59
5. Conclusions ... 60
6. References ... 61

Part II
Stomach 65
RUPERT HÖLZL

Chapter 5
Surface Gastrograms as Measures of Gastric Motility
RUPERT HÖLZL

1.	Introduction: A Short History of Gastric Motility Records	69
2.	Electromotor Activity of the Stomach	72
	2.1. The Role of Indices of Electromotor Activity	72
	2.2. Contractile Activity of the Stomach	74
	2.3. Electrical Activity of the Stomach	76
3.	Signal Parameters of Gastric Activity and Their Psychophysiological Information Content	79
4.	Electrical Recordings from the Abdominal Surface: Current Practice in Psychophysiology	82
	4.1. Apparatus and Procedures: Overview	83
	4.2. Recording Sites	86
	4.3. Signal Analysis	92
	4.4. Validity of Electrogastrograms—Critical Evaluation	105
5.	Magnetogastrography	109
	5.1. Classical Methods	109
	5.2. Three-Axes Magnetogastrogram with Freely Moving Magnet.	110
	5.3. Magnetogastrographies with Ferromagnetic Tracer Material..	111
	5.4. Signal Analysis	113
6.	Conclusion	113
7.	References	114

Chapter 6
Conjoint Gastrography: Principles and Techniques
GERHARD M. MÜLLER, RUPERT HÖLZL, AND HEINRICH A. BRÜCHLE

1.	Introduction	123
2.	Rationale of Conjoint Gastrography	124
3.	Electrogastrograms	125
	3.1. Recording Sites	125
	3.2. Electrodes and Skin Preparation	126
	3.3. Amplifiers and Filters	127

4.	Magnetogastrograms	129
	4.1. Magnetometers and Magnetic Capsules	129
	4.2. Amplifiers and Filters	130
	4.3. Procedure	130
	4.4. Procedure with Ferrite Test Meal	132
5.	General Procedure and Control Measurements	133
6.	Data Acquisition	135
	6.1. Laboratory Configuration	135
	6.2. Portable Data Logging	135
7.	Signal Analysis	136
	7.1. Overview	136
	7.2. Principles of Fourier Analysis in Gastrography	136
	7.3. Basic Fourier Mathematics	140
	7.4. Auto- and Cross-spectral Analyses of Conjoint Gastrograms	147
	7.5. Evaluation of Spectra	151
8.	Selected Results	153
	8.1. Peak Histograms	155
	8.2. Cross-Correlograms	155
	8.3. Coherence Functions	155
9.	References	158

Chapter 7
Measurement of Gastric Acid Secretion

PETER R. WELGAN

1.	Introduction	161
2.	Measurement of Gastric Acid	162
	2.1. The pH Method	162
	2.2. The pH Meter–Titration Method	163
	2.3. Titration with Chemical Indicators	163
3.	Tests of Gastric Secretory Function	164
	3.1. Basal Acid Output (BAO)	164
	3.2. Peak Acid Output (PAO), Maximal Acid Output (MAO), and Calculated Maximal Acid Output (CMAO)	164
4.	Psychophysiological Measures of Gastric Acid	164
	4.1. Intragastric Measures	165
	4.2. External Measurement of Gastric Acid	167
5.	Subject Considerations in Gastric Research	169
	5.1. Subject Selection	169
	5.2. Subject Preparation	169
	5.3. Intubation Procedure	170
6.	References	171

Chapter 8
Telemetric and Isotope Methods of Measuring Gastric Acid Secretion, Motility, and Emptying
GEORG STACHER

1.	Measurement of Gastric Acid Secretion by Intragastric Titration and a Telemetering pH Sensor	173
2.	Measurement of Intragastric Pressures by Means of a Telemetering Capsule	175
3.	Measurement of Gastric Motility and Emptying by a Radioisotope Technique	177
4.	References	177

Chapter 9
Responsiveness of the Stomach to Environmental Events
ROBERT M. STERN

1.	Introduction	181
2.	Causes for Inadequate Information about Stomach Responsiveness	181
	2.1. Unreliability of Subjective Reports	182
	2.2. Difficulties with All Known Recording Techniques	186
	2.3. Confounding by Digestive Functions	187
	2.4. Confounding by Spontaneous Activity	189
3.	Passive Responding to External Situations	191
	3.1. Temperature	191
	3.2. Tones and Lights	193
	3.3. Fear, Anger, and Other Emotional States	196
4.	Active Responding to External Stimuli	199
	4.1. Exercise	199
	4.2. Mental Arithmetic	200
	4.3. Stress and Ulceration	200
5.	Summary and Conclusions	204
6.	References	205

Chapter 10
Treating Stomach Disorders: Can We Reinstate Regulatory Processes?
BARBARA B. WALKER

1.	Introduction	209
2.	Structure, Function, and Disorders of the Stomach	210
3.	Regulation	213

	3.1.	The Role of Efferent Activity in Regulation	214
	3.2.	The Role of Afferent Activity in Regulation	215
4.	Disregulation of the Stomach		216
5.	Reinstating Regulatory Processes		219
	5.1.	The Medical Approach to Treating Stomach Disorders	219
	5.2.	The Psychoanalytic Approach to Treating Stomach Disorders	222
	5.3.	The Psychobiological Approach to Treating Stomach Disorders	223
	5.4.	Biofeedback and Gastric Activity	226
6.	Summary		228
7.	References		229

Part III
Colon 235
WILLIAM E. WHITEHEAD

Chapter 11
The Measurement of Colon Motility
MARVIN M. SCHUSTER

1.	Introduction	239
2.	Measurement of the Segmenting Contractions of the Distal Colon	239
	2.1. Concept of Paradoxical Motility	239
	2.2. Recording Techniques	240
	2.3. Stimulation Techniques	241
	2.4. Quantification Techniques	244
3.	Assessment of Compliance of the Bowel Wall	245
4.	Assessment of Evacuation	247
5.	References	249

Chapter 12
Measurement of Electrical Activity of the Colon in Man
HERBERT LIVINGSTON DUTHIE

1.	Introduction	251
2.	Methods	251
	2.1. *In Vivo*	251
	2.2. *In Vitro*	252
3.	Normal Electrical Patterns *in Vivo*	253

	3.1.	Slow Waves	253
	3.2.	Fast Activity	255
4.	Normal Electrical Patterns *in Vitro*		257
	4.1.	Longitudinal Muscle	257
	4.2.	Circular Muscle	257
5.	Abnormal Electrical Patterns		258
	5.1.	Diverticular Disease	258
	5.2.	Irritable Bowel Syndrome	258
	5.3.	Other Functional Disorders	259
6.	Summary		260
7.	References		260

Chapter 13
Colonic Psychophysiology: Implications for Functional Bowel Disorders
PAUL R. LATIMER

1.	Introduction		263
	1.1.	Early Observations on Gastrointestinal Responsiveness	263
	1.2.	Early Observations on Colonic Responsiveness	264
2.	Colonic Psychophysiology		264
	2.1.	Pioneering Experiments	264
	2.2.	Hyper- versus Hypomotor Responsiveness	266
3.	Implications for Functional Bowel Disorders		268
	3.1.	Five Hypotheses	268
	3.2.	Abnormal Colonic Responsiveness Hypothesis	268
	3.3.	Abnormal Stimulation Hypothesis	278
	3.4.	Abnormal Interoception Hypothesis	280
	3.5.	Illness Behavior Hypothesis	282
	3.6.	Heterogeneity Hypothesis	283
	3.7.	Treatment Implications	284
4.	Conclusion		285
5.	References		285

Chapter 14
Irritable Bowel Syndrome: Applications of Psychophysiological Methods to Treatment
MARVIN M. SCHUSTER

1.	Introduction	289
2.	Diagnostic Criteria for Irritable Bowel Syndrome	290

3. Psychophysiology of Irritable Bowel Syndrome 290
   3.1. Effects of Meals 291
   3.2. Psychological Characteristics of Patients with Irritable Bowel Syndrome 293
   3.3. Pain from Gas 295
4. Fiber in the Treatment of Functional Bowel Disorders 296
5. Biofeedback Training to Decrease Colonic Motility 296
6. References 297

Part IV
Anal Canal and Rectum 299
WILLIAM E. WHITEHEAD

Chapter 15
Fecal Incontinence and Encopresis: A Psychophysiological Analysis
BERNARD T. ENGEL

1. Introduction 301
2. Diagnosis 302
3. Analysis of Mechanism 305
4. Intervention 309
5. References 310

Chapter 16
Manometric and Electromyographic Techniques for Assessment of the Anorectal Mechanism for Continence and Defecation
WILLIAM E. WHITEHEAD AND MARVIN M. SCHUSTER

1. Introduction 311
2. Anatomy and Physiology 312
3. Measurement Techniques 313
   3.1. External Anal Sphincter Contraction 313
   3.2. Sensibility for Rectal Distension 318
   3.3. Internal Anal Sphincter 320
4. Applications of Psychophysiological Methods to Treatment of Incontinence 326
5. References 328

Part V
Interoception 331
WILLIAM E. WHITEHEAD

Chapter 17
Interoception: Awareness of Sensations Arising in the Gastrointestinal Tract
WILLIAM E. WHITEHEAD

1. Introduction... 333
2. Methods of Investigating Visceral Perception................... 335
   2.1. Method of Limits..................................... 335
   2.2. Signal Detection Analysis 336
   2.3. Forced Choice Procedure.............................. 336
   2.4. Confounding of Perception and Control................. 336
   2.5. Discrimination Training............................... 337
3. Behavioral Significance of Visceral Perception 337
   3.1. Cuing Function in Bowel Control...................... 338
   3.2. Hunger and Satiety 338
   3.3. Labeling of Emotions 341
   3.4. Acquisition and Retention of Voluntary Control over a Visceral Response 343
   3.5. Psychosomatic Etiology............................... 344
4. Summary and Conclusions.................................. 346
5. References.. 348

Chapter 18
Intestinal Afferent Influence on Behavior
GYÖRGY ÁDÁM

1. Introduction... 351
2. Research Strategies....................................... 352
3. Subjective Detection of Gastrointestinal Stimuli................. 355
4. Effects of Stimulus Intensity and Site of Stimulation............ 356
5. References.. 360

Index 361

PART I

ESOPHAGUS
RUPERT HÖLZL

At one time or other, most of us have felt as if we had a "lump in the throat," had a "heartburn," or experienced mild or severe sickness in fearful situations. Many people suffer from frequent pains in the chest that are not due to cardiac dysfunction but seem to be related to "stress." All these observations relate esophageal function to psychological events, and the list could be prolonged indefinitely. Apart from anecdotal information and unsystematic clinical observation (cf. Schwidders, 1965) extremely little experimental data on psychological determinants of esophageal responses are available. An earlier Russian work (cf. Bykow, 1957; Razran, 1961) generally was not followed up by American and European researchers. Esophageal psychophysiology, therefore, is still in its early stages.

The chapters by Orr and Stacher describe recent attempts to analyze some basic esophageal functions and their modification by environmental influences. Stacher's study is one of the few to demonstrate defensive reactions of the esophageal smooth muscle to external (acoustic) stimuli that are clearly separated from normal peristaltic contractions following a swallow. The classical orienting-defensive response methodology employed by Stacher has proven very valuable in other areas of psychophysiology. It should be exploited more extensively in research on esophageal reactions. Stacher also demonstrates that much methodological work and technical improvements have to be achieved to make intensive study of esophageal functions possible and to relate it to clinical notions about psychosomatic factors in functional esophagus disorders. Orr adds to this issue with a very interesting experimental paradigm. He stresses the necessity of comparing esophageal responses during waking and sleep. Especially in persons suffering from gastroesophageal reflux and consequential esophagitis, motor activity of the lower esophageal sphincter seems to be changed in a characteristic

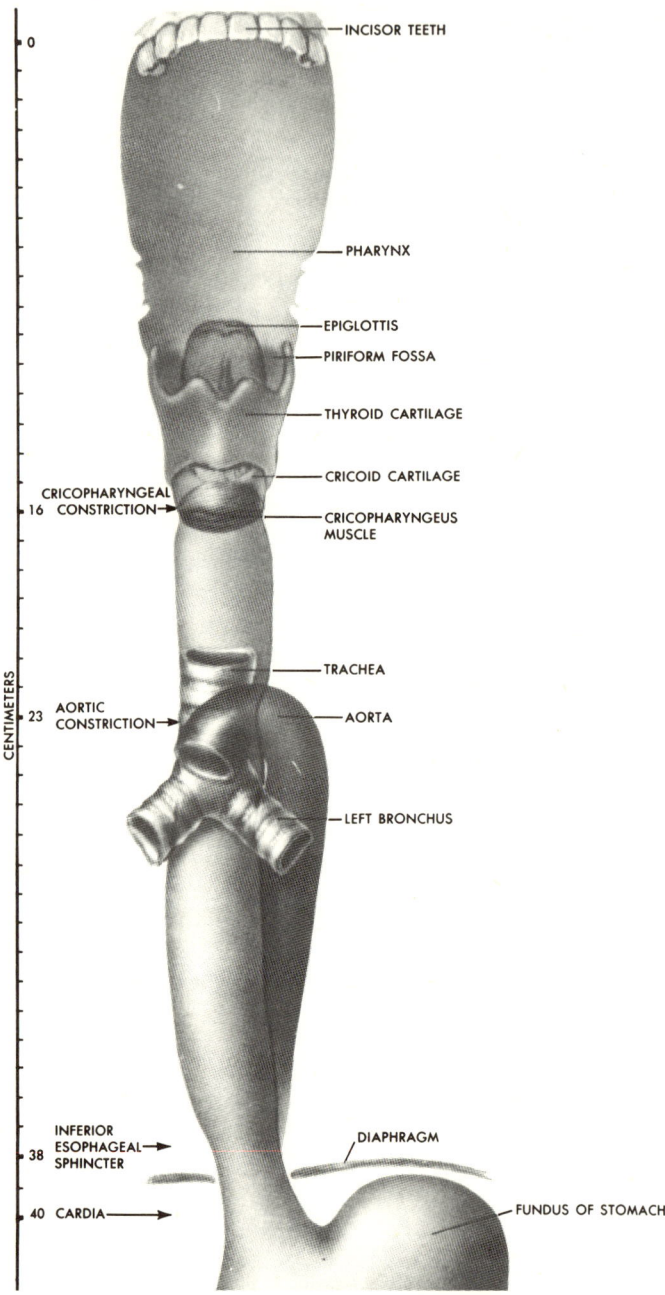

Figure 1. Anatomical main structures of esophagus. (Reproduced from F. H. Netter, 1958, with permission.)

way. This could well lead to important diagnostic improvements possibly with therapeutic consequences.

Schuster's paper amplifies this issue by demonstrating beginning psychophysiological treatment efforts for patients suffering from various functional esophageal disorders. The biofeedback treatment for insufficient lower esophageal sphincter seems very promising but needs further clinical validation. Here again technical problems so far have hindered clinical progress. No really "noninvasive" method for esophageal measurement is available or even feasible today. Therefore, not much is known about basic esophageal functions and their control by higher centers.

For instance, the mechanism of psychogenic vomiting is not well understood. Successful modification by operant techniques, however, shows the important role the central nervous system (CNS) plays in the regulation of esophageal function, despite the scarcity of data directly from psychophysiology. Pazulinek and Sajwaj review this alternative approach in some detail and connect it to the work on conditioned taste aversions (cf. Chapters 18 and 19 by Whitehead & Ádám). This chapter is particularly noteworthy for several reasons. It presents one of the most successful and well-documented behavioral approaches to functional disorders in the alimentary tract. The purely operant approach does not need bulky equipment like some of the psychophysiological methods described in the rest of the book. In this respect operant treatment of vomiting and rumination is a typical example of a group of techniques which have been subsumed under the spreading discipline of "behavioral medicine."

The impressive clinical success of operant modification of vomiting and rumination leads back to basic questions of how this is physiologically mediated. The bridge between the two research efforts must be closed by more basic psychophysiological work along the line Schuster and Orr have shown and include other physiological response systems, too. Research into the question of how nausea is related to vomiting may be a suitable starting point. The work of Cowings, Billingham, and Toscano (1977) on biofeedback and self-control in astronauts could be the beginning of this type of analysis. Labyrinthic nausea has been investigated extensively by physiologists and should provide a good experimental model to study the mechanisms by which CNS factors control esophageal functioning.

For those readers not familiar with the basic functional anatomy of the esophagus, Figure 1 summarizes the most important structures and common nomenclature.

References

Bykow, K. M. *The cerebral cortex and the internal organs* (W. H. Gantt, Trans.). New York: Chemical Publishing Co., 1957.

Cowings, P. S., Billingham, J., & Toscano, B. W. Learned control of multiple autonomic responses to compensate for the debilitating effects of motion sickness. *Theory in Psychosomatic Medicine*, 1977, *4*, 318–323.

Netter, F. H. *The Ciba collection of medical illustrations* (Vol. III, Pt. 1). New York: Ciba, 1958.

Razran, G. The observable unconscious and the inferable conscious in current Soviet psychophysiology: Interoceptive conditioning, semantic conditioning, and the orienting reflex. *Psychological Review*, 1961, *68*, 81–147.

Schwidders, W. Psychosomatic and Psychotherapie bei Störungen und Erkrankungen des Verdauungstraktes. *Acta Psychosomatica No. 7*. Basel: Geigy, 1965.

1

STUDIES OF ESOPHAGEAL FUNCTION DURING WAKING AND SLEEP

WILLIAM C. ORR

1. Introduction

Although the gut has long been recognized as the site of powerful but obscure influences from the central nervous system (CNS), interest has focused almost exclusively on CNS effects on the stomach and colon. There is a well-known and voluminous literature which has developed on the subject of the psychological influences on peptic disease, inflammatory bowel disease, and the irritible bowel syndrome, but until recently, the esophagus has been relatively ignored as an organ worthy of serious physiologic investigation, let alone scrutiny by the psychophysiologist.

Investigational efforts in esophagology have been hampered by the lack of appropriate technology to measure esophageal function. As a nonabsorptive organ in the gastrointestinal system whose function is primarily related to transport, the esophagus has not obtained the notoriety afforded the "glamor" organs of the gastrointestinal tract. Two factors have had a major influence in altering this situation: first, the brilliant efforts of Charles Code to describe the physiology of the esophagus in the 1950s; and second, the fortuitous proximity of the esophagus to the heart.

The work of Code and his colleagues (Code, Creamer, Schlegel, Olsen, Donoghue, & Anderson, 1958) at the Mayo Clinic made the esophagus accessible not only for the purpose of physiological investigation but also for diagnostic evaluation. They developed manometric techniques to describe the peristaltic

---

WILLIAM C. ORR • Department of Clinical Physiology, Presbyterian Hospital, Oklahoma City, Oklahoma 73104.

function of the esophagus as well as the physiology of the upper and lower esophageal sphincters. These sphincters serve as important barriers to the occurrence of pulmonary aspiration and gastroesophageal reflux (GER)—the reflux of acidic gastric juice into the esophagus. A codification of this work was published in the 1950s as an atlas, and this remains a benchmark in the field of normal and disordered esophageal function (Code *et al.*, 1958).

Until recently, many disorders thought to be related to the esophagus were felt to be purely functional. With the advent of more sophisticated techniques for measuring esophageal functioning a variety of specific clinical syndromes have been described which are related to identifiable organ dysfunction referable to the esophagus (Earlam, 1975; Henderson, 1976). This has resulted in a turnabout in terms of interest in the esophagus becoming oriented towards organic rather than functional etiologies.

Progress in esophagology has also been greatly aided by the fortuitous presence of the esophagus in the thoracic cavity along with the heart and thoracic aorta. The similarity of the clinical symptoms produced by these organs has long been recognized and has forced individuals concerned primarily with the heart and cardiovascular disorders to consider the esophagus in the differential diagnosis of chest pain. The coalescence of continuing growth and interest in heart and cardiovascular problems and the development of techniques allowing accurate study of the esophagus have resulted in a burgeoning interest in esophageal disorders. For example, it is becoming increasingly apparent that a wide variety of esophageal motor disorders can produce chest pain, which is in many instances virtually indistinguishable from that associated with angina and coronary artery disease (Earlam, 1975; Henderson, 1976).

In spite of this trend, and somewhat paradoxically, interest in the psychophysiological aspects of esophageal functioning has been developing rapidly. A recent study has shown clear defensive reflex responses of the esophagus to environmental stimuli (Stacher, Steinringer, Blau, & Landgraf, 1979), and Johnson has recently reported successful treatment of rumination and aerophagia with biofeedback (Johnson, DeMeester, & Haggitt, 1978). Furthermore, reports of nocturnal GER have stimulated considerable interest in esophageal functioning during sleep (Johnson & DeMeester, 1974; Orr, Robinson, & Johnson, 1981). Subsequent discussion will focus primarily on methods of evaluating esophageal function and on studies related to esophageal function during sleep.

2. Tests of Esophageal Function

2.1. Esophageal Motility

The standard clinical manometric assessment of the esophagus involves the measurement of the upper esophageal sphincter (UES) pressure, lower esophageal sphincter (LES) pressure, the relaxation of these sphincters with swallowing, and the motor functioning of the body of the esophagus. This is accomplished by passing a small tube into the body of the esophagus through the nose or mouth (usually through the nose). The tube itself is approximately 3 to 5 mm in diameter and is either a solid piece of polyethelene tubing containing three small transducers at the distal end or a collection of three (or more) 1-mm-diameter tubes glued together which allow constant water perfusion. Pressure sensors are located at 5-cm intervals. Pressure changes are conveyed to dc amplifiers via transducers located within the body of the tube or outside the body as with the infusion system. The sensing probe used in our laboratory is shown in Figure 1.

The clinical evaluation is generally carried out by passing the probe through the nose into the patient's stomach. By slowly withdrawing the probe from the stomach into the body of the esophagus each pressure sensor will pass through a high-pressure zone, the LES (Figure 2). Since the pressure measurements of the LES are extremely variable, it is best to repeat this maneuver two to three times,

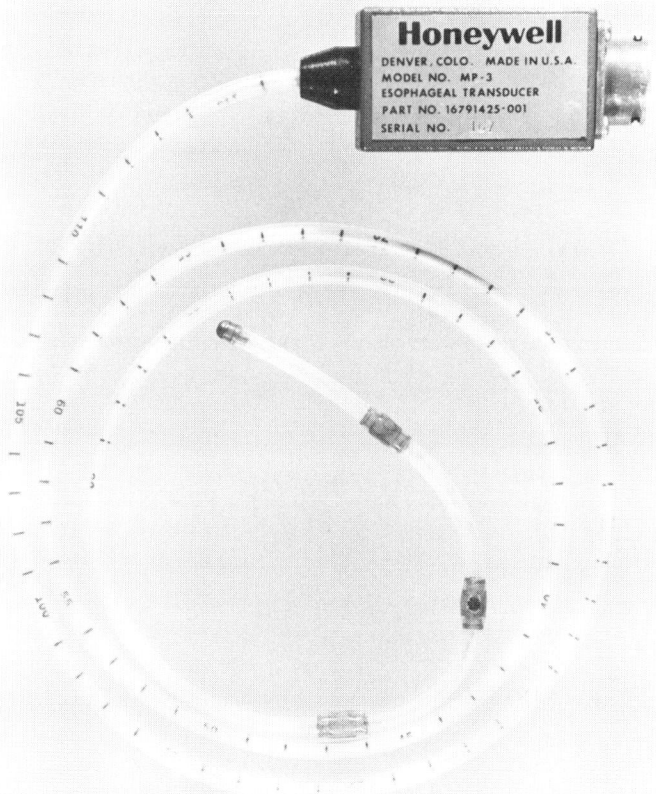

Figure 1. Standard esophageal motility probe with solid state pressure transducers. The outside diameter of the tube is 5 mm, and the pressure transducers are located at 5-cm intervals from the tip.

yielding six to nine determinations of lower esophageal sphincter pressure which can be averaged. In addition, the reflex relaxation of the LES with swallowing can be assessed easily by asking the patient to swallow when the sensing device reaches a reasonable pressure about gastric pressure. Swallows should provoke a fall in the LES pressure to intragastric pressure levels (Figure 2).

As the pressure-sensing device is brought slowly across the high-pressure zone of the LES, the relationship of the pressure excursions associated with the respiratory cycle change abruptly. This has been felt traditionally to be due to the difference in inspiratory pressure changes in the thoracic LES and the abdominal LES. However, recent studies have strongly suggested an alternative explanation of this phenomenon (Dodds, Stewart, Hogan, Steff, & Arndorfer, 1974); they have demonstrated a resting pressure gradient along the LES. Thus, as is shown in Figure 3, the pressure changes noted with the respiratory cycle alter by 180 degrees depending on whether the sensing probe is on the ascending or descending slope of the LES pressure gradient. Furthermore, these studies have brought into question the reliable measurement of LES relaxation with swallows using standard techniques. The reason is that swallowing and subsequent peristalsis cause a contraction of the longitudinal muscle of the esophagus and an oral displacement of the LES by 1–2 cm. This will usually result in the measurement probe "dropping" into the stomach and briefly recording intragastric pressure appearing as a decrease in LES pressure subsequent to swallowing, but this is not a reliable reflection of LES "relaxation."

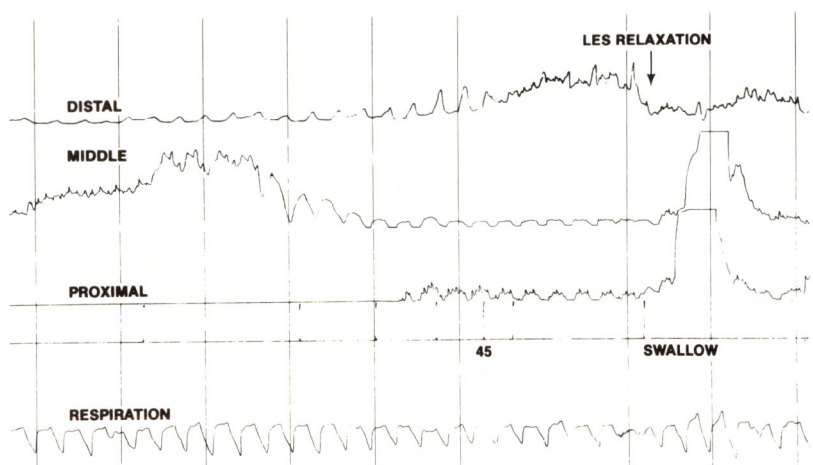

Figure 2. This tracing illustrates the elevation in pressure as the motility probe is gradually withdrawn through the lower esophageal sphincter. Pressure elevations can be appreciated in the middle and distal probes. Relaxation of the LES with swallows is shown in the distal channel. As the pressure increases to a peak, the patient is asked to swallow, and a decrease in the pressure is noted just prior to the onset of the peristaltic wave.

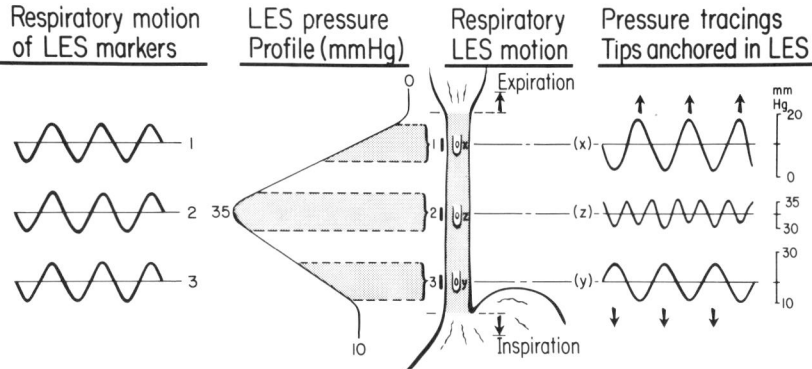

Figure 3. Schematic representation of the LES pressure profile and the pressure changes which occur at three different levels of the LES during the respiratory cycle. During expiration the LES moves orally, and aborally during inspiration. Thus, in the catheter tip labeled X, it will sense a decrease with inspiration and an increase with expiration since the LES actually moves to a point of decreased pressure from a point of increased pressure along the LES profile during the respiratory cycle. The opposite occurs at catheter tip Y (see text for explanation).

LES pressure measurements between 10 and 30 mm Hg are considered within the normal range. LES pressures below 10 mm Hg are often found in patients with severe reflux esophagitis. Pressures above 40 mm Hg, associated with the failure of LES relaxation with swallows, are characteristic of patients with achalasia. This condition precludes the normal passage of food into the esophagus and eventually results in a large, decompensated esophagus.

In order to evaluate the motor functioning of the esophagus, a series of swallows is instituted with the pressure sensors in different parts of the esophageal body. A normal peristaltic wave will produce a pressure elevation in the proximal, middle, and distal pressure sensors sequentially (Figure 4). Normal pressures of esophageal contractions range from 50 to 80 mm Hg, and the velocity ranges appreciably from the proximal (striated muscle, greater velocity) to the distal (smooth muscle, slower velocity) esophagus. This technique allows the description of numerous esophageal motor disorders ranging from aperistalsis, commonly found in patients with scleroderma (Figure 5), to diffuse esophageal spasm (Figure 6).

By continuing to slowly withdraw the probe, another high-pressure zone will be encountered, the cricopharyngeus or UES. Normal pressures here range from 40 to 80 mm Hg. The functioning of this sphincter should also be assessed by having the patient swallow when the pressure-sensing probe reaches this high-pressure zone. Again, a distinct relaxation response should be observed. In general, since the cricopharyngeus is a striated muscle, the relaxation response will be considerably faster and more abrupt than that seen with the LES (Figure 7). Evaluation of the UES completes the standard esophageal motility study.

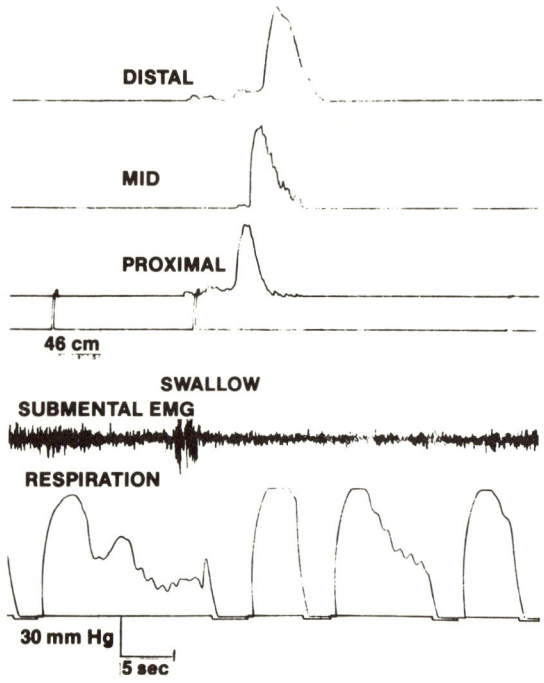

Figure 4. A normal peristaltic wave complex as recorded using the standard motility probe shown in Figure 1.

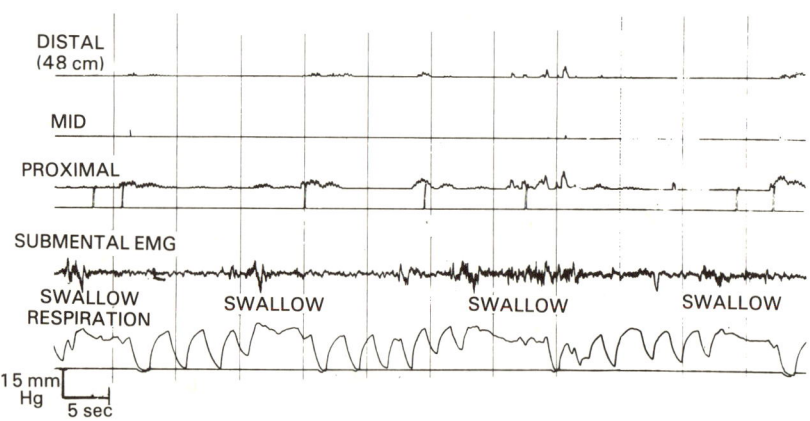

Figure 5. Complete aperistalsis associated with swallows.

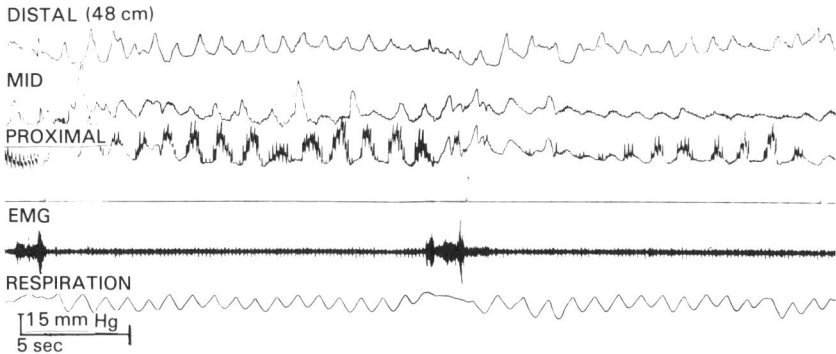

Figure 6. Diffuse esophageal spasm characterized by simultaneous and repetitive contractions in the esophagus. Swallows are identified by short bursts of activity shown in the EMG tracing.

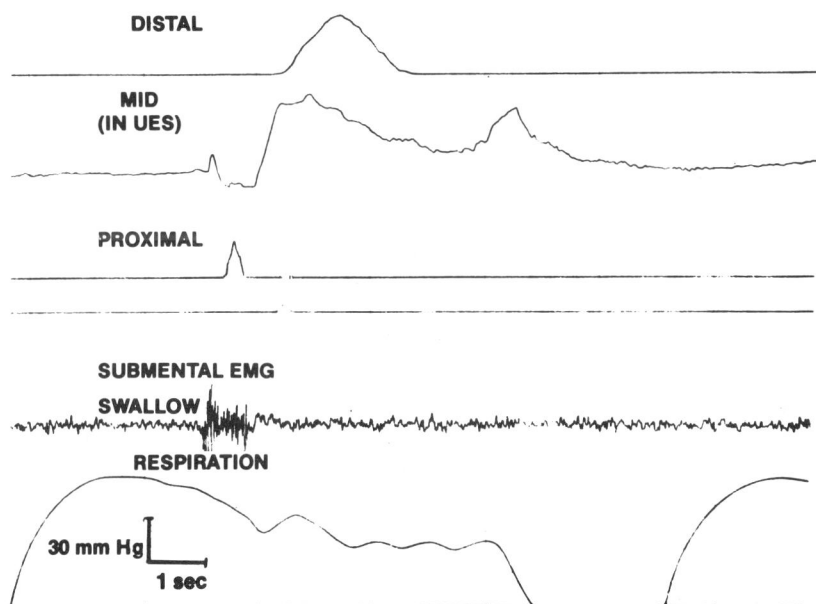

Figure 7. Relaxation of the upper esophageal sphincter (UES) associated with swallows. The middle sensing probe is in the UES, and a rapid decrease in the pressure in this tracing can be seen following the onset of a swallow. This is followed by a peristaltic wave which can be identified by successive increases in the pressure of the proximal, middle, and distal probes.

There are numerous applications of esophageal manometry to clinical investigative studies in patients with esophageal motor disorders. The availability of this tool has greatly enhanced the understanding of many disorders of the esophagus and their underlying pathophysiology.

2.2. Clinical Tests of Acid Clearance

Numerous tests are routinely used in the clinical assessment of patients suspected of having esophageal disease. Among these is the acid perfusion or Bernstein test which involves alternating the slow infusion of saline and a dilute acid solution (.1 N HCl) into the distal esophagus. In a patient whose chest pain is related to esophagitis the pain will generally be reproduced by the acid infusion and relieved by the saline infusion.

Several other tests involve monitoring the pH of the distal esophagus. The standard acid clearance test requires the infusion of 15 ml of a dilute acid solution (.1 N HCl) into the distal esophagus and an instruction to the patient to swallow every 20 sec until the pH of the esophagus returns to 5 (Earlam, 1975). This test provides a clinical assessment of esophageal acid clearance. A failure of the patient to bring the esophageal pH to 5 in approximately 10 swallows is indicative of a defective clearance mechanism.

The Standard Acid Reflux Test (SART) involves placing 300 ml of dilute acid into the stomach. The patient is then engaged in a variety of provocative maneuvers (valsalva, cough, etc.) in an effort to produce reflux. The occurrence of reflux is identified by a precipitous drop in the distal esophageal pH associated with one of the provocative maneuvers. More than two episodes of reflux would generally be considered abnormal and indicative of an imcompetent LES. More recently, prolonged monitoring (24 hr) of the distal esophagus has been used to identify reflux episodes and to assess esophageal acid clearance. By this technique the actual exposure of the esophageal mucosa to the acid contents of the stomach can be accurately measured. The present discussion will concentrate on esophageal motility and esophageal pH evaluations.

2.3. Esophageal pH Monitoring

The results of studies which have employed 24-hr monitoring of the distal esophagus have been particularly informative as to the pathophysiology of GER, reflux esophagitis, and its complications (Atkinson & VanGelder, 1977; Johnson & DeMeester, 1974; Johnson *et al.*, 1978). Johnson and DeMeester and their colleagues have demonstrated that monitoring pH from the distal esophagus allows an accurate description of the incidence of episodes of GER and the efficiency of acid clearance from the distal esophagus. These studies are accomplished with the use of a commercially available pH probe and a pH meter (Figure 8), the output of which is recorded on a standard recording device. The

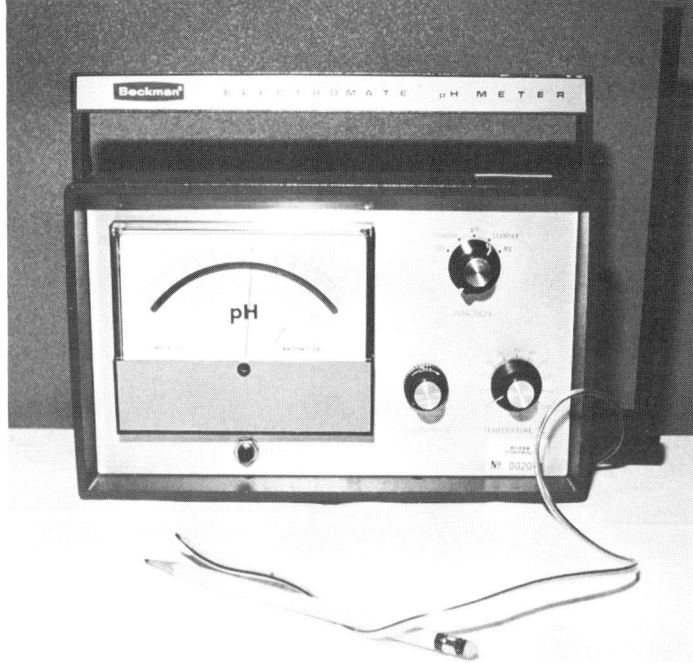

Figure 8. Standard pH meter and pH probe used in the evaluation of esophageal function.

pH probe is passed into the distal esophagus and placed 5 cm above the level of the manometrically determined LES. The patient is simply instructed to remain upright except during sleeping hours and to note any episodes of chest pain or discomfort such as heartburn.

Through the use of these techniques, three types of GER have been identified (DeMeester, Johnson, Guy, Toscano, Hall, & Skinner, 1976; Johnson et al., 1978). *Upright reflux* is characterized by multiple episodes which are rapidly cleared. *Recumbent reflux*, generally occurring during the sleeping interval, is associated with fewer episodes and more prolonged clearance times. *Combined reflux* is characterized by episodes of both recumbent and upright reflux occurring in the same individual. These data have emphasized the fact that GER occurs on a continuum and undoubtedly occurs in everyone.

Physiological or *benign reflux* is commonly seen postprandially and may involve the occurrence of multiple episodes with very prompt clearance. On the other hand, a highly symptomatic individual with esophagitis would be likely to have numerous episodes of reflux throughout the day as well as several episodes during the night. When compared with an asymptomatic individual who experiences only postprandial or physiological reflux, the total time of esophageal mucosal contact with the acid contents of the stomach is much greater in the symptomatic individual. This increase is primarily due to the occurrence of sleep-related reflux which is associated with markedly prolonged clearance. Asymptomatic individuals rarely reflux during sleep.

The development of the more severe forms of esophagitis (erosions and strictures) appears to be related to an increased incidence of recumbent reflux with its attendant prolonged acid clearance. These data have also been shown to correlate reasonably well with histologic changes compatible with esophagitis (i.e., basal zone hyperplasia and papillary elongation; Johnson et al., 1978).

3. Esophageal Function during Sleep

These results focused interest on the mechanisms of reflux and clearance during sleep. Since the series of investigations by Johnson and colleagues suggested that occurrence of GER is necessary, but not sufficient for the development of the more serious forms of esophagitis, our investigations focused initially on the issue of esophageal acid clearance during sleep. The available evidence pointed to the occurrence of prolonged acid clearance during sleep as a key factor in the pathogenesis of esophagitis. In order to examine more specifically the issue of acid clearance from the esophagus during sleep, we decided to analyze the clearance of infused bolus injections of .1 N HCl rather than spontaneously occurring episodes of GER. Briefly, the results indicated that sleep is associated with prolonged acid clearance and that esophageal acid clearance associated with arousals from sleep was significantly longer in patients with esophagitis (Orr, Robinson, & Johnson, 1981).

More specifically, the experimental protocol involved studying 13 asymptomatic normal volunteers for two successive nights in the sleep laboratory. Thirteen patients with esophagitis (defined as erythema, friability, or ulceration of the distal esophagus) were studied for one night only. All patients were quite symptomatic, having multiple daily episodes of heartburn. Sleep was polygraphically monitored via continuous recordings of the electroencephalogram (EEG), electrooculogram (EOG), and electromyogram (EMG), and esophageal pH was monitored with an electrode placed according to the previously described technique. In the normal volunteers, 15 ml of sterile water were infused on six occasions during sleep on Night 1, and on Night 2 the infusions consisted of 15 ml of .1 N HCl. The patients were studied with infusions of the .1 N HCl solution only. In addition, on the nights during which acid was infused, the .1 N HCl solution was also instilled into the distal esophagus during the presleep waking period. This was done to allow a comparison of acid clearance from the esophagus during sleep and waking.

Three primary parameters were analyzed. Referring to the schematic illustration in Figure 9, the acid clearing duration was determined by measuring the interval of time to return the esophageal pH to 5 after dropping below 4 with

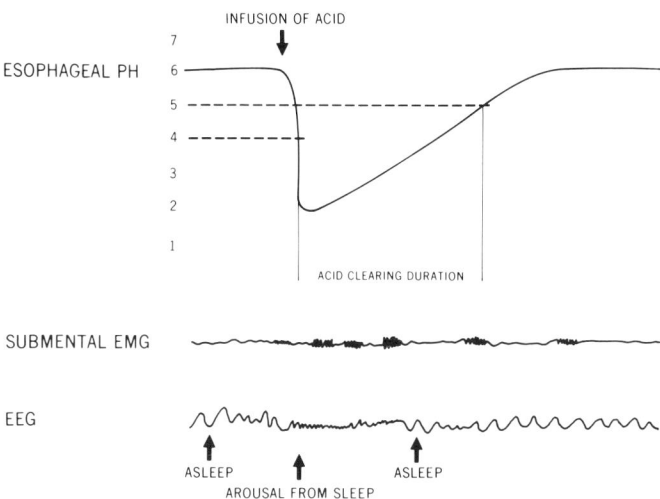

Figure 9. Schematic representation of a typical acid clearing episode (see text for explanation).

the acid infusion. The number of swallows during the acid clearing interval were computed by counting discrete bursts of EMG activity from the submental EMG. This was then converted to the number of swallows per unit time during the acid clearing interval. Since most episodes of acid infusion were associated with some degree of arousal from sleep, the actual polygraphically documented percent of wakefulness during each acid clearing interval was determined. Wakefulness, or arousal from sleep, was determined by the presence of a predominance of alpha or beta activity in the EEG and a concomitant tonic elevation in the activity of the chin EMG.

On Night 1 the introduction of sterile water into the esophagus of the normal volunteers during sleep did promote an increase ($p < .05$) in the rate of swallowing. (All comparisons were between 10 min intervals of time before and after water or acid infusion.) Thus, it appears that the introduction of a small volume of a benign liquid, resulting in minor esophageal distention, can produce a physiologic response such as swallowing. Acid infusion produced a further increase in the rate of swallowing which was a statistically significant ($p < .05$) increment when compared with the water infusion.

As can be seen in Figure 10, the introduction of acid into the distal esophagus during sleep produced significantly prolonged clearance times in both patients and controls when compared to waking (presleep) acid clearance. There was no statistically significant difference between patients and controls in terms of clearance times during sleep. It was apparent, however, that this was not an adequate analysis of these data. Since arousals from sleep have been shown to be

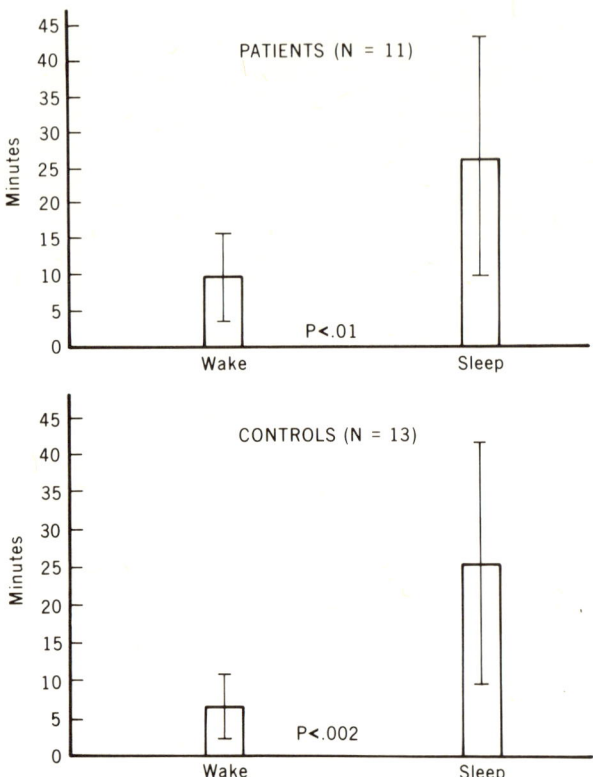

Figure 10. Acid clearing durations compared for patients and controls during waking and sleep.

associated with more frequent swallowing (Leon, Flanagan, & Moorrees, 1965), it seemed prudent to analyze these data in terms of the amount of waking occurring during the acid clearance intervals. Thus, all clearance episodes were segregated into those containing greater than 50% waking and those containing less than 50% waking. The data from this analysis are shown in Figure 11. Episodes of acid clearing associated with less than 50% waking did not reveal any significant difference in clearance times between patients and controls. On the other hand, acid clearing intervals associated with greater than 50% waking revealed significantly longer clearance in the patient group. Swallowing rate, although showing obvious increments with increases in the level of arousal, did not differentiate the patients from the control group under any circumstance (Figure 12).

Although the analysis of these data is somewhat complicated, they do reveal what might be described as a "double jeopardy" predicament for patients with esophagitis. That is, sleep-related episodes of GER are associated with markedly prolonged clearance. This was demonstrated experimentally in our study in both patients and controls. This is not a particular problem for asymptomatic individuals since they rarely reflux during sleep. The patient group, on the other hand, has been demonstrated to reflux with much greater frequency during sleep (Johnson & DeMeester, 1974; Johnson *et al.*, 1978). In addition, if the patient happens to have an arousal from sleep associated with an episode of reflux, he/she would likely demonstrate impaired clearance. The arousal from sleep associated with an episode of acid reflux or acid infusion would appear to be a normal protective mechanism against the potential complications of such an event. It might, therefore, be questioned whether the pathological defect in the patients relates to a peripheral defect in esophageal peristalsis or a central arousal dysfunction.

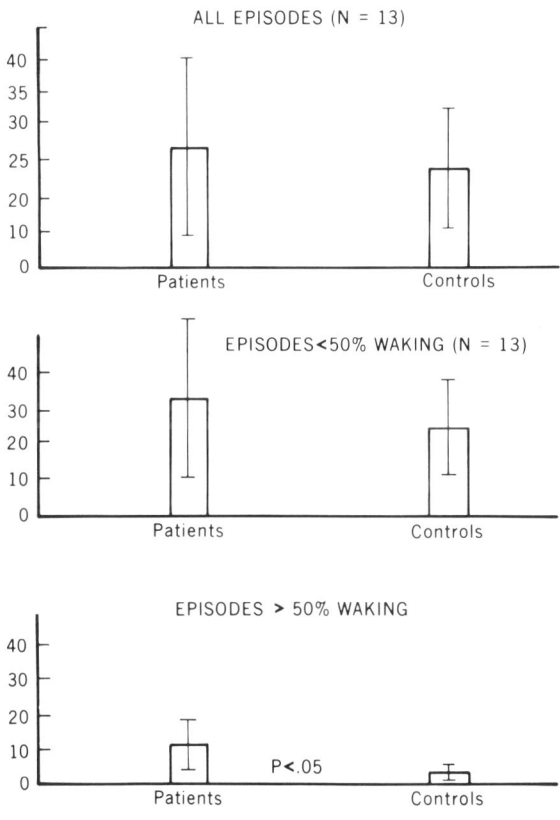

Figure 11. Acid clearing durations for different levels of waking are compared for patients and controls.

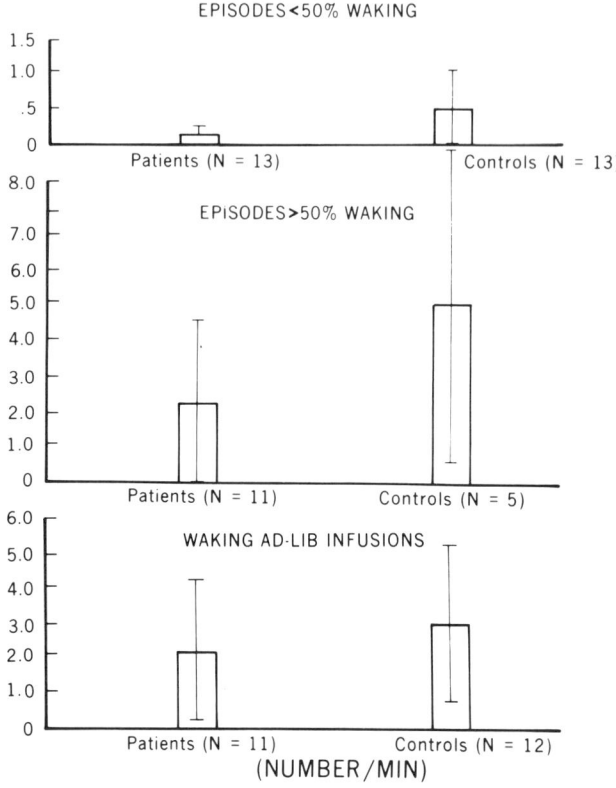

Figure 12. Rate of swallows during acid clearing intervals for patients and controls.

In order to address the issue of defective peristalsis in the patient group, a special probe was designed which included a pH sensitive tip and two pressure transducers for monitoring peristalsis. This allowed the simultaneous monitoring of both the distal esophageal pH and peristalsis. Using this probe and the exact protocol described above six normal controls were studied on two nights using sterile water and acid infusions, respectively. Peristaltic parameters analyzed were peak amplitude, velocity, and duration. Preliminary results have not shown any difference in any of these parameters between primary peristalsis occurring during wake versus sleep with the acid infusions. The incidence of secondary peristalsis (spontaneous peristalsis not preceded by a swallow) was not significantly different when acid infusions during presleep waking were compared with acid infusions during sleep.

The occurrence of secondary peristalsis with acid versus water infusions is of interest. There has been an impression among clinicians that GER promotes the occurrence of secondary peristalsis, but the mechanism for this has never been addressed. In this pilot investigation there was no significant difference between acid and water infusions in terms of the occurrence of secondary peristalsis. It would appear then that secondary peristalsis is due to the distention of the esophagus itself rather than the noxious acid stimulus.

An important study has been reported recently by Dent, Dodds, Friedman, Sekiguchi, Hogan, Arndorfer, and Petrie (1980) which involved extended (overnight) monitoring of the LES in normal, asymptomatic volunteers. They described rather remarkable variability in the minute-to-minute measures of LES pressure during sleep. Little relationship was noted between the resting LES pressure and episodes of GER, and they indicated that most reflux episodes which occurred during sleep were associated with transient arousals from sleep accompanied by inappropriate spontaneous LES relaxation. Data such as these cast some doubt on the commonly held belief that LES pressure and the occurrence of GER are related. In addition, it again raises the issue of the role of arousals from sleep in the pathogenesis of GER. Similar studies need to be conducted in patients.

4. Implications and Future Studies

These sleep studies have provided information relevant to a variety of clinical problems. They have also focused on the rather impressive complexity of the phenomenon of GER and related acid clearance from the distal esophagus. By comparing the simple response to installation of sterile water versus acid in controls and patients with esophagitis, a beginning has been made in a systematic study of the role of sleep in the pathophysiology of GER and esophagitis. These studies have raised the question of a central versus peripheral defect in the pathogenesis of esophagitis. Do patients who develop severe esophagitis do so because of a fundamental peristaltic aberration, or simply because they are unable to arouse from sleep and respond appropriately to the acid stimulus? These questions are being pursued in our laboratory by investigations such as those described above and will be continued by examining peristaltic parameters during sleep in patients with severe esophagitis.

In addition, future studies will address the issue of the monitoring of the LES during sleep in patients with esophagitis. The question must be answered as to whether the mechanism of reflux in patients with esophagitis is similar to that in the normals reported by Dent *et al.* (1980). Such studies should provide considerable information on the relevance of the LES resting pressure to the occurrence of reflux during sleep. If episodes of GER can be documented to occur without spontaneous relaxation of the LES, the LES pressure would appear to be considerably more important since it directly reflects the pressure gradient necessary to be overcome in order for GER to occur.

Pulmonary aspiration represents a logical extension of the consequences of defective clearance of refluxed gastric contents. It is felt that patients with defective acid clearance are at high risk for the development of the complications of pulmonary aspiration. Such questions raise the issue of the functioning of the UES during sleep, and this is of particular interest and potential importance since the UES is a striated muscle. The inhibition of striated muscle during rapid-eye-movement (REM) sleep has been well documented. If similar alterations can be shown in the cricopharyngeus during sleep, this would have obvious implications for the mechanism and pathophysiology of pulmonary aspiration.

5. References

Atkinson, M., & VanGelder, A. Esophageal intraluminal pH recording in assessment of gastroesophageal reflux and its consequences. *American Journal of Digestive Disease*, 1977, *22*, 365–370.

Code, C. F., Creamer, B., Schlegel, J. F., Olsen, A. M., Donoghue, F. E., & Anderson, H. A. *An atlas of esophageal motility in health and disease*. Springfield, Illinois: Charles C Thomas, 1958.

DeMeester, T. R., Johnson, L. F., Guy, J. J., Toscano, M. S., Hall, A. W., & Skinner, D. F. Patterns of gastroesophageal reflux in health and disease. *Annals of Surgery*, 1976, *184*, 459–470.

Dent, J., Dodds, W. J., Friedman, R. H., Sekiguchi, T., Hogan, W. J., Arndorfer, R. C., & Petrie, D. J. Mechanism of gastroesophageal reflux in recumbent asymptomatic human subjects. *Journal of Clinical Investigation*, 1980, *65*, 256–267.

Dodds, W. J., Stewart, E. T., Hogan, W. J., Steff, J. J., & Arndorfer, R. C. Effect of esophageal movement on intraluminal esophageal pressure recording. *Gastroenterology*, 1974, *67*, 952–960.

Earlam, R. *Clinical tests of oesophageal function*. New York: Grune & Stratton, 1975.

Henderson, R. D. *Motor disorders of the esophagus*. Baltimore, Maryland: Williams & Wilkins, 1976.

Johnson, L. F., & DeMeester, T. R. Twenty-four hour pH monitoring of the distal esophagus, a quantitative measure of gastroesophageal reflux. *American Journal of Gastroenterology*, 1974, *62*, 325–332.

Johnson, L. F., DeMeester, T. R., & Haggitt, E. C. Esophageal epithelial response to gastroesophageal reflux, a quantitative study. *American Journal of Digestive Diseases*, 1978, *23*, 498–509.

Leon, C. S. C., Flanagan, J. B., Jr., & Moorrees, C. F. A. The frequency of deglutition in man. *Archives of Oral Biology*, 1965, *10*, 83–96.

Orr, W. C., Robinson, M. G., & Johnson, L. F. Acid clearance during sleep in the pathogenesis of reflux esophagitis. *Digestive Diseases and Sciences*, 1981, *26*, 423–427.

Stacher, G., Steinringer, H., Blau, A., & Landgraf, M. Acoustically evoked esophageal contractions and defense reactions. *Psychophysiology*, 1979, *16*, 234–240.

2

THE RESPONSIVENESS OF THE ESOPHAGUS TO ENVIRONMENTAL STIMULI
GEORG STACHER

1. Introduction

The contractile activity of the esophagus is one of the bodily functions which is affected by psychological events or events in the environment of the healthy human organism. We all are familiar with expressions such as "I can't swallow that" or "There is a lump in my throat," indicating altered esophageal function in states of emotional tension or of psychic upset. Moreover, these expressions do not simply reflect subjective feelings but correspond to real changes in the pattern of esophageal motility which has been reported in a number of publications. The mechanisms by which these changes are brought about are still unclear and not much progress has been made in determining their role in the development of esophageal motor disorders.

2. Types of Esophageal Motility

Normal esophageal motor activity, by contrast, has been the subject of intense research in the past decade and is relatively well understood at present. The esophagus, in contrast to other parts of the gastrointestinal tract, has no mechanical or electrical resting activity (Diamant, 1977). When a swallow is initiated, a programmed sequence of neural discharges successively excites the muscles of the mouth, pharynx, and esophagus (Diamant & El-Sharkawy, 1977). The bolus is pushed by the contraction of the oral and pharyngeal muscles

---

GEORG STACHER • Psychophysiology Unit at the Psychiatric and at the First Surgical Clinic, University of Vienna, A-1090 Vienna, Austria.

through the relaxed upper esophageal sphincter into the esophagus and is transported downward by a peristaltic contraction wave beginning with the closure of the upper esophageal sphincter and passing through the striated and smooth muscle portions of the esophagus. The bolus finally is delivered into the stomach through the relaxed gastroesophageal sphincter, which closes after the passage.

This swallow-induced type of contractile activity has been termed *primary peristalsis* as opposed to *secondary peristalsis,* which is triggered by material which has remained within or has been refluxed into the esophagus from the stomach (Meltzer, 1899). The latter type of peristalsis is similar to the former in all aspects except that there is no swallowing in the oropharyngeal region and no relaxation of the upper esophageal sphincter.

There is good evidence that both types of activity are controlled by a complex swallowing center located in the brainstem nuclei and in the reticular formation (Doty, 1968; Jean, 1972; Sumi, 1972; Roman & Tieffenbach, 1972). In addition to this central control mechanism there is an intrinsic peripheral control mechanism in the wall of the smooth muscle portion of the esophagus which can function independently of the central mechanism (Christensen & Lund, 1969; Diamant, 1974). Thus, activation of either mechanism can produce an aborally proceeding wave of contraction.

In addition to the two types of peristaltic contractions there is a third, nonperistaltic type of activity which occurs synchronously in all parts of the esophagus. This activity, termed *tertiary,* can either represent a nonpropulsive response to swallowing or be independent of swallowing. Tertiary contractions were reported to occur spontaneously in a high proportion of healthy subjects (Ingelfinger, 1958; Nagler & Spiro, 1961b; Orlando, Bozymski, & Blaylock, 1977) and have been held to be the result either of unusual neurogenic discharges or of various distant stimuli (Ingelfinger, 1958). An increased incidence of nonpropulsive, not swallow-initiated contractions as well as of nonpropulsive esophageal responses to swallowing has been reported to be prevalent among the elderly (Ingelfinger, 1958; Soergel, Zboralske, & Amberg, 1964; Mandelstam & Lieber, 1970) and also during pregnancy (Nagler & Spiro, 1961a).

3. Relation of Tertiary Contractions to Psychological Stress

The nonpropulsive type of esophageal activity was reported by a series of authors to be the characteristic feature of esophageal motility under the influence of psychic strain. As early as 1883, Kronecker and Meltzer reported that psychic upset (*psychische Erregungen*) induced esophageal contractions. Jacobson (1927) observed spastic contractions of the esophagus during emotional stress. Other researchers found a significant relationship between nonpropulsive motor activity and the patients' emotional state (Rubin, Nagler, Spiro, & Pilot, 1962). Wolf and Almy (1949) reported that patients who had complained that swallowed food seemed to "stick" in the retrosternal region showed on X-ray examination uncoordinated rather than propulsive contractions in the lower two-thirds of the esophagus when emotionally charged situations from their lives were discussed and that the barium in the esophagus was "milked up and down."

It has been suggested that this nonpropulsive activity, which might be aimed at defending the stomach from a substance recognized as noxious only after the initiation of a swallow, represents a symbolic revulsion, referring to deep, unconscious conflict. The resulting dysphagia was interpreted as "an unconscious rejection of incorporation resulting from agressive impulses, often sexual in nature" (Kronfeld, 1934) or to be due to an ambivalent attitude towards incorporation (Alexander, 1950). These psychosomatic hypotheses, however, were not supported by subsequent research. On the contrary, they gradually were abandoned as purely somatic factors were found to be operative in a number of swallowing disorders. Cohen (1973) pointed out why psychosomatic conceptions such as *globus* or *hysterical dysphagia* (Vinson, 1922), also known as "Plummer–Vinson syndrome," had to be discarded: It could never be shown that globus patients were more hysterical than healthy subjects, and it was shown that webs and folds in the hypopharynx were present in 86% of a group of patients diagnosed as having hysterical dysphagia (Jacobs & Kilpatrick, 1964).

Similarly, *cardiospasm,* held to represent a spastic contraction of the gastroesophageal junction, was regarded purely as a form of conversion hysteria and assumed to be the somatic outcome of unconscious psychic conflict symbolized by the patient (Weiss & English, 1957). Symptom exacerbations were related to fresh psychic insults, and sexual, hostile, and self-punitive acts were felt to be operative. However, cardiospasm is no longer used as a diagnostic label since evidence has accumulated that the underlying disturbance is not a spastic contraction of the cardia but a failure of the lower esophageal sphincter to relax upon swallowing, that is, an achalasia of this structure. The sphincter represents a distinct zone at the gastroesophageal junction characterized by a relatively high resting pressure, which, upon the initiation of a swallow, relaxes to the level of intragastric pressure and contracts after the passage of the bolus (Kelley, Wilbur, Schlegel, & Code, 1960). It has become clear that achalasia is not induced by psychic factors but by a loss or absence of ganglion cells in the myenteric plexus of the sphincter and by a lesion of the extrinsic parasympathetic nerves (Smith, 1970). As to the etiology of the lesion, clinical and pathological observations tend to support an infective hypothesis. Apart from globus, hysterical dysphagia, and cardiospasm, many other esophageal symptoms and diseases were viewed as being of emotional origin. However, virtually all psychosomatic formulations of swallowing disorders have been discarded with advanced understanding of esophageal physiology.

Nevertheless, it is well documented that the esophagus reacts with nonpropulsive contractions to emotional tension and psychic strain as well as to a variety of external stimuli such as cold, hot, or burning food, and to carbonated beverages (Kronecker & Meltzer, 1883). Recently, Stacher (unpublished data) has observed that the esophageal body also responds with nonpropulsive contractions to stimuli not related to ingestion, such as the noise produced by the clapping of the hands. To investigate the responsiveness of the esophagus to such non-food-related external stimuli, a series of experiments were carried out in our laboratory.

4. Experimental Studies of Acoustically Induced Esophageal Contractions

4.1. Intensity of Stimuli Required to Produce Contractions

In a first series, the threshold intensity of an acoustical stimulus necessary to evoke a contractile response was determined (Stacher, Schmierer, & Landgraf, 1979). Twenty-two healthy young subjects were exposed, via headphones, to a sequence of 1000-Hertz (Hz) tones 1.5 seconds (sec) in duration with a rise and decay time of 5 milliseconds (msec). The intensity of the tones varied in 5-dBA steps between 70 and 125 dBA. The tones were presented in random order and at random intervals from 30 to 40 sec and each intensity was presented twice. Esophageal pressures were recorded by means of a Kulite model P 31 solid-state pressure transducer fitted with three pressure sensors spaced at 5-cm intervals and arranged radially 120 degrees apart. The transducer was passed into the esophagus via the nose and was positioned with sensors 5, 10, and 15 cm above the oral border of the gastroesophageal sphincter. An electromyogram (EMG) of the mylo-hyoid muscles was used to identify swallowing, and a strain gauge pneumograph was used to monitor respiration. All signals were processed by a Beckman R-411 Dynograph. The tones were produced by a programmable Wavetek Type 152 function generator. It was found that all of the subjects responded to the tones. The threshold intensity necessary to elicit a response ranged between 75 and 125 dBA, and the mean threshold of the subjects studied was at 86.8 ± 3.0 dBA.

In a second series the proportion of healthy subjects of a wider range of age who responded with nonpropulsive contractions to 1000-Hz 90-dBA tones (i.e., to tones of an intensity slightly above the threshold level at which the subjects of the first series showed contractile responses) was determined (Stacher *et al.*, 1979). It was found that 36 of the 40 subjects ranging in age from 19 to 74 years responded with a nonpropulsive contraction to one or more of the 40 tones presented (Figure 1).

The response-to-stimulus rate per subject, that is, the percentage of tones eliciting a tertiary contraction, varied between 2.5 and 100, and the mean percentage was 47.2 ± 5.1. None of the tones elicited a primary or secondary

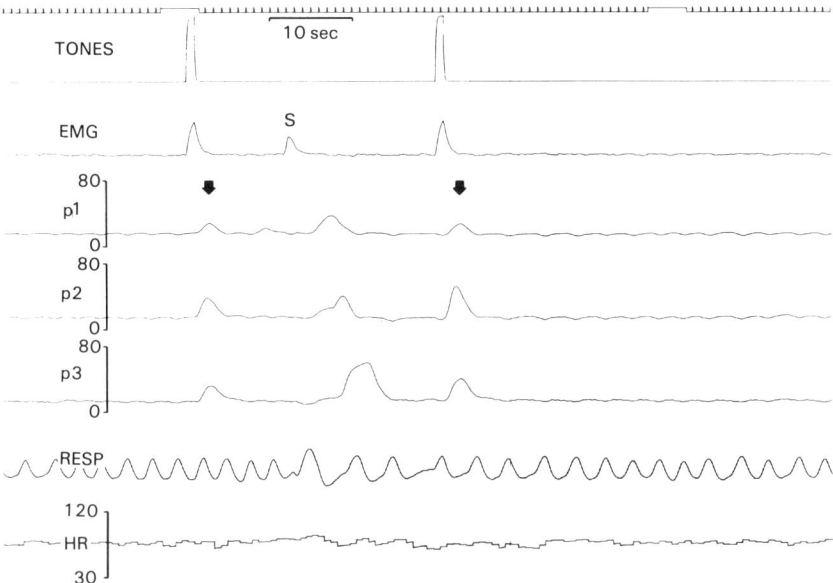

Figure 1. Esophageal motility recorded from a healthy male, 23 years old, exposed to 1000 Hz, 90 dBA tones. The polygraph tracing shows, from top to bottom: time in seconds; integrated acoustical stimuli (TONES); integrated surface electromyogram of the mylo-hyoid muscles (EMG); esophageal pressures in millimeters of mercury at 15 cm (p 1), 10 cm (p 2), and 5 cm (p 3) orad of the lower esophageal sphincter; respiration (RESP); and heart rate (HR), in beats per minute (30 to 120). Arrows indicate esophageal contractile responses to tones; "S" indicates swallowing and the subsequent peristaltic contraction wave.

contraction wave. There was a significant tendency toward fewer contractile responses with increasing number of stimuli presented. In addition, the amplitude of the contractile responses decreased, but not significantly. However, in none of the subjects with a large number of contractile responses did the response extinguish. The EMG of the mylo-hyoid muscles showed increases in activity in response to all of the stimuli presented, the amplitude of the response increasing slightly with increasing numbers of stimuli. There was no relationship between the amplitude of the EMG response and the occurrence or the amplitude of an esophageal response. The response latency of the EMG response (< 0.05 sec) was much shorter than the latency of the esophageal response (0.95 ± 0.02 sec).

4.2. Orienting versus Defense Reactions

The decrease in number and amplitude of contractile responses might indicate that with repetitive stimulation either the excitation mechanism fatigues or that inhibition obliterates any excitatory influence, reflecting an adaptation of the subject to the stimuli. Some of the subjects reported that they perceived the stimuli as startling. Since the stimuli presented were of sudden onset, that is, had rise times of 0 and 5 msec respectively, and since it has been reported that the effective stimulus for startle is the rapid rise of a sufficiently intense sound (Fleshler, 1965; Berg, 1973), an interpretation of the esophageal response as forming part of the startle reaction seemed possible. However, if startle had been the major determinant of the response, both the esophageal and the mylo-hyoid muscle responses should have disappeared after a small number of stimulus presentations since the startle reaction habituates rapidly (Landis & Hunt, 1939). Furthermore, the long latency of the response seemed not to favor an interpretation of the esophageal response as forming part of the startle reflex. Stacher, Schmierer, and Landgraf (1979), therefore, speculated that the esophageal response could be related to the "component b" response of forearm muscle action potentials (Davis, 1948), which according to Sokolov (1963) has been equated with the defense reaction. Such an interpretation also seemed compatible with the earlier reports that emotional tension or psychic strain were associated with an increased nonpropulsive contractile activity of the esophagus (Kronecker & Meltzer, 1883; Rubin et al., 1962; Wolf & Almy, 1949).

To test the hypothesis that nonpropulsive contractile responses of the esophagus to auditory stimuli form part of the defense reaction of the healthy organism, a further series of experiments was carried out (Stacher, Steinringer, Blau, & Landgraf, 1979). To distinguish defense reactions from orientation reactions, three levels of intensity of auditory stimuli were used. In addition, heart rate changes were monitored since heart rate acceleration has been reported to be indicative of a defense reaction and heart rate deceleration of an orientation reaction (Graham & Clifton, 1966). Since it was stated by Sokolov (1963) that the orientation reaction to a stimulus with signal content is stronger and more resistant to habituation than to a stimulus without signal content, stimuli of two levels of signal content were presented via headphones. To distinguish defense and orientation reactions from startle reactions, two different levels of rise and decay time of the stimuli were used—one with rapid rise time (0 msec) suited to elicit startle and the other with slow rise time (30 msec) which would preclude startle. The stimuli without signal content were 36 tones of a frequency of 1000 Hz, a duration of 2 sec, and an intensity of 65, 80, or 95 dBA. These stimuli were presented as a series of triads with each triad containing one tone of each intensity. The order of tones within each triad was constant, 65, 80, and 95 dBA. Half of the triads consisted of tones with rise and decay times of 30 msec, the other half of tones with rise and decay times of 0 msec. The order of triads with the two levels of rise times was randomized, and the interstimulus intervals varied from 20 to 40 sec.

The stimuli with signal content consisted of presentations of pairs of tones separated by 2 sec. All tones were 2 sec in duration and had rise and decay times of 30 msec. The first tone of each pair was of a constant frequency (1000 Hz) but varied in intensity (65, 80, and 95 dBA). The second was of a constant intensity (80 dBA) but varied in frequency (900, 975, 1000, 1025, and 1100 Hz). The pairs of tones were grouped in triads. The sequence of pairs within the triads was the same over the whole experiment (65, 80; 80, 80; 95, 80 dBA). Twelve pairs at each level of intensity of the first tone were presented. In four pairs the second tone was of the same frequency and in the remaining eight of a different frequency (two each of 900, 975, 1000, 1025, and 1100 Hz) with respect to the first tone. The stimulus pairings were identical for all subjects, and the interstimulus pair intervals varied randomly from 20 to 40 sec.

It was found that the number as well as the amplitude of esophageal contractile responses increased significantly with increasing stimulus intensity. While there were only a few contractile responses to 65- and 80-dBA tones, a high proportion of 95-dBA tones elicited responses (Figure 2).

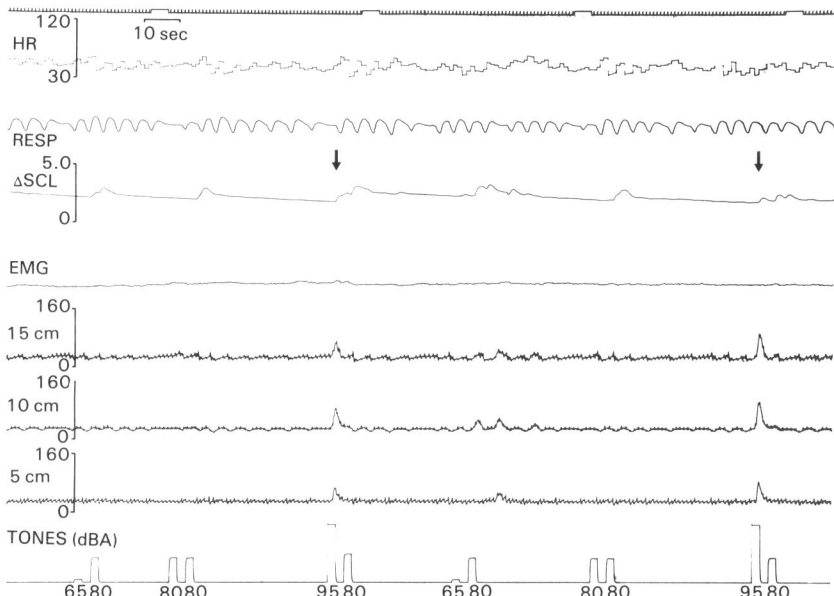

Figure 2. Esophageal motility recorded from a healthy male, 22 years old, exposed to pairs of acoustical stimuli differing in pitch and intensity. The polygraph tracing shows from top to bottom: time in seconds; heart rate (HR) in beats per minute (30 to 120); respiration (RESP); change in skin conductance level (ΔSCL) in Siemens; integrated surface electromyogram of the mylo-hyoid muscles (EMG); esophageal pressures in millimeters of mercury at 15, 10 and 5 cm orad of the lower esophageal sphincter; and integrated acoustical stimuli (TONES) with intensity in dBA. Arrows indicate contractile responses to stimuli.

The rise time to full intensity of the stimuli remained without any influence on the number and amplitude of contractile responses, and there was also no difference in number and amplitude of contractions in response to stimuli with and without signal content. The fact that most of the contractile responses occurred to stimuli with intensities beyond the range to which humans usually show the orienting response, together with the finding that stimuli with signal content did not evoke more contractions than those without signal content, suggests that the esophageal responses do not represent part of an orienting response. There was also no sign of one of the characteristic features of the orientation reaction: At no level of intensity or signal content did the esophageal contractile responses show any tendency towards habituation. The fact that contractile responses were no more frequent and no more intense to stimuli with sudden rise time than to stimuli with slow rise time speaks against an interpretation of the response as forming part of a startle reaction. Startle reactions are usually elicited by stimuli with sudden rather than with gradual rise to full intensity (Fleshler, 1965; Berg, 1973). Although the large majority of contractile responses were associated with accelerative heart rate responses, reported to be indicative of a defense reaction (Graham & Clifton, 1966), there was no one-to-one relationship between the occurrence of a nonpropulsive contraction and heart rate change. Taken together, the results of the reported study suggest that the nonpropulsive contractions of the esophagus in response to acoustical stimuli do not form part of a startle or of an orientation reaction but represent part of the defense reaction of the healthy organism to intense exogenous stimuli.

5. Implications for Understanding and Treatment of Esophageal Motor Disorders

Whether or not these findings have any relevance to normal or disordered patterns of esophageal motor activity cannot be answered from the data of the reported studies. However, contractile responses to external stimuli might be facilitated by an increased excitability of the esophagus or of the entire organism as prevails in states of emotional tension or anxiety. It is well known that emotional tension also aggravates the symptoms of dysphagia in conditions of disturbed esophageal function (Jacobson, 1927; Rubin *et al.*, 1962). On the other hand, the symptoms of such disturbances can be alleviated and the strength of contractions diminished by strategies suited to induce relaxation and relative security in the patients concerned (Jacobson, 1927). In a patient with manometrically proven diffuse esophageal spasms, spontaneous as well as diazepam-induced drowsiness was associated with a greatly diminished number of spastic contractions, and the amplitude of the contractions was reduced markedly. When the patient fell asleep, neither swallow-initiated nor "spontaneous" contractions occurred (Figure 3). On awakening, by contrast, the spastic contractions immediately set in with full intensity.

However, a diminished number or even an absence of swallows during sleep is not unique to patients with diffuse esophageal spasms but is physiological; the number of swallow-induced as well as of spontaneously occurring esophageal contractions decreases markedly in states of drowsiness and relaxation. Some years ago, we studied three healthy subjects who had learned to relax themselves using the technique of "autogenic training" (Schultz, 1970). In all of these subjects the number and amplitude of swallow-initiated as well as of tertiary contractions decreased with increasing depth of relaxation (Berner, Fink, Naske, & Stacher, 1974). However, it has not been shown as yet that manometrically proven motor disorders of the esophagus, such as diffuse spasms or achalasia, can be cured by relaxation techniques, psychotherapy, or conditioning.

One recent report (Kaplan & Evans, 1978) of the successful treatment of a case of functional dysphagia on the model of fear of fear can hardly be evaluated as the patient did not undergo any manometric investigation of esophageal function and no definition of her dysphagia was given. The case history presented,

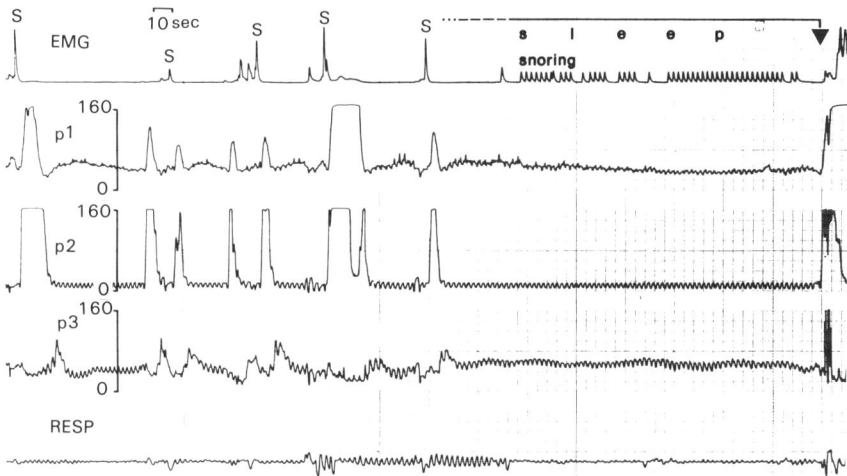

Figure 3. Esophageal motility recorded from a female, 71 years old, with diffuse esophageal spasms. The polygraph tracing shows from top to bottom: time in seconds; integrated electromyogram of the mylo-hyoid muscles (EMG); esophageal pressures in millimeters of mercury at 10 cm (p 1) and 15 cm (p 2) orad of the gastroesophageal sphincter and within the sphincter (p 3); and respiration (RESP). "S" indicates swallowing. The vigorous spastic contractions visible on the left part of the tracing disappear as the patient falls asleep and snores, as indicated by the saw-tooth like activity in the EMG. Upon awakening (arrow), spastic contractions set in with full strength.

however, seems to suggest that the patient suffered from achalasia. The symptoms were accentuated when the patient was confronted with the negative social consequences of being unable to consume food or drink in public. When she had learned socially appropriate strategies for coping with this situation, her difficulty in swallowing occurred only in very formal or crowded situations.

Notwithstanding the fact that strategies aimed at inducing relaxation and reassurance can help patients to cope with their swallowing disorders, permanent or long-lasting therapeutic effects in such conditions can still be accomplished only by pharmacological or surgical procedures in diffuse spasm and mechanical dilatation or myotomy in achalasia. Despite the well-documented reactivity of the esophagus to external and internal stimuli, the classical psychosomatic concept that functional disorders such as "exaggerated" or "inappropriate" esophageal responses can lead to organic diseases has remained purely speculative.

6. References

Alexander, F. *Psychosomatic medicine: Its principles and applications.* New York: Norton, 1950.
Berg, K. M. *Elicitation of acoustic startle in the human.* Unpublished Ph.D. thesis, University of Wisconsin, 1973.
Berner, P., Fink, G., Naske, R., & Stacher, G. Der entspannende Einfluss des autogenen Trainings auf die Motilität der Speiseröhre. *Zeitschrift für Psychosomatische Medizin und Psychoanalyse,* 1974, *20,* 384–390.
Christensen, J., & Lund, G. F. Esophageal response to distension and electrical stimulation. *Journal of Clinical Investigation,* 1969, *48,* 408–419.
Cohen, B. R. Emotional considerations in esophageal diseases. In A. E. Lindner (Ed.), *Emotional factors in gastrointestinal illness.* Amsterdam: Excerpta Medica, 1973.
Davis, R. C. Motor effects of strong auditory stimuli. *Journal of Experimental Psychology,* 1948, *38,* 257–275.
Diamant, N. E. Electrical activity of the cat smooth muscle esophagus: A study of hyperpolarizing responses. In E. E. Daniel (Ed.), *Proceedings of the Fourth International Symposium on gastrointestinal motility.* Vancouver: Mitchell Press, 1974.
Diamant, N. E. How now esophageal peristalsis? *Gastroenterology,* 1977, *73,* 1353–1354.
Diamant, N. E., & El-Sharkawy, T. Y. Neural control of esophageal peristalsis: A conceptual analysis. *Gastroenterology,* 1977, *72,* 546–556.
Doty, R. W. Neural organization of deglutition. In C. F. Code (Ed.), *Handbook of physiology. Section 6: Alimentary canal* (Vol. 4). Washington, D.C.: American Physiological Society, 1968.
Fleshler, M. Adequate acoustic stimulus for startle reaction in the rat. *Journal of Comparative Physiology and Psychology,* 1965, *60,* 200–207.
Graham, F. K., & Clifton, R. K. Heart-rate change as a component of the orienting response. *Psychological Bulletin,* 1966, *65,* 305–320.
Ingelfinger, F. J. Esophageal motility. *Physiological Reviews,* 1958, *38,* 533–583.
Jacobs, A., & Kilpatrick, G. S. The Paterson–Kelly syndrome. *British Medical Journal,* 1964, *2,* 79–82.
Jacobson, E. Spastic esophagus and mucous colitis. *Archives of Internal Medicine,* 1927, *30,* 433–445.

Jean, A. Localization and activity of medullary swallowing neurones. *Journal de Physiologie*, 1972, *64*, 227-268.
Kaplan, P. R., & Evans, I. M. A case of functional dysphagia treated on the model of fear of fear. *Journal of Behavior Therapy and Experimental Psychiatry*, 1978, *9*, 71-72.
Kelley, M. L., Jr., Wilbur, D. L., II., Schlegel, J. F., & Code, C. F. Deglutive responses in the gastroesophageal sphincter of healthy human beings. *Journal of Applied Physiology*, 1960, *15*, 483-488.
Kronecker, H., & Meltzer, S. J. Der Schluckmechanismus, seine Erregung und seine Hemmung. *Archiv für Anatomie und Physiologie, Physiologische Abteilung*, 1883, *7*, 328-362 (*Suppl. Festgabe*).
Kronfeld, A. Oesophagus-Neurosen. *Psychotherapeutische Praxis*, 1934, *1*, 21-26.
Landis, D., & Hunt, W. A. *The startle pattern*. New York: Johnson Reprint Corporation, 1968. (Originally published, 1939.)
Mandelstam, P., & Lieber, A. Cineradiographic evaluation of the esophagus in normal adults: A study of 146 subjects ranging in age from 21 through 90. *Gastroenterology*, 1970, *58*, 1045.
Meltzer, S. J. On the causes of the orderly progress of the peristalsis movements in the esophagus. *American Journal of Physiology*, 1899, *2*, 266-272.
Nagler, R., & Spiro, H. M. Heartburn in late pregnancy. Manometric studies of esophageal motor function. *Journal of Clinical Investigation*, 1961, *40*, 954-970. (a)
Nagler, R., & Spiro, H. M. Serial esophageal motility studies in asymptomatic young subjects. *Gastroenterology*, 1961, *41*, 371-379. (b)
Orlando, R. C., Bozymski, E., & Blaylock, N. B. Tertiary contractions of the esophagus: A manometric study in healthy subjects. *Gastroenterology*, 1977, *72*, 1109.
Roman, C., & Tieffenbach, L. Activity of vagal efferent fibers innervating the baboon's esophagus. *Journal de Physiologie*, 1972, *64*, 479-506.
Rubin, J., Nagler, R., Spiro, H. M., & Pilot, M. L. Measuring the effect of emotions on esophageal motility. *Psychosomatic Medicine*, 1962, *24*, 170-176.
Schultz, I. H. *Das autogene Training* (13. Auflage). Stuttgart: Thieme Verlag, 1970.
Smith, B. The neurological lesion in achalasia of the cardia. *Gut*, 1970, *11*, 388-391.
Soergel, K. H., Zboralske, F. F., & Amberg, J. R. Presbyesophagus: Esophageal motility in nonagenarians. *Journal of Clinical Investigation*, 1964, *43*, 1472-1479.
Sokolov, E. N. *Perception and the conditioned reflex*. Oxford: Pergamon, 1963.
Stacher, G., Schmierer, G., & Landgraf, M. Tertiary esophageal contractions evoked by acoustical stimuli. *Gastroenterology*, 1979, *77*, 49-54.
Stacher, G., Steinringer, H., Blau, A., & Landgraf, M. Acoustically evoked esophageal contractions and defense reaction. *Psychophysiology*, 1979, *16*, 234-241.
Sumi, T. Role of pontine reticular formation in the neural organization of deglutition. *Japanese Journal of Physiology*, 1972, *22*, 295-314.
Vinson, P. O. Hysterical dysphagia. *Minnesota Medicine*, 1922, *5*, 107.
Weiss, E., & English, O. S. *Psychosomatic medicine*. Philadelphia: Saunders, 1957.
Wolf, S., & Almy, T. P. Experimental observations on cardiospasm in man. *Gastroenterology*, 1949, *13*, 401-421.

3

DISORDERS OF THE ESOPHAGUS
Applications of Psychophysiological Methods to Treatment
MARVIN M. SCHUSTER

1. Introduction

The term *functional* has two specific definitions. One usage implies that a disorder is not physical and to many people this means that the disorder is illusionary or "only in one's head." However, to those who are involved in physiological investigations the term *functional* implies that there is no detectable primary structural abnormality and the problem is, therefore, physiological.

Functional disorders of the esophagus are disorders of motility (Schuster, 1979) since motility is the only function of the esophagus. The esophagus serves simply as a transit tube. There is no significant secretion, absorption, or digestion that takes place within the esophagus so when there is a disorder in primary physiologic function of the esophagus this is a motility disorder.

2. Disorders of the Esophagus

The esophagus can be divided into three anatomical areas: (1) the cricopharyngeus, which is the upper esophageal sphincter; (2) the body of the esophagus; and (3) the lower esophageal sphincter. The lower esophageal sphincter in the human is not an anatomical structure; it is a physiological region of constricted muscle which was described early in the 1950s by Dr. Inglefinger.

Abnormalities of esophageal motility may consist of augmented motility, decreased motility, or discordance of motility. The upper esophageal sphincter,

---

MARVIN M. SCHUSTER • The Johns Hopkins School of Medicine and the Division of Digestive Diseases, Baltimore City Hospital, Baltimore, Maryland 21224.

the cricopharyngeus, has to be precisely coordinated during swallowing so that the hypopharynx contracts exactly as the cricopharyngeus relaxes. If there is discordance between these two events, then high dysphagia ensues because contraction of the pharynx occurs against the closed cricopharyngeus (Seaman, 1976). The peristaltic wave begins in the upper, striated portion of the esophagus and progresses to the smooth muscle portion, which is the lower two-thirds of the esophagus.

2.1. Globus Hystericus

Globus hystericus does not carry with it a detectable motor disorder. The symptom is expressed as an *as if* phenomenon. Patients do not say, "There is a knot in my throat"; they say, "It feels *as if* there is a knot in my throat. Whenever I swallow even saliva, it feels *as if* there is a lump, or a knot in my throat." This lump is located in the region of the cricopharyngeus and may represent simply heightened awareness of cricopharyngeal contractions. If one becomes preoccupied with the physiological event—the cricopharyngeal opening or relaxation—a lump can be felt in the throat. There are numerous anecdotal reports of successful treatment of this disorder with various forms of psychotherapy but no systematic research has been undertaken.

2.2. Diffuse Esophageal Spasm

Diffuse esophageal spasm is associated with pain in the substernal area, but the pain may be referred to other areas of the body (Bennett & Hendrix, 1970). The areas of referred pain are similar to the areas of pain experienced in heart disease. Consequently, the distinction between the sensations produced by spasm of the coronary arteries and spasm of the esophagus is vital.

Diffuse esophageal spasm is manifested primarily by pain and by dysphagia. This is not the dysphagia in which pain is associated with swallowing. This pain is associated with reflux or with unknown events, and the pain is located in the body of the esophagus. The pathophysiology of this pain is that of spasm, which may be acid-induced, idiopathic, or perhaps stress-related. Not all spasm is acid-induced spasm. There are patients, especially among the elderly, who have what is presumed to be a neuromuscular disorder which is associated with spasm. And yet, no matter what the underlying basis, there does seem to be a fairly good response to antacids, to spasmalytic agents, and possibly to some forms of psychotherapy. Psychotherapy may help the patients cope rather than affecting their underlying pathophysiology.

2.3. Reflux Esophagitis

One of the reasons for pain in the substernal area is esophagitis which is often associated with reflux. This can lead to stricture formation with obstructive symptoms. One of the primary protective mechanisms of the esophagus in avoiding the ravages of esophagogastric reflux is peristaltic clearing. Clearing takes place as the normal "housekeeping" function of the esophagus; a peristaltic wave sweeps material out of the esophagus (Johnson & DeMeester, 1974). Primary peristalsis results from swallowing, which begins as a voluntary act. Reflux from the stomach into the esophagus induces secondary peristalsis. In all these cases the peristaltic wave has a clearing action. Normal subjects restore the pH of the esophagus from a pH of 2 caused by reflux of acid into the esophagus to a pH which is nearly neutral within 8 or 9 swallows. Patients with esophagitis require a minimum of 12 swallows and usually more than that. The acid-clearing mechanism is one which can and should be approached from a behavioral point of view which requires some degree of ingenuity and a lot of patience.

In patients with reflux esophagitis who were monitored overnight, episodes of heartburn were associated with sudden drops in pH. Much of this was postprandial, but some of it was not. After months of treating these patients with alginic acid (Gaviscon) and after the disappearance of the inflammation of the esophagus, there were fewer episodes of reflux and fewer reports of heartburn; so there does seem to be an ability to alter the motor activity of patients who have the symptom of reflux, at least by this pharmacological technique, and also, potentially by behavioral techniques.

2.4. Achalasia

Patients who have longstanding achalasia often have a massively dilated esophagus with a "bird–beak" narrowing at the sphincter. There can be three week's accumulation of food and liquid in the esophagus, with the heavy barium dripping through the less dense liquid and forming a droplike appearance. This is the end stage of achalasia. The associated motor disorder is that of the absence of a normal peristaltic wave (Vantrappen, Hellemans, Deloof, Valembois, & Vandenbroocke, 1971). The lower esophageal sphincter fails to relax. Noting this phenomena, Sir Arthur Hurst (1911) called this lack of relaxation achalasia instead of cardiospasm, a term which had been used up to that time. In the vigorous form of achalasia, intense spasm occurs above the unyielding esophageal sphincter. Patients with achalasia demonstrate Cannon's Law of denervation because if one administers a cholinergic agent such as acetylcholine or its beta analog, mecholyl, one can induce an intense spasm (Shepherd & Diamant, 1972) manifested by an alteration in tone as well as diffuse phasic contractions which are extremely painful.

Generally, the major symptom of achalasia is that of dysphagia. The pathophysiology is aganglionosis in the body of the esophagus, and perhaps also in the sphincter. The sphincter fails to relax to normal levels. The treatment for this malady is pneumostatic dilation which is designed to rupture the esophageal sphincter. Since one cannot restore the normal motility pattern to the denervated body of the esophagus, the goal instead is to remove the functional (not anatomical) obstruction by rupturing the lower esophageal sphincter with brusque pneumostatic dilation. Alternatively, one can use surgery. This is the second order of treatment and is used only if the pneumostatic dilation fails. Achalasia has not been successfully treated by means of biofeedback or other behavioral techniques, but that does not mean that it cannot be treated by these methods.

3. Physiology of the Lower Esophageal Sphincter

3.1. Reflex Motor Responses

The *lower esophageal sphincter* (*LES*) is defined as an area of elevated resting tone. As a perfused catheter is pulled through the sphincter, one sees first a rise in pressure, then a drop in pressure as the instrument comes out of the sphincter and moves into the esophagus because intrathoracic pressure is lower than intragastric pressure. With deglutition (swallowing) there is a reflex relaxation in the lower esophageal sphincter. In scleroderma there is no high pressure zone and no relaxation with deglutition (Cohen, Fisher, Lipshutz, Tumer, Myers, & Shomacher, 1972). That same situation usually exists in patients with reflux esophagitis who do not have scleroderma (Dodds, Hogan, & Miller, 1976), although there are patients with reflux who have normal resting pressures in their lower esophageal sphincter.

Reflux is not simply a matter of an inadequate basal resting tone in the sphincter because the lower esophageal sphincter, like other sphincters in the body, does not remain in a steady state. It has to contend with increased forces. This can be illustrated by the effects of increasing intragastric pressure produced by leg-raising, bending, coughing, or placing a blood pressure cuff around the abdomen. As pressures increase within the abdomen of normal subjects, intrasphincteric pressure increases in order to maintain the barrier ratio. In patients who have reflux, however, increases in intragastric pressure do not result in appropriate increases in sphincteric pressure. The sphincter is not a static but a functioning, physiologic organ (a concept basic to any understanding of the sphincter's physiologic role).

3.2. Pharmacology of the LES

There are a number of agents (Nebel, Fornes, & Castell, 1976) which affect the lower esophageal sphincter pressure: cholinergic, adrenergic, dopaminergic, or peptidergic, and gastrointestinal hormones. Gastrin is one of the hormones released when acid reaches the duodenum or when the stomach is distended. Metoclopramide, methylcholine, beta-methylcholine, and urecholine are drugs which increase lower esophageal sphincter resting pressure and have been used for the treatment of reflux. On the other hand, secretin decreases lower esophageal sphincter resting pressure, predominantly by inhibiting the action of gastrin. Smoking of tobacco, especially cigars, drinking of alcohol, or using anticholinergics decreases lower esophageal sphincter pressure. This fact is important because many physicians treat reflux by giving anticholinergic drugs in order to decrease the acid output of the stomach. However, this treatment may aggravate the symptoms because the antisecretory activity of the anticholinergic drugs is not as strong as the antispasmodic activity. The spasmolytic activity of the drug reduces the resting activity of the lower esophageal sphincter and relaxes the stomach so that the acid which is produced in the stomach remains there and therefore may reflux and augment the symptoms. Essence of peppermint (a supposed antacid), which is one of the age-old remedies for dyspepsia, does the opposite of what it was thought to do. It relaxes the sphincter and predisposes to reflux. Until recently researchers thought that pregnant women had so much trouble with reflux esophagitis because pressures within the abdomen were augmented. Although this concept may be true, reflux esophagitis also occurs because estrogens and progesterone decrease the resting pressure of the lower esophageal sphincter.

4. Biofeedback Training to Raise Lower Esophageal Sphincter Pressure

Using the presented background on esophageal disorders, I would now like to describe some of the experiments done in our laboratory using biofeedback to control lower esophageal sphincter (LES) resting pressure (Schuster, Nikoomanesh, & Wells, 1973). Biofeedback should be added to the list of remedies which can increase LES resting pressures. This was the first area to which we applied biofeedback techniques. The reasons for selecting the lower esophageal sphincter were these:

1. There is more accumulated physiological data on the resting pressure of the lower esophageal sphincter than on any other part of the gastrointestinal tract.
2. The LES is a muscle that is exclusively smooth muscle with only autonomic innervation.
3. The LES is in a relatively steady resting state.
4. There are known disorders associated with abnormal resting pressures—decreased pressure associated with reflux esophagitis and increased pressure associated with achalasia.

The technique (Figure 1) that we used for biofeedback training involved placing a triple-lumen catheter so that the distal tip was in the stomach and the middle tip was in the LES (positioned at the zone of highest resting pressure) so

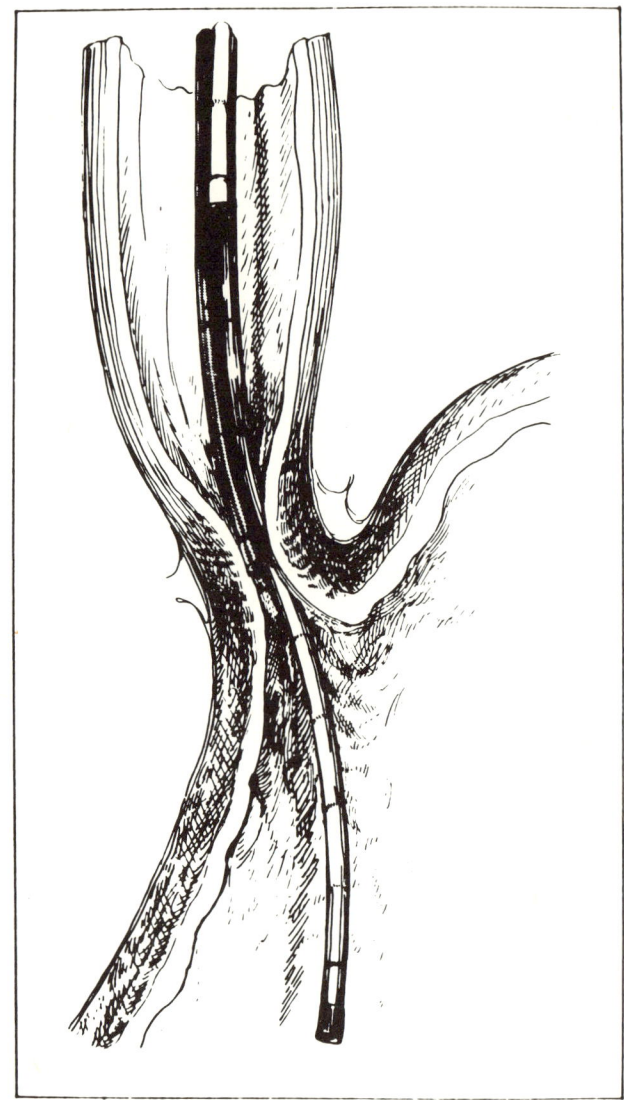

Figure 1. Tandem 3 catheter assembly used to measure pressures from esophagus, lower esophageal sphincter, and stomach (from Schuster, Nikoomanesh, & Wells, 1973).

that if there were any movements of the catheter up or down, a decrease rather than increase of pressure would occur. The goal was to try to get the patients to increase resting pressure. Any inadvertent movement would have had the opposite effect. The proximal tip of the catheter was in the esophagus. While the tracings of pressure were being made the patient was shown a meter which

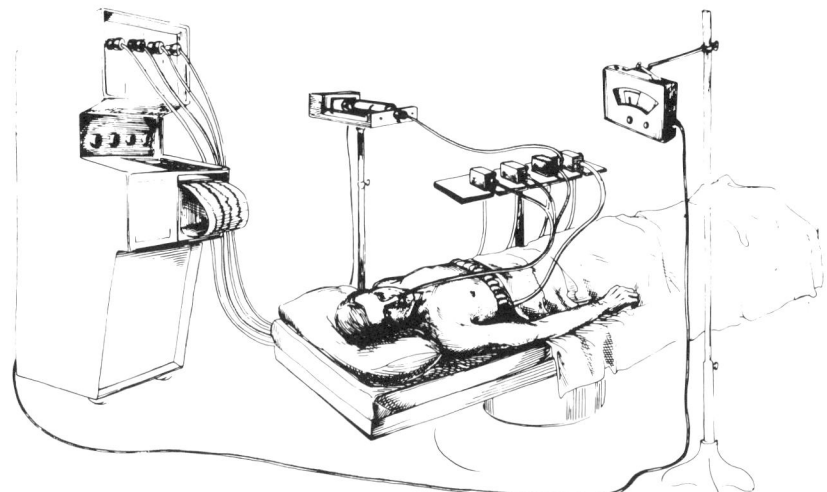

Figure 2. Biofeedback technique with pressure from lower esophageal sphincter (middle catheter) displayed on a meter which could be observed by the subject (from Schuster, Nikoomanesh, & Wells, 1973).

recorded pressure at the middle tip (the one in the LES, Figure 2). This meter could be turned on and off without the patient knowing. The instructions to patients and normal subjects were to look at the needle of the meter and to make the needle move up by any technique available to him or her which did not alter respiration or involve contracting abdominal or any voluntary muscles. We monitored respiration and movement with a bellows pneumograph and in some instances with surface electrodes for striated muscle electromyography.

Figure 3 shows tracings of respiration, intraesophageal pressures, intrasphincteric pressures, and intragastric pressures. At a given point the meter was turned on without the subject's knowledge, and then the subject was asked to increase the pressure (i.e., to make the needle go up). Normal subjects and patients with reflux esophagitis were able to effectively do this without altering respiration, intraesophageal pressure, or intragastric pressure. One of our concerns was that we might induce an achalasia-like state. If the person contracted the sphincter and maintained the contraction, deglutition might not produce the normal reflex relaxation. However, this did not occur; deglutition did induce normal relaxation during a time when the patient was contracting the sphincter. If anything, the relaxation was increased because it started from a higher resting level and moved down to intragastric levels. Rarely in basal studies does one see sphincter relaxations as profound as we encountered.

An interesting phenomena we observed was that of an anticipatory response (Figure 4). We noted that after subjects had been trained to contract the LES on

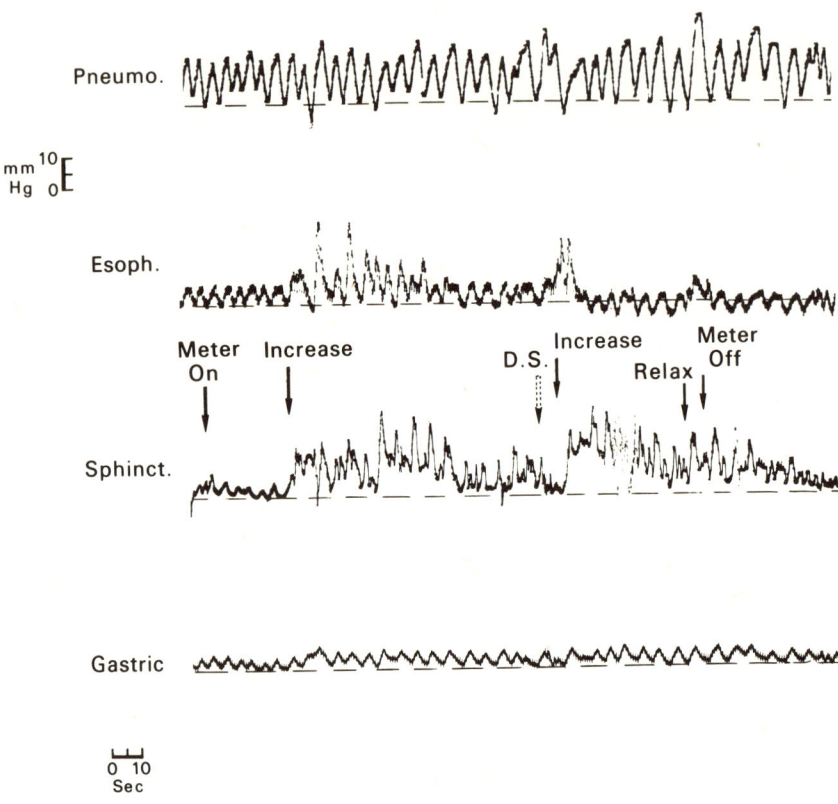

Figure 3. Tracings during biofeedback training session directed towards increasing lower esophageal sphincter pressures (from Schuster, Nikoomanesh, & Wells, 1973).

command, simply instructing them to observe the meter, even though the meter was still off, resulted in an increase in sphincter pressure. When the patient would recognize this was going on and the pressure decreased, we would switch the meter on (still there would be no command to increase) and yet another increase would occur. When sphincter pressure came back down to baseline again, the patient would be commanded to increase the sphincter pressure, and he would do so. This is an illustration of an anticipatory response, and it suggests that there are associated phenomena similar to those described by Pavlov and others in classical conditioning; when the experimenter simply walked into the room, a conditional stimulus would produce the response.

Figure 5 compares increases in intrasphincter pressure to intraesophageal pressures and intragastric pressures during attempts to increase intrasphincteric

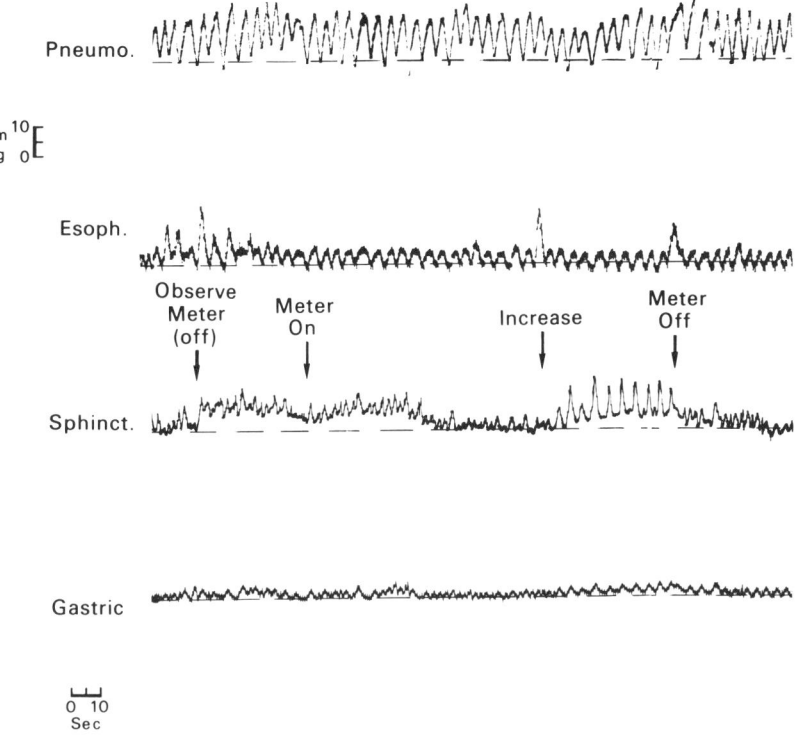

Figure 4. Anticipatory response after successful biofeedback training (from Schuster, Nikoomanesh, & Wells, 1973).

pressure. In our laboratory the normal resting pressures are at 14 to 16 mm Hg. The subject, whose results are shown in Figure 5, doubled the resting pressures without altering intraesophageal or intragastric pressures. Of our patients 70% with reflux esophagitis have also been able to double their resting esophageal sphincter pressures. We have so far studied 10 subjects. The problem is that doubling the LES pressure for a patient who starts out with a resting pressure of 2 mm Hg and brings it up to 4 mm Hg still does not result in an effective barrier or an effective LES. Much work needs to be done to determine whether biofeedback will be an effective clinical tool. However, two of our patients who had extremely severe symptoms of reflux esophagitis and were not amenable to any form of medical treatment have had excellent clinical results. Biofeedback, in the future, may be one of the therapeutic techniques which can be applied to the treatment of gastroesophageal reflux.

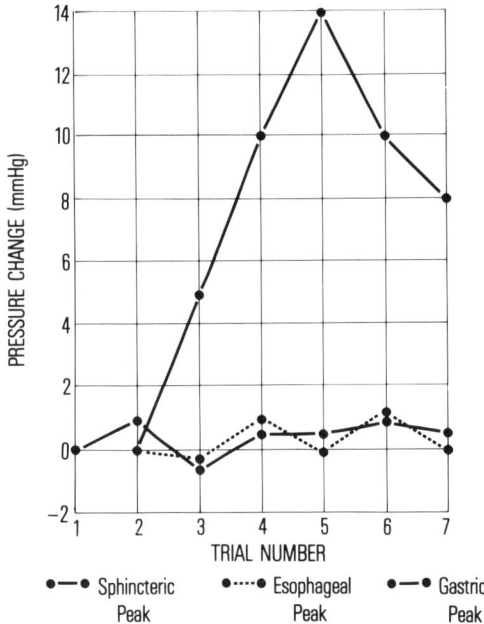

Figure 5. Graphic depiction of pressure tracing from sphincter, esophagus, and stomach over seven trials during a single training session in one subject (from Schuster, Nikoomanesh, & Wells, 1973).

5. References

Bennett, J. R., & Hendrix, T. R. Diffuse esophageal spasm: A disorder with more than one cause. *Gastroenterology*, 1970, *59*, 273–279.

Cohen, S., Fisher, R., Lipshutz, W., Tumer, R., Myers, A., & Shomacher, R. The pathogenesis of esophageal dysfunction in scleroderma and Raynaud's disease. *Journal of Clinical Investigations*, 1972, *51*, 2663–2668.

Dodds, W. J., Hogan, W. J., & Miller, W. N. Reflux esophagitis. *American Journal of Digestive Diseases*, 1976, *21*, 49–67.

Hurst, A. F. *The sensibility of the alimentary canal*. London: Oxford University Press, 1911.

Johnson, L. F., & DeMeester, T. R. Twenty-four hour pH monitoring of the distal esophagus. *American Journal of Gastroenterology*, 1974, *62*, 325–332.

Nebel, O. T., Fornes, M. F., & Castell, D. O. Symptomatic gastroesophageal reflux: Incidence and precipitating factors. *American Journal of Digestive Diseases*, 1976, *21*, 953–956.

Schuster, M. M. Disorders of motility. In P. B. Beeson, W. McDermott, & J. B. Wyngaarden (Eds.), *Cecil textbook of medicine*. Philadelphia: W. B. Saunders, 1979.

Schuster, M. M., Nikoomanesh, P., & Wells, D. Biofeedback control of lower esophageal sphincter contraction. *Rendiconti di Gastroenterologia*, 1973, *5*, 14–18.

Seaman, W. B. Pharyngeal and upper esophageal disphagia. *Journal of the American Medical Association*, 1976, *235*, 2643–2646.

Shepherd, J. K., & Diamant, N. E. Mecholyl test: Comparison of balloon kymography and intraluminal pressure measurement. *Gastroenterology*, 1972, *63*, 557–563.

Vantrappen, G., Hellemans, J., Deloof, W., Valembois, P., & Vandenbroocke, J. Treatment of achalasia with pneumatic dilatation. *Gut*, 1971, *12*, 268–275.

4

PSYCHOLOGICAL TREATMENT APPROACHES TO PSYCHOGENIC VOMITING AND RUMINATION

ROBERT PAZULINEC and THOMAS SAJWAJ

1. Introduction

Vomiting or emesis is a common physiological malady which may have many causes (Feldman & Fordtran, 1978). One etiological factor which is gaining increasing attention in the literature is the possible psychogenic basis for emesis (Hill, 1968; Hoyt & Stickler, 1960; Kanner, 1972; Leibovich, 1973; Reinhart, Evans, & McFadden, 1977). Attempts have been made to distinguish three unique types of psychogenic vomiting: (1) chronic vomiting; (2) rumination; and (3) cyclic vomiting (Feldman & Fordtran, 1978; Kanner, 1972). Each is believed to present a different clinical picture and different etiology.

The term *chronic vomiting* is sometimes used interchangeably with psychogenic vomiting and can be defined as recurrent regurgitation of stomach contents, usually during or after meals. Chronic vomiters generally have a history of vomiting for many years, often beginning in childhood. Kanner (1972) notes that their vomiting may be part of a general hypochondriacal pattern and is often self-induced. As is the case in all three of these disorders, there appears to be no organic basis for the symptoms.

Rumination (or *merycism*) is a voluntary process whereby food is brought

---

ROBERT PAZULINEC • Department of Human Development Counseling, George Peabody College of Vanderbilt University, Nashville, Tennessee 37240. THOMAS SAJWAJ • Behavioral Medicine Program, Lamar Medical Center, Vernon, Alabama 355921.

from the stomach into the mouth. Some of this food is ejected from the mouth while some is rechewed and reswallowed (Kanner, 1972). The rumination process is unique in that it entails the regurgitation of food one mouthful at a time, episodes of which typically occur after every meal and occasionally between meals. It is seen as voluntary because individuals actively engage in behaviors such as putting fingers into their throat or contracting their abdominal muscles to bring the food back to their mouth. This syndrome seems to be primarily associated with infants and retarded individuals, although it has also been noted in adults of normal intelligence.

Cyclic vomiting involves prolonged vomiting episodes which last from two to five days without any apparent organic basis. These attacks have both a sudden onset and a spontaneous recovery (Davenport, Zrull, Kuhn, & Harrison, 1972). The episodes recur at varying intervals ranging from every few weeks, to once a month, to only three or four times a year.

The actual incidence and prevalence of psychogenic vomiting disorders are unknown. This is attributable to the failure of many health professionals to consider psychological factors when dealing with physiological symptoms. In many instances vomiting and rumination may be associated with and mistaken for other disorders such as food allergies (Sajwaj, Libet, & Agras, 1974).

Historically, vomiting has been attributed to numerous organic causes. However, in many instances where no physical etiology could be found, further investigation uncovered a common group of psychological problems which appeared to be functionally related to vomiting (Richmond, Eddy, & Green, 1958). Explanations for the psychological etiology of chronic, ruminative, and cyclical vomiting differ, not only between syndromes, but also vary for each disorder, depending on one's theoretical position. The prevailing opinion on the origin of these disorders is that they are either a result of a functional neurosis or a conditioned, pathological response. There is agreement that psychogenic vomiting usually has its onset during childhood, a time when psychiatric disturbances tend to be somaticized because of the individual's limited behavioral repertoire (Ferholt & Provence, 1976; Stein, Rausen, & Blau, 1959).

2. Clinical Syndrome

For operational purposes chronic, ruminative, and cyclical vomiting will be considered as subtypes of psychogenic vomiting. Attention will be given to the clinical consequences of the syndromes together with treatment approaches.

2.1. Topography

The topography of rumination has several behavioral variants. Fullerton (1963), Menking, Wagnitz, Burton, Coddington, and Sotos (1969), Murray,

Keele, and McCarver (1977), and Sajwaj et al. (1974) report that vomiting and subsequent rumination is preceded by vigorous lip and tongue movements. The individual typically folds or curves his/her tongue in a spoonlike fashion, protruding it in and out of the mouth. This action is accompanied by lip smacking and chewing movements (Becker, Turner, & Sajwaj, 1978). Stein et al. (1959) liken the entire process to a reverse sucking movement with the mouth.

Richmond et al. (1958), Fullerton (1963), Menking et al. (1969), and O'Neil, White, King, and Carek (1979) note that their clinical subjects utilized abdominal muscular contractions to induce regurgitation. For some subjects, abdominal contractions accompanied tongue and lip movements (Fullerton, 1963; Menking et al., 1969). Other studies found that some individuals induce vomiting through digital stimulation of the mouth and throat, either alone or in conjunction with some of the above-mentioned behaviors (Toister, Condron, Wosley, & Arthur, 1975; O'Neil et al., 1979; Marholin, Luiselli, Robinson, & Lott, 1980).

Vomiting and rumination occur either during or after meals for a duration of 20–60 min or until all food is lost (Marholin et al., 1980; Sajwaj et al., 1974). The individual regurgitates food one mouthful at a time, some of which is ejected and the remainder chewed and reswallowed. The act of rumination is usually done when the person is alone (Fleisher, 1979; Gaddini & Gaddini, 1959). Throughout the process the subject appears engrossed in the behavior, often exhibiting pleasure and enjoyment, and typically resists efforts at distraction (Kanner, 1972; Menking et al., 1969). There is no evidence of pain or discomfort. In addition, the subject will often appear irritated if his/her efforts to ruminate are unsuccessful. This is particularly true of infants (Richmond et al., 1958).

Behaviorally, infant ruminators exhibit considerable anxiety and tension, and they appear sullen, worried, insecure, and reluctant to smile. They are withdrawn and unresponsive (Cunningham & Linscheid, 1976) and cry constantly (Sajwaj et al., 1974). Some ruminating infants resist physical contact (i.e., being picked up) by crying or fidgeting when contact is attempted (O'Neil et al., 1979). Others, when held, cling desparately to the adult. These are the only periods when the crying ceases (Fullerton, 1963).

Older ruminators behave in a similar fashion. They are withdrawn, depressed, and appear anxious. Most of these individuals have limited social behavior (Luckey, Watson, & Musick, 1968).

The topography of behaviors presented by chronic vomiters is different from that exhibited by ruminators. Similar to the rumination syndrome, chronic vomiters usually regurgitate during or after meals (Duker & Seys, 1977; Feldman & Fordtran, 1978; Hill, 1968; Kohlenberg, 1970). In many instances the episode is self-induced either digitally or through abdominal contractions (Kanner, 1972; Watkins, 1972). Other studies, however, have reported the involuntary nature of the regurgitation (Munford & Pally, 1979). Hill (1968) noted that, unlike rumination, chronic vomiting episodes are more often accompanied by nausea. The episodes appear to occur regardless of physical position (Ferholt & Provence, 1976), and the frequency varies from two to three times to as many as 10 times daily (Munford & Pally, 1979; Watkins, 1972). Clinical observations in several studies have led to the conclusion that the vomiting has no visible impact on the individual (Alford, Blanchard, & Buckley, 1972; Feldman & Fordtran, 1978; Ferholt & Provence, 1976). The subjects exhibited no distress about vomiting, either before or after it occurred.

Chronic vomiters often have a history of this disorder ranging anywhere from several months to many years. Hill (1968) indicates that the onset generally is in early childhood. Other studies report onsets during adolescence and early adulthood (Burgess, 1969; Ingersoll & Curry, 1977; Kohlenberg, 1970; Rich, 1978).

Cyclic vomiting presents a different clinical picture. The episodes range from 2-6 days with a sudden onset and an abrupt end (Feldman & Fordtran, 1978; Kanner, 1972). There appears to be no discernible cause for the attack. Throughout its course, nothing is retained. Medication appears to have little impact on stopping the episode, nor have surgical interventions been successful (Reinhart et al., 1977). The attacks recur at intervals of several weeks or months. Feldman and Fordtran (1978) state that the onset for the syndrome is during early childhood, while the episodes usually end at puberty. Some studies have reported onsets during adolescence (Sperling, 1968).

Immediately prior to the episode, the individual acts lethargic and complains of feeling ill. During the attack he/she exhibits a distinct personality change, becoming hostile, irritable, withdrawn, and depressed. The person also frequently displays regressive behavior (Davenport et al., 1972). The vomiting episodes seem to be precipitated by the subject becoming disappointed or angry when they do not get their way. Kanner (1972) believes that any event of considerable excitation may trigger the attacks.

2.2. Etiology

There is disagreement about the etiology of the various psychogenic vomiting disorders. Regardless of the subtype of psychogenic vomiting syndrome, the literature is divided into two primary camps with regard to the etiology for these disorders. Advocates of learning theory attribute the origin and maintenance of the vomiting to conditioning principles. The behavioral hypothesis is that initially the child vomits within normal limits. This behavior is then inadvertantly conditioned by a respondent conditioning process so that new stimuli and situations elicit vomiting or by an operant conditioning process where vomiting is reinforced and shaped by the primary caretaker through his/her attention (Toister et al., 1975; Wright, Brown, & Andrews, 1978). Consequently rumination becomes a conditioned response as a function of parental attention (Linscheid & Cunningham, 1977).

Similar behavioral hypotheses are proposed for chronic vomiting. Burgess (1969), Ingersoll and Curry (1977), and Wright and Thalassinos (1973) hypothesize that chronic vomiting is a learned habit. Munford and Pally (1979) suggest that, in their study, chronic vomiting was initially a conditioned response to stress and anxiety and later to family attention. Watkins (1972) indicates that chronic vomiting is an avoidance response; the individual learns to vomit to avoid and/or escape tasks or situations he/she dislikes.

Generally the psychiatric, pediatric, and psychotherapy literatures attribute these disorders to a dysfunctional mother–child relationship. Fleisher (1979) proposes that rumination is the result of either a neglectful or overattending mother. Typically these mothers are immature, dependent, and unable to provide the nurturance, physical intimacy, and comforting the infant needs (Gaddini & Gaddini, 1959; Richmond et al., 1958). They tend to be preoccupied with their own needs and experience considerable psychiatric problems. Fullerton (1963) states that many mothers of ruminating infants had inadequate mothers themselves. Menking et al. (1969) note that the mothers of ruminating infants tend to hold these children both mechanically and infrequently. There is a general ambivalence displayed toward the child.

Fleisher (1979) believes that by three months of age, the child realizes his/her separateness and dependence upon the primary caretaker. Because of the dysfunctional relationship between the mother and child, the mother is often not responsive to her child's needs. In these instances, the child feels helpless. The infant's only recourse is to seek more attention from his/her mother or entertain himself/herself. As the mother's unresponsiveness continues, the child resorts to increasing amounts of self-stimulation, in this case rumination. Fullerton (1963) proposes a similar hypothesis and adds that as the infants become aware of their mothers' attitudes about them, they respond out of immaturity through physiological processes. The mother's emotional problems are manifested by the child in gastrointestinal disturbances because of the symbiotic nature of the relationship (Stein et al., 1959).

The medical and psychotherapeutic literature reaches similar conclusions on the genesis of chronic vomiting. Ferholt and Provence (1976) suggest that the infant triggers strong feelings from the past in his/her mother, and these feelings inhibit her ability to be nurturant. The mothers are seen as unresponsive to their children and often feel that their child is rejecting them, intentionally, through their vomiting. Berlin, McCullough, Liska, and Szurek (1957) suggest that the origins of chronic vomiting include the entire family's interactional patterns and relationships. Of particular importance to these authors is the impact of the father, as well as the mother, on the child's vomiting. Hill (1968) found three common features in a study of adult chronic vomiters. These individuals had an unusually high number of antagonistic, hostile relationships with a significant other with whom they were living. More importantly, they felt trapped in these relationships. Second, the vomiters had a much higher incidence of parental loss during childhood as a result of death, divorce, or separation, than did a control group. Finally, chronic vomiters tended to have parents, and in some cases grandparents, with extended histories of vomiting.

A review of cases of cyclical vomiting and its origin also stresses the mother–child relationship. Reinhart *et al.* (1977) report that cyclical vomiting is a function of a prolonged symbiotic relationship between mother and child. These mothers are described as dependency-provoking, and their children are described as passive and masochistic. Other studies have noted that cyclical vomiters appear high-strung, nervous, and emotionally unstable (Kanner, 1972). Davenport *et al.* (1972) suggest that the mother–child conflicts interfere with the child's initial process of identification. Rinehart *et al.* (1977) list three necessary factors for the emergence and continuance of cyclical vomiting: (1) a child with sensitive physiological mechanisms, (2) a symbiotic mother–child relationship, and (3) a stressful event.

The learning and psychodynamic theories of the etiology of psychogenic vomiting are not necessarily incompatible. Both approaches emphasize patterns of inappropriate or insufficient interactions between the environment, typically the mother, and the child. The behavioral approach emphasizes the nature of the specific episodes of adult–child interaction (e.g., providing attention when the child ruminates), while the dynamic approach stresses the nature of the broader pattern of adult–child interaction and the factors prompting the adult to behave in inappropriate ways toward the child. The case of rumination reported by Sajwaj *et al.* (1974) supports both approaches. While the authors used a behavioral technique to eliminate rumination permanently in an infant girl, there was considerable evidence that marital difficulties and the mother's own serious emotional problems had severely impaired her relationship with the child.

2.3. Clinical Consequences

The clinical consequences of chronic psychogenic vomiting include malnutrition, dehydration, electrolyte imbalance, and severe weight loss. The individual gradually suffers from inanition. Recurrent vomiting also increases the possibility of secondary medical complications due to the person's lowered resistance to disease. At its extremes, the vomiting can become life threatening. Stein *et al.* (1959) and Sajwaj *et al.* (1974) estimate a mortality rate between 15% and 20%.

In addition to its life-threatening aspects, psychogenic vomiting can result in considerable developmental retardation and regression. Typically as ruminators/vomiters become more obsessed with this behavior, they tend to exclude other people and environmental activities and become unresponsive to the environment. The vomiting behavior interferes not only with normal activities but also with learning. An example is the Sajwaj *et al.* (1974) study which shows that the social, emotional, and language development of an infant increased rapidly once rumination was stopped. Similarly, O'Neil *et al.* (1979) report that a 26-month-old child stopped walking, talking, and playing with toys after the onset of vomiting. In general, psychogenic vomiters have a much more limited behavioral and emotional repertoire than their normal counterparts.

A third clinical consequence associated with psychogenic vomiting/ruminating is that the afflicted individuals come to be avoided by other people, which may exacerbate the disorder. Toister *et al.* (1975) observed that the mother of a 7-month-old chronic vomiter reduced her interactions with the infant because she did not want the infant to vomit on her. This avoidance resulted in minimal attention for appropriate behavior and intermittent reinforcement for vomiting. The latter, unfortunately, was one of the few times the mother actively responded to the baby. Marholin *et al.* (1980) observed that, because of the constant vomiting of a 16-year-old, mentally retarded patient, the boy was avoided by both staff and peers. As a consequence, his involvement in daily programming was often interrupted. Sajwaj and Meyerrose (1980) reported a large increase in interactions between institutional ward staff and ruminators when rumination was reduced to very low levels.

3. Treatment Approaches

The procedures used to treat the various psychogenic vomiting disorders fall into six main categories. In the pediatric and psychiatric literature, three approaches are reported: medical interventions, massive attention, and psychotherapy. More recently, two other general categories of treatment approaches have evolved from the behavior therapy area. These are peripheral electric shock and taste aversion techniques. Also drawn from the behavioral literature is a category of miscellaneous behavioral interventions (e.g., differential reinforcement of other behaviors, extinction, positive reinforcement, and overcorrection). Each major area will be reviewed with regard to the specific treatment techniques involved, their effectiveness, and their advantages and limitations.

3.1. Medical Interventions

Some medical interventions involve making alterations in the individual's eating regimen. These have included thickened foods, dietary changes, smaller amounts of food, and changes in posture, both during and after feeding (Lang & Melamed, 1969; Toister *et al.*, 1975; Cunningham & Linscheid, 1976). A second type of medical intervention has involved the use of chemotherapy. Numerous kinds of antinausea drugs and antiemetics have been used (Stein et al., 1959). A third type of intervention revolves around the use of various mechanical restraints (Kanner, 1972). These restraints include a device known as a *ruminator cap*, which effectively keeps the individual's jaws shut. The cap is placed on the patient after meals, during the time the person usually ruminates. Another technique has been to plug the nostrils or block the esophagus. Still another restraint is the use of arm splints for those patients who digitally induce vomiting. As a last resort, nasogastric feeding tubes and surgery have been used.

The effectiveness of these various interventions is not clear. Several reports note negative results (e.g., Kanner, 1972; Lang & Melamed, 1969; O'Neil et al., 1979; Stein et al., 1959; Toister et al., 1975). Marholin et al. (1980) notes that although some of the mechanical restraints have been effective in reducing or extinguishing vomiting and/or ruminating, there is no generalization of effect after the devices have been discontinued. In a discussion of rumination, Kanner (1972) recommends thickened foods and increased attention instead of drugs, mechanical devices, and surgery for the treatment of psychogenic vomiting.

3.2. Massive Attention

One of the more frequently used therapeutic techniques for psychogenic vomiting has been massive attention. This technique is utilized primarily with infants and has been coupled at times with therapy for the infant's parents. *Massive attention* involves assigning surrogate caretakers to be with the infant throughout the day. Their role is to provide the child with as much attention, nurturance, comforting, and physical stimulation as possible. This approach is viewed as a way to interrupt the unpleasant and dysfunctional mother–child interaction (Richmond et al., 1958). The use of massive attention has been shown to be an effective treatment technique (Fleisher, 1979; Gaddini & Gaddini, 1959; Hallowell & Gardner, 1965; Kanner, 1972; Menking et al., 1969).

Ferholt and Provence (1976) used massive attention with a 10-month-old infant who had a history of chronic vomiting since birth. In prior hospitalizations, no organic etiology had been found. In his last hospitalization, at 10 months, changes in feeding practices and mild sedation were unsuccessful. The child was then transferred to a pediatric research unit.

Both parents exhibited psychiatric symptoms (anxiety, depression, etc). Also, the infant's mother was ambivalent about being a parent. Observations of the mother–child interaction revealed a mother who provided an insufficient caring environment for her son. She had minimal interactions with the child, and these involved little warmth or nurturance. The baby appeared upset and anxious. He displayed little attachment to his mother and did not engage others in social contact. The child vomited small amounts of food approximately 30 times a day. He exhibited little distress during his vomiting episodes.

Treatment involved assigning a nurse to spend a majority of the day with the child. The goal was to help the infant develop a specific object relationship through the provision of comfort and need gratification. Simultaneously, a therapist worked with the child's parents. The focus was on events in the past which interfered with the mother's current ability as a parent. Eventually the couple decided that they were not ready to be parents and gave the baby up for adoption.

The use of massive attention was associated with gradual decreases in vomiting and increases in weight gain while the child was in the hospital. As treatment progressed, the baby also began to vocalize more and appeared happier. After approximately two months of treatment, vomiting had subsided and the child was adopted. A follow-up at 39 months showed a normal child with no recurrence of vomiting.

Stein *et al.* (1959) found similar results using massive attention with an 8-month-old ruminator. Treatment was twofold: (1) A nurse was assigned to spend eight hours a day with the infant, and (2) the mother was provided psychotherapy. Therapy focused on her guilt feelings about being a poor parent. In addition, she was instructed in appropriate parenting skills. The use of massive attention resulted in a cessation of ruminating after one month with corresponding weight gains.

One of the most effective uses of massive attention was reported by Fullerton (1963) in his work with a 7-month-old ruminator. The child had had a history of vomiting after every meal since birth and weighed 4.8 kg on admission to a hospital. A nurse was assigned to the child for eight hours each day. Within four days, the infant's ruminations had ceased, even in the nurse's absence. The elimination of rumination resulted in the emergence of more vocalizations and smiling. The baby was discharged after three weeks of hospitalization with a weight of 5.7 kg.

While massive attention appears to be an effective technique in treating vomiting/ruminating behaviors, there are some limitations inherent in this approach. With the exception of the Fullerton (1963) study, massive attention results in a gradual elimination of vomiting. Total elimination appears to gake from three to eight weeks. Therefore, in life-threatening cases, this approach would seem to be contraindicated. A second limitation is that assignment of a staff person to the child for the entire day is costly and impractical in many instances. Finally, all of the reported successful cases involved infant ruminators, not adults or children.

3.3. Psychotherapy

Often therapists have attempted to use psychotherapy as the primary treatment intervention with chronic and cyclic vomiters. The literature reports favorable results (Berlin *et al.*, 1957; Reinhart *et al.*, 1977; Rich, 1978; Sperling, 1968).

Davenport *et al.* (1972) used psychotherapy to treat three children suffering from cyclic vomiting. The illustrative subject had a history of vomiting since three months of age. Episodes had increased from approximately six times a year to about every three weeks and culminated in hospitalization. The episodes lasted five to seven days, and attacks appeared to be precipitated by the child being disappointed or not getting her way. Before onset she would exhibit a drastic change in personality with hostility and regressive behavior. Direct anger was never observed between episodes.

The child's parents had a history of psychosomatic complaints. She acted seductively toward her father, and this behavior was reciprocated by him. She was negativistic with her mother and would not follow her mother's instructions.

Therapy, at first, attempted to help the client become aware of the considerable anger which appeared during her attacks and to whom it was directed. In the second phase of therapy, staff attempted to minimize the child's inappropriate anger. This approach resulted in anger being directed at the therapist. The child was then placed on imipramine and soon thereafter vomiting ceased. Therapy continued throughout her hospitalization and focused upon the child's jealousy of her brother and her feelings of rejection by her mother. Treatment lasted approximately one year.

Leibovich (1973) believes that a variety of personality and psychiatric disorders may lead to functional vomiting. Consequently the therapist must first determine the nature of the vomiting, as well as the individual's personality and psychodynamic structure. Leibovich (1973) suggests three different types of therapeutic interventions depending on the person's psychiatric disorder. Treatment for neurotics should focus primarily on ventilation. Therapy with psychotics, borderlines, and severely depressed individuals must focus primary attention on their symptoms with a gradual effort at rebuilding ego functions. Treatment for resistive clients entails first forming a trusting relationship with the person. Then, the therapist should attend to the psychosomatic symptom by exploring the stressful events precipitating the symptom and the feelings arising from these events.

The primary feature of psychotherapy, as a treatment for psychogenic vomiting, is a focus on broadly defined personality and family structures. Although the authors of the studies cited in this section believe that the technique is effective, treatment appears to take nine months or longer. Thus, this approach is of limited value in cases where the vomiting is life-threatening. Psychotherapy would also not be indicated for infants or retarded individuals.

3.4. Peripheral Electric Shock Therapy

As an alternative to the more traditional approaches to psychogenic vomiting and rumination, aversive conditioning has been utilized as a technique to inhibit these behaviors. A number of studies have reported a cessation of vomiting after the use of contingent peripheral electric shock (e.g., Bright & Whaley, 1968; Galbraith, Byrick, & Rutledge, 1970; Linscheid & Cunningham, 1977; Watkins, 1972; White & Taylor, 1967). This technique involves administering a brief but painful shock to the individual's arms or legs when psychogenic vomiting or rumination begin. Shock usually has the effect of eliminating the vomiting or ruminative behavior within four days (Luckey et al., 1968; Toister et al., 1975; Wright & Thalassinos, 1973). Watkins's (1972) treatment of a severely retarded, institutionalized 14-year-old male is an exception. In this case, electric shock, given contingently over an 11-hr period each day whenever the subject attempted to induce vomiting, required eight weeks of treatment before vomiting stopped.

The case study provided by Lang and Melamed (1969) is more typical. They stopped ruminative vomiting by contingently shocking the behavioral antecedents of the regurgitation. Their subject was a 9-month-old male, who had a history of ruminating after every meal for the prior four months. Since the disorder's onset, the child had been hospitalized on three different occasions during which no organic causes were found. Various treatments (dietary changes, drug therapy, different feeding positions, and massive attention) were tried without success. The child's weight was 5.4 kg when treatment began, and he was being fed with a nasogastric pump.

Electromyographic readings showed that the onset of rumination was associated with considerable throat movements. Electrodes were placed on the child's thigh, and he was shocked for 1 sec at 1-sec intervals whenever the vigorous throat movements occurred. Sessions after each feeding lasted one hour. The initiation of shock therapy quickly reduced ruminative behavior. It was totally eliminated by the sixth session. Within one month, the infant had gained 453 g. Follow-up evaluations at one month and one year revealed no recurrence of rumination. As ruminative behavior was reduced, there was a corresponding increase in the child's responsiveness to the environment.

Similar to Lang and Melamed (1969), Kohlenberg (1970) also chose to aversively condition the antecedents of emetic behavior, but without the encumbrance of the electromyographic apparatus. He designated overt abdominal contractions as the target behavior to be shocked. The subject was a 21-year-old, severely retarded female who had been vomiting after meals for three months. Treatment sessions lasted for 80 min after each meal. Shock threapy greatly reduced both abdominal contractions and regurgitation and totally eliminated the behavior within three days. A one-year follow-up showed that vomiting had reemerged and again had become a problem. Kohlenberg concluded that, while peripheral shock may be an effective technique in suppressing psychogenic vomiting, a maintenance program using shock may be necessary to ensure continued elimination of the target behavior.

Cunningham and Linscheid (1976) enhanced treatment generalization by using contingent shock in a variety of locations at different times of the day. They reported the elimination of ruminative vomiting in a 9-month-old boy as a result of this technique. More importantly, at six-month follow-up, no further ruminative behavior was evident.

Given these findings, it is apparent that electric shock therapy can be an effective tool for the quick elimination of psychogenic vomiting. The use of shock would be especially helpful in life-threatening cases. There are, however, considerable ethical, legal, and humanitarian concerns that must be considered before electric shock is used. In addition, any severe punishment procedure, such as electric shock, has the potential for serious abuse. As a result, the usage of electric shock has been curtailed severely. When it is used, the guidelines of May, Risley, Twardosz, Friedman, Bijou, Wexler et al. (1975) should be followed meticulously.

3.5. Taste Aversion Methods

In an effort to capitalize on the effectiveness of aversive conditioning but avoid some of the limitations and hazards associated with electric shock, several authors have utilized the contingent application of aversive tastes to treat psychogenic vomiting. This method typically involves injecting lemon juice or tabasco sauce into the child's mouth when emesis or its antecedents occur. From 5 to 10 ml of lemon juice or 2 to 3 drops of tabasco sauce are squirted into the subject's mouth whenever he/she exhibits the various tongue and mouth movements identified as the beginning of emetic behavior. The taste-aversion studies have reported promising results (Becker et al., 1978; Bright & Whaley, 1968; Marholin et al., 1980; Murray et al., 1977; Sajwaj et al., 1974).

Sajwaj et al. (1974) first demonstrated the use of lemon juice therapy with a 6-month-old female whose health was rapidly declining because of her rumination. The child was unresponsive to the environment, displaying clear symptoms of inanition. Rumination occurred after every meal and was preceded by vigorous tongue and lip movements. Rumination continued for approximately 20 to 40 min after feeding. Treatment involved the squirting of 5–10 ml of lemon juice into the child's mouth whenever she displayed the antecedent lip and mouth movements. There were 30–60-sec intervals between administrations. The lemon juice would continue to be reapplied as long as the emetic behaviors were observed during the 20-min sessions.

The experimental design included baseline and reversal conditions as well as two treatment conditions. The use of lemon juice resulted in rapid declines in ruminative behaviors. Complete elimination of rumination was achieved by the 12th day of the last condition. Concurrent with the reductions in rumination, the infant became more responsive and attentive. Long-term follow-up (up to seven years) showed no recurrence of rumination. The authors noted two side effects resulting from the use of lemon juice. Frequent use of the lemon juice would irritate the mouth. Also there was the potential for aspiration if lemon juice should get into a baby's lungs. These difficulties can be minimized if the infant's head is held upright. Other precautions would be to reduce the amount of juice and/or decrease the force with which it is squirted.

Murray et al. (1978) used a combination of techniques, with tabasco sauce being the major intervention, with a ruminating infant. The subject was a 6-month-old boy who had been ruminating after meals for two weeks. The infant induced rumination through tongue and mouth movements. The treatment program involved both aversive conditioning and positive reinforcement. The child was held during feeding. If the mouth and tongue movements associated with rumination appeared, he was placed in his crib and several drops of tabasco sauce were put in his mouth. This procedure was repeated as long as emetic behaviors were observed. Upon cessation of rumination the child was held for about 20 min. This combination of taste aversion and positive reinforcement techniques effectively reduced rumination by Day 3 of treatment and totally suppressed it by Day 10 of the study. A follow-up at 10 months revealed no further episodes of rumination.

Becker et al. (1978) were able to substantially reduce rumination within two weeks in a 3-year-old retarded girl using lemon juice therapy in a day-treatment program. Becker et al. also reported the appearance of prosocial and self-stimulatory behavior when rumination was reduced. The toddler's mother was then taught the aversive procedure. Follow-up visits were made over a six-month period to ensure continuation of the treatment. However, approximately one year after treatment the child was rehospitalized for rumination. At that time, the family admitted to using the lemon juice only in the presence of a doctor or other hospital staff.

The Marholin et al. (1980) study is the only one in the literature which has used both lemon juice and tabasco sauce. Marholin et al. successfully treated a 16-year-old profoundly retarded male with a 5-year history of rumination using contingent lemon juice. Treatment lasted a total of 62 days, but rumination was actually eliminated by the second week of therapy. The reduction of rumination was associated with large weight gains and an increase in social and communication skills. Lemon juice treatment of the second subject, an 11-year-old profoundly retarded male, was not as successful. Lemon juice initially reduced ruminative behavior for the first 11 days of treatment. The behavior then reappeared and approximated base-line levels. Contingent tabasco sauce was substituted, and this resulted in immediate reductions of rumination and associated behaviors. At 1-month follow-up no ruminative behavior was evident. Marholin et al. suggest that the effectiveness of lemon juice or tabasco sauce may be due to the fact that it is "topographically related" to ruminative behavior, that is, both behavior and treatment involved substances in the client's mouth.

Sajwaj and Meyerrose (1980) reported an analysis of the effectiveness of lemon juice for three profoundly retarded, institutionalized individuals. Rumination histories were 4, 15, and 33 years in length. All three individuals did little other than ruminate. One was considered deaf because he was not observed to respond to sounds. Lemon juice was applied for every observed episode of rumination. Although the ward staff were inconsistent in following this instruction, rumination was decreased to a low level in all individuals but was not eliminated. Water, when substituted for the lemon juice was ineffective. With rumination reduced, many new behaviors suddenly appeared, some appropriate and some self-stimulatory. All new behaviors tended to decrease over time. The individual considered deaf began to respond to sounds, particularly human voices. At the 6-year follow-up, two of the individuals were ruminating at rates well below pretreatment levels. The other individual had completely reverted to rumination. No episode of abusing the use of the lemon juice by ward staff was noted.

Clark (1956) reported positive results with a ruminating infant by placing a quinine tablet in her formula. His hypothesis was that the child would experience the aversive bitter taste of her vomitus and extinguish her rumination. A decrease in rumination and a corresponding increase in weight were associated with the onset and maintenance of this treatment.

The use of the taste-aversion technique in the treatment of psychogenic vomiting has several advantages. These interventions reduce and/or eliminate vomiting/rumination in a relatively short amount of time. This factor makes the technique amenable for treatment in serious cases. Also, there are few ethical and humanistic objections to taste-aversion. Lemon juice and/or tabasco sauce involve little encumbrances, and their use is practical in many settings. Lastly, taste-aversion does not appear to be as abusable as electric shock.

There are several limitations to the use of taste-aversion methods. To date, these methods have only been applied with infants, children, and mentally-retarded individuals. Also, the use of lemon juice and tabasco sauce has shown mixed results in treating vomiting in severely and profoundly retarded persons. Because this is a punishment procedure, there is the possibility that there will not be a treatment generalization unless the technique is employed in a variety of environments. In a similar fashion, the technique may be contraindicated for use in the home by families who lack the motivation or ability to use it consistently. As with all aversive conditioning, taste-aversion should only be approached carefully (May *et al.*, 1975).

3.6. Differential Reinforcement and Other Behavioral Techniques

To avoid the obvious limitations of electric shock therapy, many behaviorally oriented therapists have opted for alternative treatment approaches. Several studies have utilized differential reinforcement either alone or in conjunction with other techniques and have reported favorable results (Ingersoll & Curry, 1977; Munford & Pally, 1979; O'Neil *et al.*, 1979; Wright *et al.*, 1978).

Differential reinforcement of other behaviors can be operationally defined as the reinforcement of appropriate nonvomiting behaviors while simultaneously imposing extinction on the targeted behavior (vomiting). Wright *et al.* (1978) used this technique to treat a 9-month-old female who had regurgitated and ruminated since she was three weeks old. The child was eager to eat at feedings but ruminated soon thereafter. The infant's mother was observed to give the child considerable attention after she had ruminated. Thereafter, treatment consisted of giving the child attention whenever she exhibited appropriate behavior and giving no attention following ruminative behavior. The implementation of differential reinforcement procedures resulted in a gradual but consistent decline in rumination. The child was discharged from the hospital after 56 days of treatment. At that time, her rumination was at minimal levels. Follow-up evaluations at 7 and 13 months revealed no further ruminating.

O'Neil *et al.* (1979) compared differential reinforcement, taste aversion, and massive attention in the treatment of a ruminating, 26-month-old female. Differential reinforcement was more effective than either taste-aversion or massive attention in eliminating ruminative behavior. While lemon juice (taste-aversion method) reduced ruminating, this decline was not as significant as the decrease attributed to differential reinforcement. O'Neil *et al.* noted that a limitation of their findings was that the study did not allow for the assessment of differential reinforcement prior to the initiation of punishment.

Munford and Pally (1979) demonstrated that differential reinforcement could be applied effectively on an outpatient basis. They treated an 11-year-old boy who had vomited for eight years. His relatives were instructed to ignore the boy whenever he vomited, offering no help or sympathy; but to praise him and give physical affection whenever he did his homework or chores. The vomiting rate declined from 29 instances during a one-week base line to none by the third week. Follow-up at three months and one year showed no further emesis.

A variation on the use of differential reinforcement is the use of extinction procedures alone to treat vomiting. Alford *et al.* (1972) used extinction with a 17-year-old female chronic vomiter who was hospitalized after a suicide gesture. The patient frequently sought staff attention in inappropriate ways. Her treatment consisted of meals six times a day with a staff member present. Upon emesis the staff person immediately left the room and did not return for the remainder of the meal. The patient was not told that the staff member would leave if she vomited. A reversal condition was utilized to demonstrate the effectiveness of the extinction procedures. When the extinction methods were observed to be effective in suppressing the patient's vomiting, attempts were made to generalize the treatment results. The client was returned to a regular meal schedule. Only then was she told about the research findings up till that time. In addition, staff and other patients were told to ignore the client whenever she talked about regurgitation. The patient was also told she would receive a 30-min isolation period for vomiting. The overall results indicated that extinction procedures effectively suppressed vomiting after the first day of treatment. A 7-month follow-up revealed only one vomiting incident. Wolf, Birnbrauer, Williams, and Lawler (1965) also used an extinction technique to eliminate vomiting in an institutionalized 9-year-old retarded girl. Wolf et al. observed that, when vomiting occurred in school, the girl would be sent back to her dormitory, and this appeared to reinforce the vomiting behavior. When she was made to remain in class after episodes (extinction), vomiting ceased.

Correction and overcorrection procedures were used by Azrin and Wesolowski (1975) and Duker and Seys (1977) to treat vomiting. *Correction* is the procedure whereby an individual is required to correct the results of his/her actions. In addition, he/she may be required to perform other behaviors (*overcorrection*) which are closely associated with the results of their behavior. Duker and Seys (1977) implemented overcorrection procedures with a 19-year-old, profoundly retarded female after the patient's vomiting proved resistant to differential reinforcement procedures and taste-aversion methods. Whenever the patient vomited she was instructed to first wash herself, then clean up the vomitus, and finally to overcorrect by cleaning portions of the wall and floor. A reversal design was used, and positive reinforcement was provided throughout for non-vomiting behaviors. The results indicated that the overcorrection procedures effectively reduced vomiting behavior.

In a similar fashion Azrin and Wesolowski (1975) coupled a positive practice procedure with self-correction in treating a profoundly retarded, 36-year-old female. The positive practice procedure entailed having the patient repeatedly practice the appropriate way to vomit (i.e., going to the restroom) whenever the target behavior was exhibited. She also was required to clean up her vomitus (self-correction). The treatment procedures eliminated vomiting one week after their introduction.

Several other behavioral interventions for psychogenic vomiting have been reported. Jackson, Johnson, Ackron, and Crowley (1975) used food satiation to reduce vomiting behavior. Their assumption was that satiation would reduce the probability of the vomiting response from reoccurring. They allowed the individual to eat until satiated at every meal (*satiation* being defined as a complete refusal to eat more food). The treatment approach was used with two profoundly retarded adults and resulted in 94% and 50% reductions in vomiting behavior, respectively. Spergel (1975) used induced vomiting to treat chronic emesis in a 10-year-old child. The patient was forced to vomit by a staff member who placed a finger down the patient's throat. The subject's vomiting ceased after five trials. Although these interventions were successful, the obvious medical complications associated with forced vomiting severely curtail this procedure's use.

Burgess (1969) treated a case of episodic vomiting by changing the events that preceded vomiting. In this case, a young woman's vomiting episode always occurred on the morning after a date the prior evening. Burgess drastically altered the circumstances of evening dating and then gradually returned them to those circumstances typical for the woman prior to the appearance of vomiting. At 1-year follow-up the client was still free of the vomiting. Using a similar concept, Katahn (1967) used a combination of desensitization and counseling to reduce episodic vomiting in a college basketball player.

As noted earlier, these behavioral interventions are effective treatments for vomiting disorders. They are applicable to a variety of populations (infants, children, adolescents, and retardates) and can eliminate vomiting within a relatively short period of time. One of the more promising aspects of the behavioral interventions is their compatibility with outpatient treatment. Because the techniques are relatively simple, they can be taught to parents or staff, thus reducing treatment time and increasing cost effectiveness.

Inherent in the advantages of the behavioral techniques are their limitations. At times, social reinforcement contingencies can be difficult to detect, thereby reducing the utility of the extinction aspects of differential reinforcement procedures. In life-threatening cases, there is often not enough time to extinguish the vomiting behavior solely through changes in positive reinforcement contingencies. Some studies have reported treatment of one to two months before extinction was completed. Overcorrection procedures necessitate staff working with only one patient for considerable periods of time. In many situations, this amount of time will be logistically impossible. Also, satiation and induced vomiting procedures raise ethical and health-related issues.

4. Comparison of Treatment Approaches

The effectiveness of the various medical interventions is not clear. Although several of the studies reported in this review found little or no success with these methods, it may well be that their successful usage is not being reported in the published literature. These medical procedures seem to be regarded as standard or generally accepted treatments which do not need to be subjected to clinical trials. Furthermore, these techniques are often used concurrently with other interventions, such as increased attention (Kanner, 1972).

The effectiveness of psychotherapy for psychogenic vomiting is also difficult to assess. The published reports are anecdotal case studies which provide little quantitative data. The intervention itself is poorly specified, so that the exact nature of the interactions between the therapist and client is unknown. Given the poor specification of the psychotherapeutic procedures, it is possible that components of massive attention and behavioral procedures are actually being used, thereby confounding any conclusions about the effectiveness of psychotherapy.

The evidence for the effectiveness of massive attention is more substantial. Although quantitative data on rumination are generally lacking, most of the studies report weight data. Further, a cessation of rumination is reported within a three to eight week period, with one case (Fullerton, 1963) reporting success within four days. Although these studies are weak by strict scientific standards, there seems to be a consensus in the pediatric and psychiatric literature that increases in overall attention are correlated with the reduction of rumination in infants. Whether massive attention can be effective with other forms of psychogenic vomiting or with rumination in retarded individuals has not been demonstrated.

The evidence for the effectiveness of the various techniques derived from behavior therapy is compelling. Most of the studies quantify the measurement of psychogenic vomiting and describe precisely the intervention procedures. Further, several of the studies employ a reversal of treatment procedures, that is, treatment is started, temporarily withdrawn, and then restarted. The use of this tactic controls for time-related confounding events and considerably strengthens the demonstration of the treatment technique.

Most of the behavioral treatment techniques, especially those using electric shock and taste-aversion, report reduction and elimination within a few days of treatment. While several of these studies report relapses after treatment is discontinued, others report continued success at long-term follow-up. It should also be noted that the failures at follow-up occur with institutionalized, severely or profoundly retarded individuals with long histories of psychogenic vomiting; these cases are the most difficult populations with which to carry out any behavior change program.

Although the behavioral interventions appear to be better validated than the other treatment techniques discussed, one must be cautious in interpreting these research reports. The entire literature on psychogenic vomiting is small, and the number of cases reported on its subcategories, especially chronic and cyclical vomiting, are very few.

5. Conclusions

The study of psychogenic vomiting is in its infancy. Well-documented cases of successful treatment are not plentiful and have only appeared in the last few years. Little is known about the etiology of these disorders, even though a great deal of theoretical speculation has been offered, and the physiological mechanism of psychogenic vomiting has not been systematically studied. In fact, the categorization of psychogenic vomiting into chronic vomiting, cyclical vomiting, and rumination may be premature given the sparseness of the literature.

Several of the cases cited in this review are difficult to place neatly into one of these three categories. Even an estimate of the incidence of this disorder, in the general population, is unknown.

Progress in understanding and treating psychogenic vomiting will depend on three factors. First, more cases of psychogenic vomiting will need to be reported so that the range, diversity, and incidence of the disorder can be better described. Most helpful would be reports on large groups of patients studied and treated in the same way. Second, the scientific quality of the evaluation of the various treatment approaches must be improved. Uncontrolled case studies will not add extensively to the understanding of these disorders. Perhaps the most significant contribution of the behavioral approaches is their emphasis on scientific vigor and unequivocal demonstration of the effectiveness of the treatment. Finally, the physiology of psychogenic vomiting must be investigated. Only then can the effects of the environment on psychogenic vomiting be understood and treatment approaches be improved.

Despite these limitations, the study of rumination has grown considerably in recent years. Since the evaluation by Kanner (1972) of the state of the art in treating rumination, a range of promising behavioral techniques have appeared, not only for rumination but also for other forms of psychogenic vomiting. Now practicing clinicians have a wide array of treatment techniques available. As the knowledge of the psychophysiology of the digestive tract increases, one can expect greater advances in treating psychogenic vomiting.

6. References

Alford, G., Blanchard, E., & Buckley, T. M. Treatment of hysterical vomiting by modification of social contingencies: A case study. *Journal of Behavior Therapy and Experimental Psychiatry*, 1972, *3*, 209–212.

Azrin, N. H., & Wesolowski, M. D. Eliminating habitual vomiting in a retarded adult by positive practice and self correction. *Journal of Behavior Therapy and Experimental Psychiatry*, 1975, *6*, 145–148.

Becker, J., Turner, S., & Sajwaj, T. Multiple behavioral effects of the use of lemon juice with a ruminating toddler-age child. *Behavior Modification*, 1978, *2*, 267–278.

Berlin, I. N., McCullough, J., Liska, E. S., & Szurek, S. A. Intractabile episodic vomiting in a three-year-old child. *Psychiatric Quarterly*, 1957, *31*, 228–249.

Bright, C. O., & Whaley, D. L. Suppression of regurgitation and rumination with aversive events. *Michigan Mental Health Research Bulletin*, 1968, *11*, 17–20.

Burgess, E. Elimination of vomiting behavior. *Behavior Research and Therapy*, 1969, *7*, 173–176.

Clark, F. H. Rumination. *Archives of Pediatrics*, 1956, *73*, 12–19.

Cunningham, C., & Linscheid, T. Elimination of chronic infant ruminating by electric shock. *Behavior Therapy*, 1976, *7*, 231–234.

Davenport, C., Zrull, J., Kuhn, C., & Harrison, S. Cyclic vomiting. *Journal of American Academy of Child Psychiatry*, 1972, *11*, 66–87.

Duker, P., & Seys, D. Elimination of vomiting in a retarded female using restitutional overcorrection. *Behavior Therapy*, 1977, *8*, 225–257.

Feldman, M., & Fordtran, J. Vomiting. In M. S. Sleisenger & J. S. Fordtran (Eds.), *Gastrointestinal disease: Pathophysiology, diagnosis, management* (2nd Edition). Philadelphia: W. Saunders, 1978.

Ferholt, J., & Provence, S. Diagnosis and treatment of an infant with psychophysiological vomiting. *Psychoanalytic Study of the Child*, 1976, *31*, 439–459.

Fleisher, D. R. Infantile rumination syndrome. *American Journal of Diseases of Children*, 1979, *133*, 266–269.

Fullerton, D. T. Infantile rumination: A case report. *Archives of General Psychiatry*, 1963, *9*, 593–600.

Gaddini, R., & Gaddini, E. Rumination in infancy. In L. Jessner & E. Pavenstadt (Eds.), *Dynamic psychopathology in childhood*. New York: Grune & Stratton, 1959.

Galbraith, D., Byrick, R., & Rutledge, J. An aversive conditioning approach to the inhibition of chronic vomiting. *Canadian Psychiatric Association Journal*, 1970, *15*, 311–313.

Hallowell, J., & Gardner, L. Rumination and growth failure in a male fraternal twin. *Pediatrics*, 1965, *36*, 565–571.

Hill, O. Psychogenic vomiting. *Gut*, 1968, *9*, 348–352.

Hoyt, C., & Stickler, G. A study of 44 children with the syndrome of recurrent (cyclic) vomiting. *Pediatrics*, 1960, *25*, 775–779.

Ingersoll, B., & Curry, F. Rapid treatment of persistent vomiting in a 14-year-old female by shaping and time out. *Journal of Behavior Therapy and Experimental Psychiatry*, 1977, *8*, 305–307.

Jackson, G., Johnson, C., Ackron, G., & Crowley, R. Food satiation as a procedure to decelerate vomiting. *American Journal of Mental Deficiency*, 1975, *80*, 223–227.

Kanner, L. *Child psychiatry* (4th Edition). Springfield: Charles C Thomas, 1972.

Katahn, M. Systematic desensitization and counseling for anxiety in a college basketball player. *Journal of Special Education*, 1967, *1*, 309–314.

Kohlenberg, R. J. The punishment of persistent vomiting: A case study. *Journal of Applied Behavioral Analysis*, 1970, *3*, 241–245.

Lang, P., & Melamed, B. Case report: Avoidance conditioning therapy of an infant with chronic ruminative vomiting. *Journal of Abnormal Psychology*, 1969, *74*, 1–8.

Leibovich, M. A. Psychogenic vomiting. *Psychotherapy and Psychosomatics*, 1973, *22*, 263–268.

Linscheid, T., & Cunningham, C. A controlled demonstration of the effectiveness of electric shock in the elimination of chronic infant rumination. *Journal of Applied Behavior Analysis*, 1977, *10*, 500.

Luckey, R., Watson, C., & Musick, J. Aversive conditioning as a means of inhibiting vomiting and rumination. *American Journal of Mental Deficiency*, 1968, *73*, 139–142.

Marholin II, D., Luiselli, J. K., Robinson, M., & Lott, I. T. Response-contingent taste-aversion in treating chronic ruminative vomiting of institutionalized profoundly retarded children. *Journal of Mental Deficiency Research*, 1980, *24*, 47–56.

May, J. G., Risley, T. R., Twardosz, S., Friedman, P., Bijou, S. W., Wexler, D., et al. Guidelines for the use of behavioral procedures in state programs for retarded persons. *M. R. Research*, 1975, *1*. (Monograph)

Menking, M., Wagnitz, J., Burton, J., Coddington, R. D., & Sotos, J. F. Rumination—A near fatal psychiatric disease of infancy. *The New England Journal of Medicine*, 1969, *280*, 802–804.

Munford, P., & Pally, R. Outpatient contingency management of operant vomiting. *Journal of Behavior Therapy and Experimental Psychiatry*, 1979, *10*, 135–137.

Murray, M., Keele, D., & McCarver, J. Treatment of rumination with behavioral techniques: A case report. *Behavior Therapy*, 1977, *8*, 999–1003.

O'Neil, P., White, J., King, Jr., C., & Carek, D. Controlling childhood rumination through differential reinforcement of other behavior. *Behavior Modification*, 1979, *3*, 352–372.

Reinhart, J., Evans, S., & McFadden, D. Cyclic vomiting in children: Seen through the psychiatrist's eye. *Pediatrics,* 1977, *59,* 371–377.

Rich, C. L. Self-induced vomiting, psychiatric considerations. *Journal of the American Medical Association,* 1978, *239,* 2688–2689.

Richmond, J., Eddy, E., & Green, M. Rumination: A psychosomatic syndrome of infancy. *Pediatrics,* 1958, *22,* 49–54.

Sajwaj, T., Libet, J., & Agras, S. Lemon juice therapy: The control of life-threatening rumination in a six-month-old infant. *Journal of Applied Behavior Analysis,* 1974, *7,* 557–563.

Sajwaj, T. E., & Meyerrose, M. *The treatment of life-threatening rumination with the contingent use of lemon juice.* Paper presented at the International Symposium on the Psychophysiology of the Gut: Experimental and Clinical Aspects, Munich, June 1980.

Spergel, S. Induced vomiting treatment of acute compulsive vomiting. *Journal of Behavior Therapy and Experimental Psychiatry,* 1975, *6,* 85–86.

Sperling, M. Trichotillomania, trichophagy and cyclic vomiting. *International Journal of Psychoanalysis,* 1968, *49,* 682–689.

Stein, M., Rausen, A., & Blau, A. Psychotherapy of an infant with rumination. *Journal of the American Medical Association,* 1959, *171,* 2309–2312.

Toister, R. P., Condron, C. J., Worley, L., & Arthur, D. Faradic therapy of chronic vomiting in infancy: A case study. *Journal of Behavior Therapy and Experimental Psychiatry,* 1975, *6,* 55–59.

Watkins, J. T. Treatment of chronic vomiting and extreme emaciation by an aversive stimulus: Case study. *Psychological Reports,* 1972, *31,* 803–805.

White, J. C., Jr., & Taylor, D. Noxious conditioning as a treatment for rumination. *Mental Retardation,* 1967, *5,* 30–33.

Wolf, M., Birnbrauer, J., Williams, T., & Lawler, J. A note on apparent extinction of vomiting behavior of a retarded child. In L. Ullmann & L. Krasner (Eds.), *Case studies in behavior modification.* New York: Holt, Rinehart & Winston, 1965.

Wright, D. F., Brown, R., & Andrews, M. Remission of chronic ruminative vomiting through a reversal of social contingencies. *Behavior Research and Therapy,* 1978, *16,* 134–136.

Wright, L., & Thalassinos, P. Success with electric shock in habitual vomiting: Report of two cases in young children. *Clinical Pediatrics,* 1973, *12,* 594–597.

PART II

STOMACH
RUPERT HÖLZL

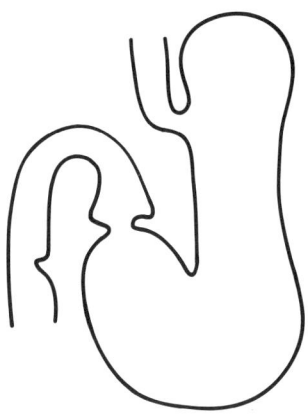

The stomach seems to be that part of the gastrointestinal tract which received most attention by psychophysiologically orientated investigators. This may be due in part to the relatively high prevalence of functional stomach disorders and their early identification as stress-related diseases. Although it is difficult to arrive at reliable figures because of frequently lacking clinical symptoms, current estimates state that about 10% to 20% of the population get peptic ulcers (ventriculi duodeni) at least once during their life. At any given time, 1% to 2% of the population suffer from an active ulcer verifiable by radiological examination (Wenderoth, 1978). For men aged 40 to 55, the figure is even higher (6%).

The peptic ulcer for some time was seen as *the* psychosomatic disorder by both psychoanalysts and gastroenterologists. Since Beaumont's pioneering observations (Beaumont, 1833) and the well-known physiological experiments by Cannon (1909) many reports appeared demonstrating psychological influences on stomach acid production and contractile activity.

The basic functions of the gastric organ are to receive and store what we eat and drink, to produce digestive juice mainly consisting of the enzyme pepsin, hydrochloric acid, and mucus, and to mix and transport stomach contents by proper movements, finally releasing the resulting chymus through the pylorus into the duodenum, well broken down and mixed with acid and enzymes for the following stages of digestion.

The nervous system modulates the secretory and motor functions of the stomach. Under physiological conditions, this is a necessary regulatory process and ensures that alimentary and other biological functions like mating, fight, or flight remain well-coordinated and do not interfere with each other. When these regulatory processes, however, meet their limits, as in overwhelming or unduely prolonged *stress*, gastric dysfunction (secretory and motoric) will be the consequence. A chronic dysfunction, like a peptic ulcer, eventually leads to tissue damage of the stomach. Barbara Walker in Chapter 10 analyzes this process in some depth. She summarizes current knowledge about the psychophysiological *interface* to primary stomach functions. Much gastroenterological research pertinent to the local pathogenesis in peptic ulcer formation has been done. At least some information on psychological conditions leading to ulceration is available from animal experiments done in Brady's and Weiss's group (cf. Chapter 10). But almost nothing is known about the psychophysiological mechanisms, the "interface" connecting psychological conditions, neurophysiological correlates, and local stomach variables. The problem is made even worse by the fact that experimental ulcers produced in the typical animal study are not good equivalents of peptic ulcers in humans, neither in localization nor in histology (Bykow & Kurzin, 1966; Oi, Toriumi, Miho, & Kijima, 1971; cf. Hölzl, Schröder, & Kiefer, 1979). Obviously direct psychophysiological studies with human subjects on gastric changes under specified stimulus conditions, instrumental learning procedures, and achievement and social situations are needed. Robert M. Stern (Chapter 9) collected available data on this issue and related it to the problem of perception of gastric reactions to external stimulation. Walker's and Stern's reviews make it clear that despite some quite promising reports in the psychophysiological literature much more research in the laboratory with healthy *and* diseased people is needed for a more detailed picture of that "interface" to emerge.

Given the practical relevance of the question (exactly how psychological factors cause pathological and finally ulcerative changes in stomach functions) the relative scarcity of data is astonishing. One important reason may be found in the difficulty of performing experimental studies in this area. For instance, there is the variance stemming from prior alimentation and similar factors (cf. Chapter 9). But already at the very basis of psychophysiological investigation into stomach reactions almost insurmountable obstacles have to be overcome: In contrast to the study of, for example, cardiovascular psychophysiology, measurement of relevant physiological variables of the organ under investigation in a nondisturbing way, is difficult, and until recently satisfactory methods were not available. Because much effort went into important methodological work, Chapters 5 by Hölzl, 7 by Welgan, and 8 by Stacher deal with the issue of measuring gastric motility and secretion in more detail.

It is hoped that the advent of noninvasive methods for studying the stomach will stimulate more psychophysiological studies of that organ, but will perhaps also lead to similar developments for other parts of the gut which lack these techniques consequently hindering research on psychological determinants of function. Complicated technological tasks arise when smooth muscle activity must be evaluated from the body surface. Involved methods of analysis, originally invented by communication engineers for noisy physical signals, have been used on gastrointestinal activity by several research groups. It is sometimes difficult for the psychologist to evaluate studies using these methods if their basic assumptions are not reported. Chapter 6 by Müller, Hölzl, and Brüchle, therefore, apart from reporting on a special example of noninvasive gastrography, includes some elementary information on Fourier techniques which often have been used in the analysis of gastrographic records.

In recent years, self-control of gastrointestinal responses has received increasing attention. If successful biofeedback training of gastric motor and/or secretory function could be demonstrated, alternative treatments for ulcer patients instead of surgical intervention, prolonged drug therapy, or nonspecific psychotherapy could be devised. The chapters by Barbara Walker and Peter Welgan also report on instrumental learning of gastric motor and secretory responses which could possibly lead to the development of therapeutic biofeedback procedures. Their work also shows the major technical and methodological problems encountered by such an approach. Not only is training difficult but also one has to deal with the problem of carefully defining what really is learned in the training. Better specification of response classes reinforced by the feedback signal leads back to the basic measurement problem. It is considered to be

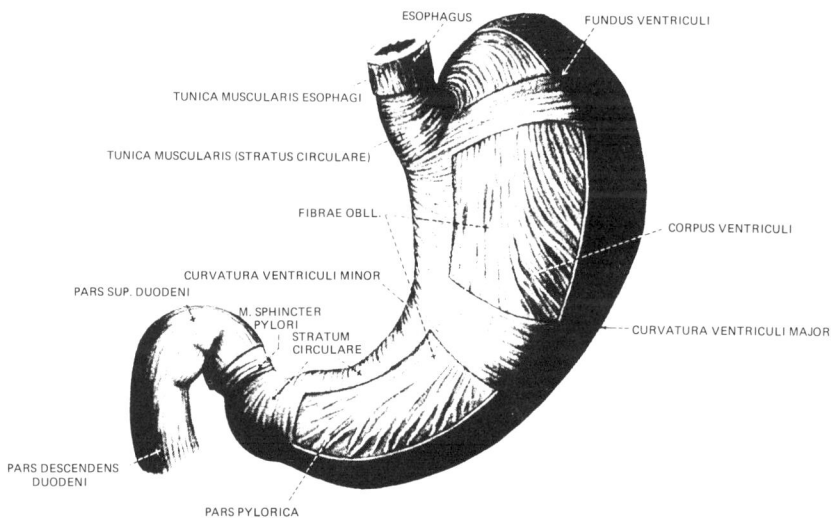

Figure 1. Major anatomical parts and landmarks of stomach. Circular and oblique muscle fibers are shown by superficial dissection. The "pars pylorica" is also called "pyloric antrum." In another more usual nomenclature the term "antrum" denotes to total lower third of the corpus including the pars pylorica. The so-called "cardia" is the entrance of the esophagus into the stomach. (Figure reproduced from Kiss & Szentágothai, 1971, with permission.)

solvable, however, along the lines several psychophysiological and gastroenterological research groups have been working along during the last years (Smout, 1980).

In the following chapters many technical terms of anatomy and physiology will be used. Not all of them could be explained in detail by the authors for lack of space. Figure 1 may help the reader identify the gross-anatomical parts of the organ we are dealing with in this section.

References

Beaumont, W. *Experiments and observations on the gastric juice and the physiology of digestion.* Plattburgh: Allen, 1833. (Facsimile: Cambridge, Massachusetts: Harvard University Press, 1929.)

Cannon, W. B. The influence of emotional states on the functions of the alimentary canal. *American Journal of Medical Sciences,* 1909, *137,* 480–487.

Hölzl, R., Schröder, G., & Kiefer, H. Indirect gastrointestinal motility measurement for use in experimental psychosomatics: A new method and some data. *Behavior Analysis and Modification,* 1979, *3,* 77–97.

Kiss, F., & Szentágothai, J. *Anatomischer Atlas des menschlichen Körpers* (Vol. II). Stuttgart: G. Fischer, 1971.

Oi, M., Toriumi, T., Miho, O., & Kijima, M. Location of experimental ulcers as compared with that of human peptic ulcer. In C. J. Pfeiffer (Ed.), *Peptic ulcer.* Kopenhagen: Munksgaard, 1971.

Smout, A. J. P. M. *Myoelectric activity of the stomach: Gastroelectromyography and electrogastrography.* Delft: University Press, 1980.

Wenderoth, H. Ulkuskrankheit. In H. Hornbostel, W. Kaufmann, & Siegenthaler (Eds.), *Innere Medizin in Praxis und Klinik. Verdauungstrakt* (Vol. 4). Stuttgart: Thieme, 1978.

5

SURFACE GASTROGRAMS AS MEASURES OF GASTRIC MOTILITY

RUPERT HÖLZL

1. Introduction: A Short History of Gastric Motility Records

Since the early observations by Beaumont (1833), a number of studies have been reported on the psychophysiology of stomach secretory and electromotor activity. The latter, which serves as the necessary mixing and transport functions of the stomach for digestion, has been evaluated by various techniques. Beaumont used *direct observation* of a part of the stomach wall in a patient with a large fistula and found marked changes in secretory and contractile activity of the stomach under psychological influences including strong emotions and anticipation of meals. A century later Wolf and Wolff (1943) used this method in a more systematic study of their famous patient, Tom, to show that the motor activity of the fistulated stomach section changed with different emotional states. Whether hyper- or hypomotility was observed depended on the kind of emotion elicited (cf. Stern, Chapter 9, this volume).

Cannon (1909) seems to have been the first to use *fluoroscopic examination* to evaluate stomach motility in animals during states of rage, distress, or fear. Since then, this method has been used to observe, both clinically and experimentally, the motor response of the stomach to various stimuli ranging from meals to psychoanalytic "conflict interviews" (Zander, 1976, 1977).

Early on, *intragastric pressure recordings* were used to obtain more quantitative and reliable measures of gastric motor activity under a variety of experimental conditions. In this way, Cannon and Washburn (1912) and Carlson

---

RUPERT HÖLZL • Department of Psychology, Max Planck Institute of Psychiatry, 8000 Munich 40, The Federal Republic of Germany.

(1912a,b) found strong contractions of the empty stomach after long fasting periods which they believed were related to feelings of hunger ("hunger pangs"). These authors used an air-filled balloon on an intragastric tube. The catheter was connected to a pressure-sensitive device, the Marey capsule, to indicate contractions as rises in intragastric pressure. Later, use of water-filled tubing, constant perfusion of the catheters, and more precise pressure transducers improved the frequency response and sensitivity of the system.

At present, direct sensing pressure catheters with subminiaturized pressure sensitive elements are available which do not need extracorporal pressure transducers or perfusion pumps. However, the basic method is still the same as that developed by Cannon and Washburn and Carlson and is widely used in experimental and clinical gastroenterology. Because of the aversive properties of the procedure, psychophysiological studies only rarely have used the technique (i.e., Griggs & Stunkard, 1964; Stunkard & Koch, 1964; Whitehead & Drescher, 1980).

As early as 1922, Alvarez published *electrical recordings* from the abdomen of a cachexic woman in which peristaltic movements of the stomach could be palpated through the extremely thin abdominal wall. The potentials measured with D'Arsonvaal's galvanometer could be related to stomach movements (Alvarez, 1922; Alvarez & Mahoney, 1922). The recordings were called *electrogastrograms* (EGG). Much later, Davis and his co-workers introduced them into psychophysiology to study the influence of various stimuli on gastric electromotor activity (Davis, Garafolo, & Gault, 1957; Davis, Garafolo, & Kveim, 1959).

The technique seemed promising by the time it was first reviewed (Russell & Stern, 1967), but the EGG was not developed further or even used much after 1967. At about the same time as these psychophysiological studies, a new series of gastroenterological studies were published which attempted to record the electrical activity of the gastrointestinal tract from the abdominal surface of animal and human subjects (cf. Tiemann & Reichertz, 1959a,b). Pharmacological conditions and motility changes under certain pathological conditions were found in those early experiments. Another group of indirect techniques, the *magnetogastrogram* (MGG), were introduced by Wenger and his co-workers (Engel & McFall, 1959; Wenger, Engel, & Clemens, 1955; Wenger, Henderson, & Dinning, 1957; Wenger, Engel, Clemens, & Cullen, 1961). This technique involved measuring stomach contractions by using a small iron rod or magnet which the subject swallowed (sometimes sutured to the stomach walls). Afterwards, a magnetic field probe was placed over the abdomen to pick up magnet movements. This method, also, was not followed up by psychophysiologists.

In addition to the well-established effects of hypersecretion, changes in gastric motor functions play an important part in the production of peptic ulcers.

Some of those changes can be brought about by psychological variables such as strong emotions and stressful situations (cf. Stern, Chapter 9, this volume). Disturbance of gastric emptying or gastroduodenal reflux of chymus for instance are incorporated into several models of gastroduodenal ulcerogenesis, for example George (1968); Rhodes, Bernando, Phillips, Rovelstad, and Hofman (1969); or Bonfils (cited by Zander, 1976; cf. the short reviews in Hölzl, 1979; and Hölzl, Schröder, & Kiefer, 1979). Hunger-related stomach contractions and their perception have been related to disordered regulation of food intake in obese or anorexic patients by Stunkard and Fox (1971), and Bruch (1973). Generally, gastrointestinal motility, its perception, and consequent psychological events are thought to be important causative or concomitant variables in psychosomatics or in basic psychophysiological research. In some instances, modification by operant learning procedures and biofeedback was attempted (Deckner, Hill, & Bourne, 1972; Smith, 1972; Smith, Renault, & Schuster, 1973; Walker, Lawton, & Sandman, 1978; Whitehead & Drescher, 1980). Success in this area would be of clinical importance also (cf. Walker, Chapter 10, this volume). Given this background, the scarcity of psychophysiological investigations into gut motility is astonishing. Walker and Sandman (1977) suspected that "the wide-spread belief that a valid technique for studying the gastrointestinal tract does not exist" (p. 393) might be one reason for this unsatisfying state of affairs.

The only noninvasive techniques for measuring gastric motility, which would be acceptable to psychophysiologists in terms of minimal distress to the subject and the possibility of continuous recording over long periods, are the electrogastrogram (EGG) and the magnetogastrogram (MGG) which measure from the abdominal surface (see p. 82). Unfortunately both techniques yield results difficult to quantify, and there is doubt about their physiological meaning. Although Walker and Sandman (1977) criticized the neglect of the EGG by psychophysiologists (e.g., during experimental analyses of stress responses in ulcer patients), the rational bases for being sceptical about naive use of surface gastrography still exist. One problem is to identify the sources of the electrical signals recorded from the abdominal area. Another is that a general solution for the task of quantifying and extracting the relevant information content of the gastrographic record has not been found. Similar problems exist *mutatis mutandis* with the MGG.

This chapter reviews the evidence on what is being measured by surface gastrograms and how they can be reliably and economically analyzed. Two other noninvasive techniques, telemetric intraluminal pressure recordings and the analysis of abdominal sounds, are not considered here. The latter method provides only a qualitative index of large gut movements and has no physically well-defined relationship to stomach contractions (Furman, 1973). Telemetry, on the other hand, although producing reliable pressure recordings, presents certain problems of apparatus and application which have so far prevented its more general use in psychophysiology. For special applications, however, it is the method of choice (Fink & Stacher, 1972).

2. Electromotor Activity of the Stomach

2.1. The Role of Indices of Electromotor Activity

In a review on biofeedback training of gastric motility, Hubel (1974) rightly criticized the naive use of the electrogastrogram as a measure of motility by Deckner *et al.* (1972). *Motility,* if one means contraction and peristalsis, is a mechanical variable whereas the EGG is an electrical one. When interpreting the EGG as a correlate of contractions of the smooth muscles in the stomach walls, two problems are encountered.

The EGG records not only the projections of the summated action potentials of the gastric muscles, but a compound signal from different electrical sources in the internal organs. Signal analysis, therefore, must attempt to separate the gastric component. Secondly, "the electrogastrogram measures the frequency of the gastric pacemaker potential (gastric slow wave) rather than motility . . . , although slow wave frequency determines the maximal contraction rate" (Hubel, 1974, p. 1086). This means that not only is the electrogastrogram an indirect measure of the electrical activity of the smooth muscles, but there also is no one-to-one relation between these electrical potentials of the smooth muscles and mechanical contractions. In evaluating psychophysiological or gastroenterological studies using the EGG as a motility measure, it is essential to discuss the solutions these studies offer to those questions.

Unfortunately, this applies also to the direct measurement of intragastric pressure by open-tipped catheters and similar devices, which have sometimes been used as validation criteria against which noninvasive motility indices were evaluated (Davis *et al.,* 1959). Intragastric pressure variations are themselves consequences of motility but are not to be confused with motility itself. The correlations between localized mechanical events (i.e., muscle contractions) and overall changes of intragastric pressures are far from clear. An early study by Quigley and Brody (1952) severely criticized manometric methods on technical grounds. Some improvements have been made by using open-tipped catheter techniques, but problems remain.

For the sake of terminological clarity, therefore, the term *motility* is reserved here only for the mechanical variable of localized or generalized movement of stomach walls, well-coordinated or not. It is not used for manometric, electrical, magnetic, or other measurements (indices) of these movements, whether they are invasive or noninvasive. Pressure changes, for instance, are not smooth muscle movements albeit closely related to them. *Electromotor activity,* on the other hand, covers the whole complex of electrical and mechanical events observable in smooth muscles of the gastrum or their surroundings, which serve the biological functions of mixing and/or transport (emptying) when working in a well-coordinated fashion.

Three groups of physical variables are involved in electromotor activity.

1. The membranes of the smooth muscle fibers show changes in electrical potential which summate to mass potentials which in turn show as potential changes on the abdominal surface.
2. By a process which the physiologists call *electromechanical coupling* these electrical potentials are accompanied or followed by contraction of the muscles leading to localized or generalized movements of the stomach walls. These movements can be detected by implanted movement detectors like strain gauges or by magnets either fixed to the stomach wall or loosely lying on the stomach ground or some mucous fold. The movements of the magnets may be detected outside (Wenger et al., 1957, 1961). These magnetic changes, of course, are only indices of motility, not motility itself.
3. The contractions of the stomach lead eventually to intragastric pressure changes, but this is only the case as long as reductions in total volume are effected. Therefore, not every contraction is followed by intragastric pressure change. Elastic properties of the stomach and/or its partial filling with air or gas further modify the relation between the mechanical events of the wall contractions and subsequent pressure changes (Texter, Smith, Moeller, & Borborka, 1957; Truelove, 1968).

Gastroenterologists have done extensive work on the mechanism of these three physical indicators of gastric activity and their interrelations. It is strange that psychophysiologists only rarely have made use of this information to clarify the meaning of the indirect recording techniques they use in their experiments on psychological influences of gastrointestinal activity. To my knowledge, no serious attempt at discussion of the signal sources in the electrogastrogram has appeared in the literature since Russell and Stern's (1967) comprehensive and still classic review in Venables and Martin (1967), until a recent monograph by Smout (1980). Since then a great number of gastroenterological investigations have become available which clarify and also complicate this issue. In particular Nelsen's group (Nelsen & Kohatsu, 1968) and Duthie and Smallwood (e.g., Brown, Smallwood, Duthie, & Stoddard, 1975) have contributed greatly to the understanding of the information content of surface gastrograms.

To evaluate studies on indirect indices of gastric electromotor activity, an initial characterization of the underlying physiologic process being indexed by those various measures is essential.

2.2. Contractile Activity of the Stomach

Leaving aside for the moment the differences between intragastric pressure recordings and direct force transducers in the stomach wall, the mechanical events in the human stomach may be summarized according to Konturek and Rösch (1976) as follows: The orad portion of the stomach shows little or no contractile activity as evaluated by direct observation or by intraluminal pressure recording via small balloon probes or open-tipped catheters. Small phasic pressure changes of low amplitude and long duration are superimposed on the basal pressure. In contrast to the orad portions, the antrum, that is the caudal section, shows pronounced tonic and peristaltic contractions. The antral activity is basically what intragastric pressure probes record.

In the resting state, practically the same pressure prevails in the caudal stomach as in the rest of the abdomen, but in the contraction phase, various types of pressure waves may be recorded. They have been classified into three categories—Types I, II, and III (Code & Carlson, 1968; Davenport, 1971; Weisbrodt, 1974; cf. also Code, Hightower, & Morlock, 1952, cited in Russell & Stern, 1967, p. 226). Typical gastric pressure waves are shown in Figure 1.

Type I and Type II waves are rhythmic rises in pressure with a frequency of about 2–4 contractions per min and a duration of 2–20 sec (Figure 1). Simultaneous cineradiographic and manometric observations have shown that the waves of Types I and II correspond to visible ringlike contractions which migrate as peristaltic waves from the antrum to the pylorus. The primary function of these waves seems to be the propulsion and mixing of the stomach contents. Code *et al.* (1952) gave a slightly different description: Type I waves were characterized as monophasic waves of low amplitude with frequencies of 1–2 per

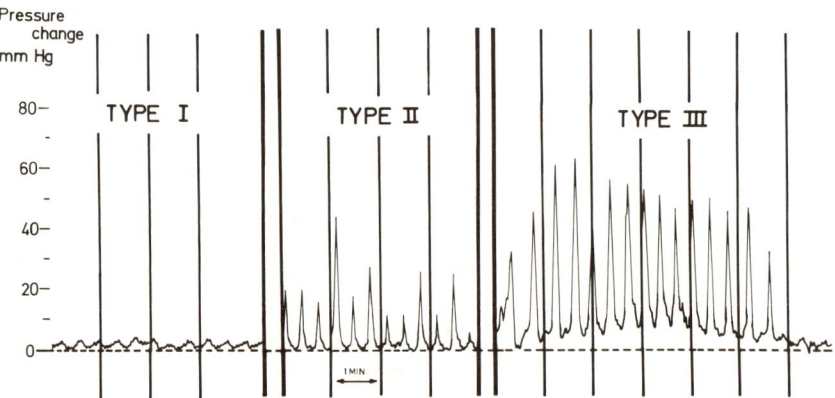

Figure 1. Types of gastric pressure waves. Modified from Code *et al.* (1952).

min in the fundus of the stomach and of 3–4 in the antrum. Type II waves, while also described as simple and monophasic, were described as having greater amplitude and frequencies in the range of 2–5 per min when appearing in a nonrhythmic pattern and of 3 per min when in a rhythmic pattern.

According to Hightower (1962), Type I waves should represent the mixing type of motor activity, while Type II stands for peristalsis which in the antrum "creates the pressure gradient that effects gastric evacuation into the duodenum" (p. 42). Both wave types coincide with the "20 second rhythm" described earlier by Carlson (1912a), if they occur in a rhythmic fashion. This is the case only in 30 to 50% of their total incidence.

Type III waves are more complex and characterized by a rise over the resting pressure for about one min. Rhythmic Type I and Type II waves are superimposed on this Type III curve, which appears seldom and irregular. The function of Type III waves is unknown but believed to be related to changes in tonus or alteration of the diameter of the lumen (Hightower, 1962).

Other authors (Rudick & Janowitz, 1974; Wolf & Welsh, 1972) give similar classifications with slight differences in characterization of wave types. For instance, Type III is said to occur predominantly near the end of an activity period or at the beginning of a rest period and to consist of an increase of basal pressure for about 1–5 min ("incomplete tetanus").

Originally this system of nomenclature was introduced by Adler, Atkinson, and Ivy (1941; cf. Hightower, 1962, p. 11). Their system contained a fourth wave type which is of lesser importance and not found in the stomach.

According to Konturek and Rösch (1976) the empty stomach shows no contractile activity 60% of the time. The rest of the time is occupied by Type I waves (25%) and Type II waves (15%), while Type III waves occur very rarely. After a long fasting period, frequency and amplitude of Type I and Type II waves increase until they occur 60% of the time. The characteristics of these contractions during a hunger period do not differ from those in the earlier interdigestive phase. Contrary to earlier authors (Cannon, 1909; Cannon, 1939; Cannon & Washburn, 1912; Carlson, 1912b). Konturek and Rösch (1976) maintain that there are no special hunger contractions. Hunger sensations are said to be uncorrelated with the strong contractions which can be recorded during a prolonged fasting period (cf. Russell & Stern, 1967, p. 222; and Chapter 17, this volume, for a fuller discussion of the sources of artifacts encountered in the earlier studies on hunger contractions). In the light of the experiments of Stunkard and his co-workers (Griggs & Stunkard, 1964; Stunkard & Koch, 1964; Stunkard & Fox, 1971), however, there has been a revival of interest in this question, and the advent of more precise and less disturbing methods of measurement may result in a more differentiated picture of the correlations between gastrointestinal motility and hunger.

When the stomach is filled, propulsive motoric activity starts almost immediately. Some authors (Cannon & Lieb, 1911; Cragg & Evans, 1960; Ganong, 1972; Jansson, 1969) maintain that it is preceded by a "receptive relaxation" of the fundus. In the beginning, the contractions are weak. After a few minutes they grow stronger, and the three types of waves mentioned above appear. The frequency of the peristaltic contractions follows the basal electrical rhythm (BER), which spreads from a center in the middle part of the stomach towards the antrum (Alvarez & Mahoney, 1922; Daniel & Irvin, 1968). These rhythmic contractions in the caudal part of the stomach have a frequency of 3 per min.

Frequency and duration of propulsive and retropulsive movements in the distal section of the stomach are determined in large part by the consistency of the food ingested. At a later stage, the peristaltic contractions become stronger and stronger and may eventually involve a total occlusion of the antral lumen. The distal stomach contracts almost simultaneously resulting in a pressure rise of about 10–25 mm Hg over the initial value. This causes "systolic contractions" which reappear cyclically and propel the stomach content through the pyloric sphincter into the duodenum. This emptying process is a coordinated sequence of electrical and mechanical events and cannot be fully understood by the simplified model of the stomach as a pump suggested by Nelsen and Kohatsu (1971) and others. The "complex" nature of the stomach movements has been substantiated by detailed fluoroscopic descriptions of the antropyloric emptying sequence (Torgersen, 1942; cited by Kramer, 1972, p. 87).

2.3. Electrical Activity of the Stomach

Direct electromyographic recordings from the gastric smooth muscles have recently produced a number of new findings on the deep signal source for the surface gastrograms (Cooke & Christensen, 1973; Daniel & Irwin, 1969; Konturek & Rösch, 1976; Rudick & Janowitz, 1974; Wolf & Welsh, 1972).

Basically two kinds of electrical activity of the smooth gastric musculature have been distinguished: an electrical base rhythm (BER) or electrical slow waves, and fast activity or action potentials.

The electrical slow waves sometimes have been called pacesetter potentials or electrical control activity (ECA; see Aeberhard, 1977, and Duthie, 1974, for definitions). The form of the ECA may vary. When occurring in a rhythmic fashion, usually the waves are nearly sinusoidal with a very stable frequency of 3 cpm (Figure 2A), but they may also occur as single, monophasic waves (Figure 2B). The slow waves start with a peak lasting several seconds and are followed by a slow repolarization. They originate from the outer layer of longitudinal muscle fibers at a pacemaker area in the middle part of the stomach on the great curvature (Weber & Kohatsu, 1970). The pacemaker zone depolarizes every 20 sec and this electrical activity spreads to the antrum.

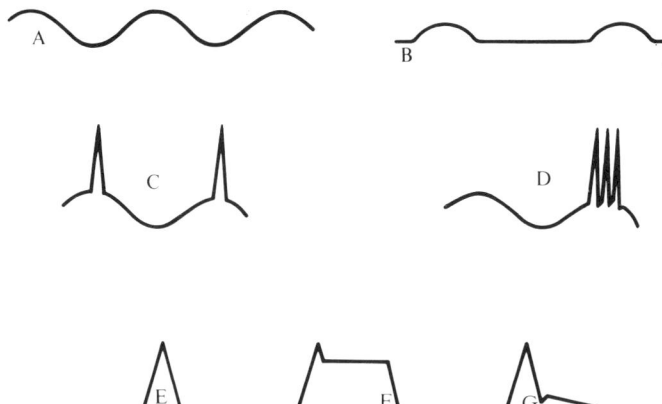

Figure 2. Types of potential changes of the gastric smooth muscle fibers. (A) Electrical slow waves or control activity (ECA): Sinusoidal waves at 3 cpm. (B) Discontinuous monophasic slow waves. (C) Slow waves with single "spikes" or action potentials on top. (D) Slow wave with a "spike burst." (E)–(G) Various forms of action potentials of gastrointestinal smooth muscle cells. (Modified from Burnstock et al. [1963].)

Presently, according to Konturek and Rösch (1976), the nature and function of slow waves are not fully understood. Their main task seems to be the integration of muscle contractions in the caudal position of the stomach. A number of operations like transsection, pyloroplasty, and vagotomy change the spreading of slow waves. Some authors (Duthie, Brown, Robertson-Dunn, Kwong, & Whittaker, 1972; Sarna, Daniel, & Kingma, 1972; see also Daniel, 1977) have proposed a model of chained relaxation oscillators, each consisting of some hundred smooth muscle cells coupled together electrically, to explain the coordinated travel of the ECA over the gastric smooth muscle. The longitudinal muscle fibers are said to be the site of these oscillators. The single oscillator is supposed to have a constant frequency on its own but may be synchronized by an oscillator of a higher frequency. The oscillators with the highest frequencies are localized near the pacemaker area, while oscillators with lower frequencies are found in more distal parts of the stomach. This ensures that the pacemaker area in the middle part "dictates to" the oscillating frequency of the oscillators near the pylorus, and the waves normally travel from proximal to distal segments of the stomach.

The second type of electrical activity of the stomach is called spike or action potentials. They may be superimposed on the slow waves as single pulses or multiple trains (Figure 2C, 2D). This fast activity consists of rapid oscillations each 5 to 10 msec in duration and lasting for up to 3 sec (Duthie, 1974). Spike potentials accompany the slow waves and show specific phase relations to them.

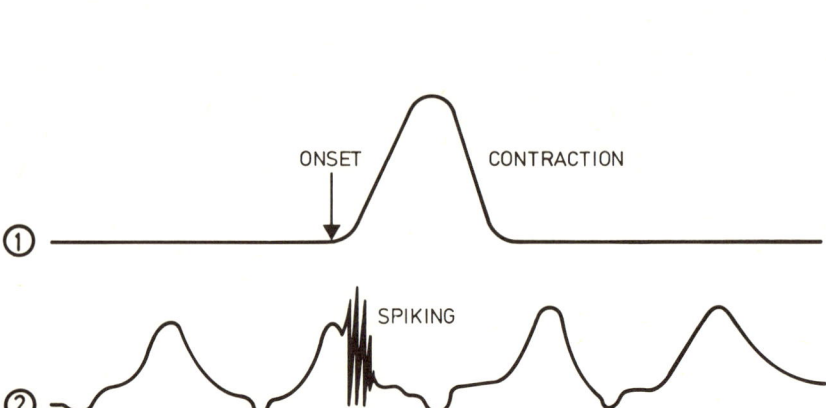

Figure 3. Relation of electrical and mechanical events at gastrointestinal muscles. (1) Mechanical record (strain gauge or manometric device). (2) Electrical potentials: Slow waves with a burst of spikes. The onset of the latter is correlated with the onset of the contraction. (Modified from Aeberhard, 1974).

While slow waves may be present without contractions, spikes are believed by many investigators always to be associated with actual stomach contractions (Konturek & Rösch, 1976; Daniel, 1977).

Figure 3 illustrates schematically the relation of ECA, spikes, and contractions. The distribution of spike potentials and, therefore, peristaltic contractions is determined by the rhythm of the slow waves. The latter is said to be endogenous. Changes in mechanical contractions by neuronal and humoral factors are mediated by this coupling of the electrical and mechanical activity.

Not all authors agree with this relatively clearcut picture. Daniel (1977), for instance, relates the so-called electrical response activity (ERA) to mechanical contractions. ERA follows after an electrical control potential (ECA) and is manifested as an increased second (plateau) potential. It is always associated with mechanical responses according to Daniel, but need not contain action potentials. The second potentials (ERA) are controlled by neural commands, mainly vagal release of acetylcholine. The intrinsic ECA determines when and where these second potentials and consequently contractions can appear.[1]

Although generally assumed, no study has demonstrated that there is CNS or autonomic modulation of the basic slow wave frequency (BER) and amplitude. In fact, there is some supporting evidence for influence of higher centers

---

[1] A similar classification is given by Smouts (1980), pp. 23 and 74, Fig. 7.

from physiological and psychophysiological experimentation (e.g., Davis et al., 1959; Hölzl et al., 1979; Kohatsu, 1970).

3. Signal Parameters of Gastric Activity and Their Psychophysiological Information Content

In summarizing, we may specify the following properties of the electromotor behavior of the stomach (which also will be the features to look for in surface gastrograms): Periodic processes are present in mechanical as well as electrical activities in the range of 1–5 cpm. They may be characterized by frequency (or its inverse period) and by amplitude. These parameters should be obtained in a wave-to-wave fashion or averaged over a certain time.

In addition, aperiodic events are present in the electromotor activity of the stomach. In the case of the mechanical activity, they take the form of singular contractions. These may be characterized by amplitude, average frequency (or intercontraction intervals) over a certain period of time, and by the phase relationships to the periodic phenomena. Duration or half-time duration would be another possible signal parameter. Spike potentials are the corresponding singular electrical events. As illustrated in Figure 2E–G, the electrical events take more complex forms, but the basic signal parameters mentioned before apply to them as well. Regular but discontinuous slow waves may be treated in a similar way. The interrelationship between slow waves and spike potentials is of special importance when analyzing the electrical activity of the stomach. According to the gastrophysiological evidence cited, one has to look for spike potentials or Daniel's ERA in electrical records when correlates of mechanical contractions are under investigation.

A third kind of parameter may be extracted from electrical and mechanical records—the very slow changes in basal tonus (pressure) or electrical potential. These changes seem to be aperiodic in nature. However, to our knowledge, no systematic investigation of this question is available, so the possibility exists that an extremely low periodic component underlies the activity. If this ultraslow component existed, period and amplitude would be its describing parameters. From the aperiodic part of these slow changes trend-in-time information may be drawn in conventional ways (e.g., with orthogonal polynomials). For certain questions, simple differences from original baseline at the beginning of the measurement, that is some kind of "displacement" measure, could be sufficient (e.g., Russell & Stern, 1967).

Finally, as a measure of total motility, especially for quantifying intraluminal pressure recordings, a so-called motility index (MI) has been defined according to one form or the other of the following formula:

$$MI = \frac{1}{T} \sum_{i=1}^{n} a_i d_i$$

where T is the time of recording, a_i is the amplitude, and d_i is the duration of the ith contraction wave; n is the number of recorded waves in interval T (e.g., Deller & Wangel, 1965; similarly in Duret & Arguello, 1969; Schütze, Wiedemann, Hanf, Lorenzen, & Emmonegger, 1979; and Stacher & Fink, 1974).

This index is somewhat arbitrarily defined to reflect "density" of smooth muscle "work" in time. Obviously it is unequivocal only as long as only one type of activity is present.

From the descriptions of patterns of gastric electromotor activity, it becomes clear that the signals are composed of several components, whether measured directly by strain gauges and extracellular electrical recordings, indirectly with intraluminal manometric devices or surface methods. Because more than one component can be present at a time, some adequate technique of decomposition must be used. The different parameters mentioned above have been defined with this intent. Other techniques derived from principles of signal analysis in communication engineering, for example, spectral analysis, have also been used (cf. Section 4.3).

Tables 1 and 2 summarize the different identifiable components of contractile and electrical stomach activity and their quantifying parameters. Each requires its special analysis method depending on whether transient, periodic, or tonic components are to be evaluated. These parameters of electromotor activity

Table 1
Overview of Common Electrical and Contractile Activity of Gastric Muscle: Electrical Activity (Electromyograms)

Event	Formal description	Parameters
Slow waves, electrical control activity (ECA), basic electric rhythm (BER)	Periodic (3 cpm), sinusoidal	Frequency or period amplitude
Second potential, electrical response activity (ERA)	Transient or periodic (if coupled with ECA), nonsinusoidal	Duration, amplitude, counts, density, (in time or relative to slow wave number), MI-like compound measure
Spikes, action potentials, electrical response activity (ERA)	Transient pulses	Duration, amplitude, counts, density, MI (see text)
Prolonged ERA, spike bursts, "tetanus"	Transient pulse trains with or without tonic components	Duration of train, average amplitude, MI (see text)
Very slow waves of unknown origin	Transient or periodic (1 cpm), sinusoidal or monophasic	Frequency or duration, amplitude
DC potentials of unknown origin	Tonic, slow shifts	Size, trend

Table 2
Overview of Common Electrical and Contractile Activity of Gastric Muscle: Contractile Activity (Strain Gauge or Manometry)

Event	Formal description	Parameters
Type I waves	Periodic or transient, sinusoidal, low amplitude	Frequency or period, amplitude, counts (if nonperiodic), MI
Type II waves	Perodic or transient, pulses, high amplitude	Frequency or period, amplitude, counts, MI
Type III waves	Transient, slow, monophasic waves with superimposed Type II waves	Duration, amplitude, trend
Basal tonus or pressure	Tonic, slow shifts	Size, trend

will have to be directly related to features of surface recordings of gastric motility (electrical or otherwise) in correlational studies over long periods and with large samples of subjects. Such studies could identify what part of and to what extent the signals from the deep source are reflected in the surface recordings. Examples of parallel records of intragastric pressure and abdominal potentials as Russell and Stern (1967) have done, are not conclusive, nor are successful demonstrations of loose correlations (albeit significant) between empirically but arbitrarily defined parameters of direct and indirect recordings. It is *not sufficient* to find features in surface recordings reminiscent of Types I, II, or III waves in manometric recordings if no actual quantitative correlation is demonstrated by simultaneous measurements.

This problem of the *physiological* information content of surface gastrograms has *not* yet been solved (this statement contradicts a few recent publications in the psychophysiological literature) and it will be dealt with more extensively in later sections (Sections 4.3 and 4.4).

The statements about coordination of fast electrical activity of stomach and duodenum pertain to contractile activity as well because of the close relationship between contraction and fast potentials. The activity sequence described mediates the coordinated transport of gastric content from the antrum through the pylorus into the duodenum. It is important also for the evaluation of feeding responses in surface gastrograms.

A second problem is posed by difficulties in the psychophysiological interpretation of changes in signal parameters in experiments on the effect of psychological stress manipulations on gastric activity and on biofeedback. Especially in biofeedback experiments, we must solve this problem if we do not want to reinforce changes in irrelevant response classes, possibly not even of a gastrointestinal origin.

Cannon's original simple notion of sympathetic-parasympathetic antagonism implied that activation of fight-flight responses inhibits gastrointestinal activity in general. The empirical data mostly contradict this simplified description (Weltz, 1940; Wolf & Wolff, 1942). When the different signal parameters of transient, periodic, and tonic components in various kinds of gastrograms are taken into account the procedure is even more complicated and the evidence is conflicting. Frequency and amplitude measures of periodic activity in surface recordings behave differently in experiments manipulating the autonomic arousal of subjects (e.g., Davis et al., 1959; Hölzl, 1979a; Hölzl et al., 1979; cf. Stern, Chapter 9, this volume).

Similar problems exist with other motility measures, if information on the meaning of changes in them is at all available. Thus to make any kind of motility records useful psychophysiologically, the following issues have to be considered: (1) the relation of a certain parameter of the particular gastrogram in question to the actual electrical and mechanical events in the longitudinal and circular layers of stomach smooth muscles; (2) the relation of these electrical and mechanical events to mixing and emptying functions; (3) the psychophysiological meaning of changes in these functions under experimental manipulations, and, therefore, (4) how and to what degree these changes are reflected in those gastrographic parameters.

Most of these issues are unresolved but for some points in the list at least partial information is available. In the following paragraphs, current gastrographic practice is discussed under these headings. Additional information on problems 3 and 4 is contained in Stern's chapter (Chapter 9).

4. Electrical Recordings from the Abdominal Surface: Current Practice in Psychophysiology

Davis and his co-workers (Davis & Berry, 1963; Davis et al., 1957, 1959; Fedor & Russell, 1965; Stern, 1964, 1965a,b) introduced surface electrogastrography to psychophysiology. Although there had been earlier studies showing the possibility of obtaining gastrointestinal electric activity from the abdominal surface going back in fact to Alvarez (1922), Davis's studies were the first systematic attempts to describe abdominal potentials in relation to their gastrointestinal sources, to prove the correlation between them, to define a suitable scoring system, and to show the influence of various psychological stress manipulations and avoidance procedures on these parameters. Ten years after the first "exploration of abdominal potentials" by Davis and his co-workers, Russell and Stern (1967) published a comprehensive overview of the recording method, the scoring system, and the then available validation data. In recent years, a few studies have appeared which revived the classic method as a tool in the clinical psychophysiological study of ulcer patients (Walker & Sandman,

1977; cf. Hölzl et al., 1979a,b) and in experiments trying to modify stomach motility by biofeedback training (Deckner et al., 1972; Smith et al., 1973; Walker et al., 1978). Therefore, this system of recording and scoring of abdominal potentials will be considered first.

4.1. Apparatus and Procedures: Overview

4.1.1. Technical Requirements

Recording of electrogastrograms from the abdominal surface requires differential amplifiers and recorders which meet the criteria set by the following properties of the signals: (1) Gut-related potentials on the abdomen are in the range of 50 to several hundred microvolts. (2) Amplification ratios, therefore, should be 10^5 or better with enough intermediate steps to 10^3 for optimal choice of amplification. (3) The frequency range extends from dc up to the higher components of the electrocardiogram ($\sim$ 40 Hz).

The most significant periodic components of the electrogastrograms lie in the frequency band from 1 to 16 cpm (or 17–270 MHz). The gastrograph, therefore, must be equipped with suitable filters to selectively amplify this frequency band which is important because the EKG and large standing potentials (dc components) present in the abdominal potentials sometimes are larger than the gastric signals by one order of magnitude. Compensation of dc potentials by "bucking circuits" has also been employed.

Because of the necessity for low-frequency recording, nonpolarizable electrodes must be used. Standard silver–silver-chloride skin electrodes are sufficient. Input impedance of the amplifier should be better than 1 MΩ. A number of research groups have described special operational recording systems for surface gastrography, the best known probably being the Russian and French ones (Krasil'nikov, 1960, 1971; Thouvenot & Martin, 1967; Thouvenot, Tonković, & Penaud, 1973).

However, any amplifier system meeting the above-mentioned requirements is suitable. Standard polygraphs with dc amplifiers, well known in psychophysiology laboratories, can be used if appropriate time constants or dc compensation and low-pass filters are provided or added. A time constant of 10–20 sec, for instance, is fully sufficient to record periodic activity ("slow waves" at the surface) in the range from 0.5 cpm upwards.[2] These time constants are easily incorporated into standard voltage input couplers of commercial polygraphs. A low-pass filter with cut-off frequency at 0.3 Hz (18 dB/octave or better) eliminates enough EKG from the record.

Attention should be paid also to the so-called common mode rejection of the

---

[2]For T_c = 10 sec, for instance, the 3-dB cutoff frequency f_c = 15.9 MHz $\approx$ 1 cpm; for T_c = 20 sec: f_c = 7.95 MHz $\approx$ 0.5 cpm.

differential amplifiers employed. This refers to the capacity of the amplifier to reject "noise" common to both differential leads. This common mode rejection is not independent of the frequencies of interest. Thus, while protecting fairly well against line interference and similar ac noise, an amplifier with theoretically high common mode rejection may have difficulties with low-frequency noise from movement or electrode artifacts. This kind of difficulty interacts with electrode impedance or grounding (see Section 4.1.2).

A practical solution for standard electrogastrography as well as a special amplifier system developed in the author's laboratory for more advanced research purposes is described in the next chapter (Chapter 6, Müller, Hölzl, & Brüchle).

These systems also provide for multichannel recordings which are usually necessary because of unavoidable anatomical variations between subjects and the resulting difficulty in defining comparable recording sites by gross-anatomical reference points (see Section 4.2).

4.1.2. Recording Procedures

The recording of EGGs in general does not differ from the recording procedure for other biosignals picked up from the body surface. Because of the very low frequency band of gastric signals, however, some of the problems encountered in recording and amplification of biopotentials in the microvolt range are to be considered more carefully than usual.

For instance, mechanical shape of electrodes and configuration of the recording field on the abdomen become quite important because dislocation of electrodes by movements or changes of position, however slight, produces low-frequency artifacts of considerable size (up to 10 times the signal amplitude) and, in contrast to recording of biopotentials with higher frequency bands, these artifacts cannot be filtered out. Therefore, small, flat, or flexible electrodes recessed in their cups, careful attention to the configuration of recording sites, and taping down the electrode wires to minimize mechanical forces on the electrode are extremely important.

The higher the input impedance of the amplifier, the lower the electrode resistance, and the better the grounding of the subject, the less severe become these problems. Therefore, careful preparation of skin sites (see Chapter 6 by Müller *et al.*), especially the grounding site, is strongly recommended. Because the situation improves further with osmotic stabilization between electrode, conduction jelly, and skin tissues, enough adaptation time (30 min or longer) should be allowed before the actual measurement. This requirement often is easily met by applying the electrodes immediately after arrival of the subject and only later finishing the other preparations including instructions, filling out questionnaires, giving a standard meal, and making final adjustment.

When using true dc amplification this situation requires special attention. No nonpolarizable electrode protects against slow drifting "contact potentials" which stem from the osmotic differences in the system of silver–silver-chloride, conduction jelly, skin, and body fluid. These drifts may be observed sometimes for hours depending on the electrochemical particulars at each stage of the system and even after abrasion of skin sites. It may be mentioned in this connection that measurement of electrode impedances with an ohmmeter containing a dc voltage source also produces strong drifts for considerable time,[3] and, therefore, should not be done close to the actual recording period. Avoiding the problem altogether by ac measurements of impedance is recommended.

With bipolar recordings (that is, with both differential leads on the abdomen and the grounding site elsewhere) considerable dc to low-frequency artifacts are produced when the subject touches the ground or metal case of the subject's chair. Only very low impedance of the ground electrode (< 2 kΩ) eliminates this effect. Since this may be difficult, especially in clinical applications with adverse recording conditions and limited preparation time, it is generally good policy to prevent adventitious subject contacts with grounded metal parts.

Another source of low-frequency artifacts comes from temperature changes at the electrode site either by changes in air cooling or—more likely—in vascular and resulting blood flow changes below the electrode.[4] For biofeedback experiments this may pose a difficult problem.

Low-frequency artifacts are also caused by changes in body position. Even when direct mechanical effects on the electrode are excluded, changes in electrode distances and in the geometrical relation of the electrodes to the stomach location may be brought about when the subject leans forward or backward only slightly. Good definition of body position is essential, therefore, especially when repeated measures are used. Mostly a semireclining sitting position is used, but this might not be optimal. Only anecdotes on this question are available from some EGG laboratories.

Last but not least, an even more exotic source of interference will be mentioned because it posed a severe problem in a clinical study by the author and was solved only because, for different reasons (see Section 6), magnetic field measurements in the vicinity of the electrode field were made at the same time: Low-frequency magnetic field interference is easily picked up in electrogastrograms when electromagnetic devices of different kinds like electric motors,

---

[3] R. M. Stern commented on this during this symposium with the words: "I discovered that all the graduate students in Davis's Lab before I came along used to check the electrode resistance with an ohmmeter and insured that you got a very nice "displacement" over about 10 min. And stating it more seriously, I find, the more careful I am with the electrodes and the kind of recording the less of this slow drift I see." (Cf. Section 4.3.1.d on the "displacement" measure.)

[4] I am indebted to Joe Kamiya, who first drew my attention to this source of artifacts while he put our laboratory to a severe test during summer 1980.

power relays, or elevators are in operation in close proximity. Even good Faraday cages are no protection against these magnetic noise signals of low frequency. Only very expensive magnetically shielded chambers will eliminate these artifacts.

4.2. Recording Sites

In the earliest report, Davis et al. (1957) stated that they had used bipolar[5] recording from one point of the abdomen to another as Alvarez had done, and later "adopted the practice of recording from an abdominal point to the dorsal surface of the right arm." They give no skeletal or other anatomical reference points, but from later reports (Russell & Stern, 1967, p. 233) it seems that the "active" electrode was usually placed on the upper left abdominal quadrant, 2.5 cm above and 5 cm to the left of the navel. This location is said to provide "the most representative recordings of the EGG" (Russell & Stern, 1967). Unipolar recordings from other abdominal quadrants and multiple channel EGGs have been obtained also. The "neutral" electrode for these unipolar recording is now usually attached to the lateral surface of the lower (right) leg (Russell & Stern, 1967). The position of the ground electrodes is not indicated in the original reports.

No systematic study of the differences between different electrode localizations and different recording schemes (unipolar versus bipolar, etc.) have been reported. A number of typical recording conventions and their relation to gross abdominal anatomy (shown in Figure 4) are illustrated in Figure 5A–5D. Figure 4 may be used as a reference for stomach and colon positions relative to the skeletal fix points which are used to define the various electrode configurations below. It should be kept in mind, however, that skeletal references and location of viscera can be quite different from individual to individual, and strong sex differences exist. Typological differences of body appearance and correlated differences in stomach form are a further source of variance (cf. Martin & Saller, 1962, p. 2207). Figure 5A shows Davis's original electrode positions in his unipolar recording together with Alvarez's sites, which he believed to be over the pars pylorica of the stomach (Alvarez, 1922, pp. 1116–1119, and his Figure 4B). The Tiemann and Reichertz (1959a) positions were quite similar. They also used a leg reference.

---

[5]"Bipolar" refers to a recording configuration where both differential leads of the input amplifier come from the active area where the signal presumably arises, that is, the abdomen. "Unipolar" recordings, on the other hand, are done with only *one* differential lead on the abdomen and the other at a "neutral" or "reference" site, for example, the leg. In both cases an additional ground electrode in the center of the recording field is recommended to fully exploit the common mode rejection capacity of the amplifier. "Unipolar" recordings are not to be mixed up with "single-ended," that is, nondifferential measurement.

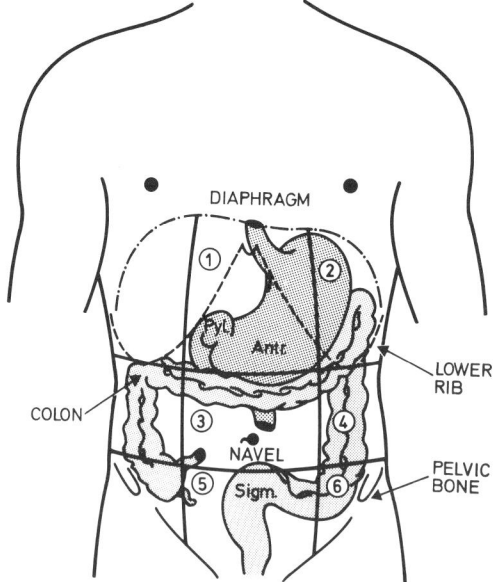

Figure 4. Schematic representation of gross abdominal anatomy in relation to position of viscera and sceletal landmarks. (1) Epigastric; (2) hypochondriac; (3) umbilical; (4) lumbar; (5) hypogastric; and (6) inguinal or iliac region.

Smith and Hain (1970) used bipolar recordings from the upper left abdominal quadrant. Their electrode positions are shown in Figure 5B. Again the navel is used as anatomical reference. The rationale of using bipolar recordings instead of unipolar recordings in the study is somewhat unclear, but from their description of the "propagation of wave forms," one may deduce that the authors believed the bipolar recordings would directly reflect more peristaltic action. From the four electrodes they selected one pair, usually Electrodes I and II or I and III, which "yielded the best 20 sec cycle Type II wave form," presumably according to a subjective criterion.

Nelsen and Kohatsu (1968) also used an array of abdominal electrodes, but in unipolar recordings against the left leg. They state that 90% of the cutaneous electrodes gave undisturbed segments of slow wave signal sufficiently long for analysis (6 min or longer). Precise electrode positions were not specified.

Among the various bipolar recording conventions the oblique "ladder" configuration used by Brown *et al.* (1975) is of special interest (Figure 5C). It allows rudimentary mapping of horizontal potential vectors over the antropyloric region and the analysis of caudally propagated waves by cross-correlational techniques (see Section 4.3). Unfortunately, the anatomical relations are no better defined than with other placements.

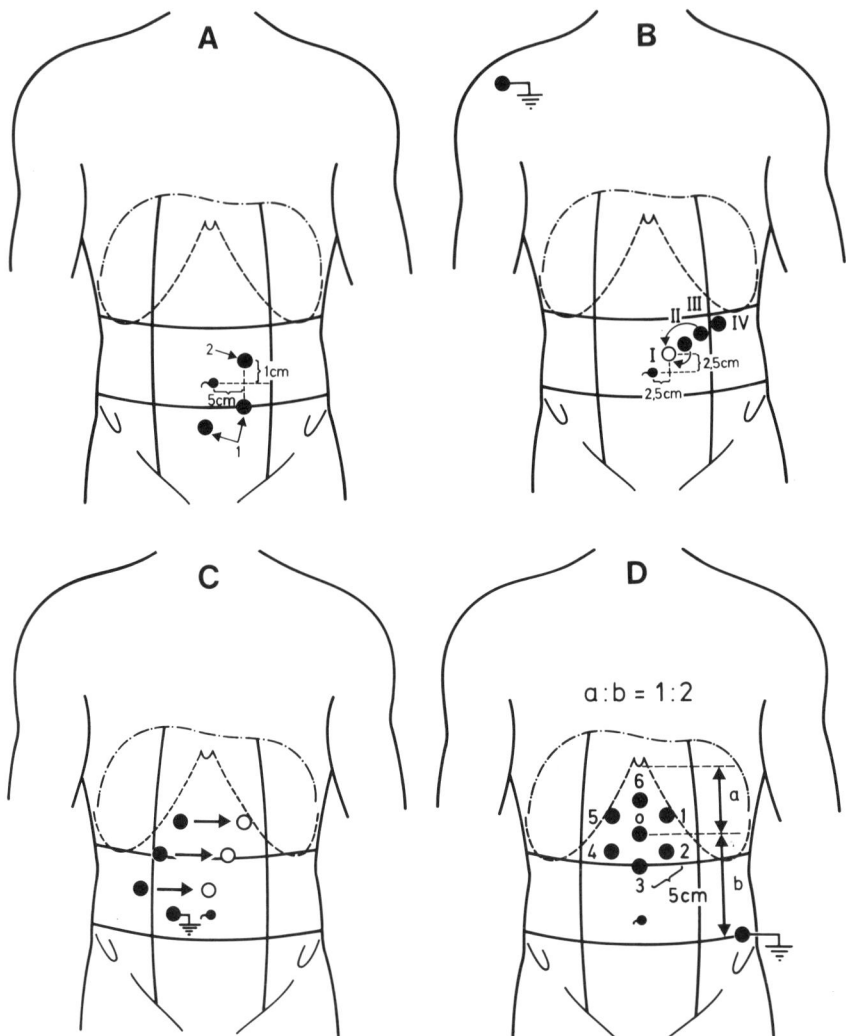

Figure 5. (A) Davis's and Alvarez's original electrode positions for surface gastrograms. (1) Alvarez's bipolar sites; (2) Davis's unipolar active site. Explanation in test. (B) Electrode array for EGG by Smith and Hain (1970). Explanation in text. (C) "Ladder" configuration by Brown et al. (1975). Explanation in text. (D) "Rosette" of bipolar recordings according to Schröder (1977) and Hölzl et al. (1979), modified from Martin's and Schultz's configuration.

This configuration seems to produce very good gastric potentials, although the procedure may be suspected to be sensitive to variations in the direction of the gastric "vector" (Martin & Thillier, 1972). These authors (Martin, Moline,

& Murat, 1971; Martin, Thouvenot, & Touron, 1967) tried to overcome this problem with a special version of bipolar electrogastrograms which they call the "rosette method." With this method six electrodes are placed around a central seventh one in a rosettelike fashion (each spaced 1 cm apart). The hexagonal configuration is placed centrally over the epigastric region for detection of gastric activity. The EGGs are obtained as bipolar recordings of the outer electrodes against the middle one. Colonic potentials seemed to be obtained with other placements of the little rosette. Martin and Thillier (1971) compared this type of abdominal potential with recordings from electrodes on the extremities (similar to conventional EKG leads) and with an umbilical site for grounding. The authors prefer this so-called "electro-gastroentero-gram" (EGEG) over the rosette method in clinical applications.

Schulz, Reitzig, Schulze, Bärsch, Etzold, and Lisewski (1973) came to different conclusions. In a direct comparison of peripheral (extremity) and local bipolar rosette recordings they found a considerably higher percentage of interpretable electrogastrograms with visually detectable slow wave patterns in the rosette recording rather than in peripheral derivations. In this report, the rosette method was said to cover a large area of the organ under investigation. Schulz and co-workers also state that with this method it is not necessary to know the exact position of the stomach because of the partial mapping of the epigastric area. In addition, they state that superposition of gastric potentials by electrical signals from other sources is less frequent and not so strong. Furthermore, the effects of experimental variables like drugs or eating are said to be reflected more sensitively in the bipolar rosette leads. In an earlier investigation in our laboratory (Hölzl et al., 1979; Schröder, 1977) similar results were found. The clearest BER components were obtained at Electrode Positions 1 and 2 of the rosette (Figure 5D) in 48% (el. 1) and 44% (el. 2), that is, in 92% of all recordings in that study or in 216 epochs of 10-min recording. The rosette in these studies was larger than in Martin's work and similar to Schulz's positioning (Figure 5D).

A number of authors have realized that more reliable data on these questions are necessary. Brown (1972, p. 176), in reviewing psychophysiologically oriented literature on the electrogastrogram, commented on the typical placement of the active electrode in unipolar recordings like Russell and Stern (1967): "None of the active locations seems to have been centered over the stomach and consequently may reflect a major component of intestinal activity." This criticism is valid even though it is generally believed that the slow wave rhythm of about 3 cycles per min is typical for the stomach (Thouvenot et al., 1973) because other parts of the gastrointestinal tract, the colon in particular, may show similar rhythms (cf. Section 4.4 on validity of EGG).

X-ray control seems to be the only safe way of defining the relationship between the positions of the surface electrodes and anatomical parts of the stomach. This has been used by Russian researchers, for example, by Krasil'ni-

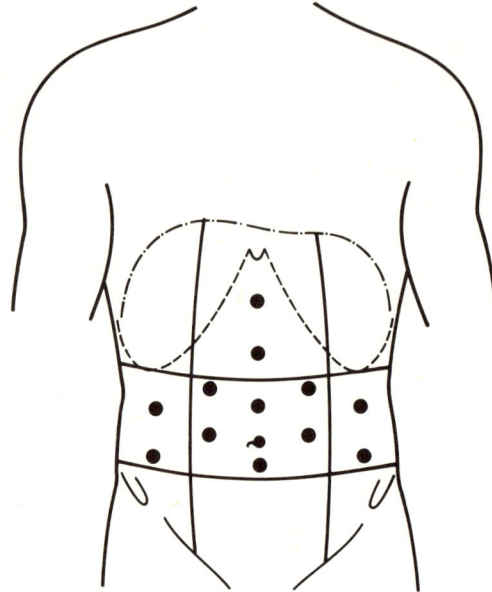

Figure 6. Monopolar mapping of abdominal area according to Thouvenot *et al.* (1973). Explanation in text.

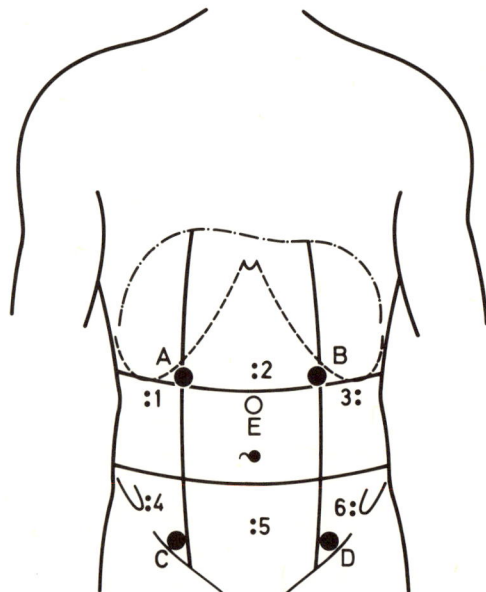

Figure 7. Combined monopolar (A–D) and bipolar mapping (1–6) of abdominal area by Tonković *et al.* (1975). Explanation in text.

kow (1971) in a modification of Sobakin's routine (Sobakin, Smirnow, & Mishin, 1962). In this study, unipolar recordings were used. The active electrode was placed exactly over the antro-pyloric region of the stomach under X-ray control. Because of X-ray hazards, the procedure of ensuring correct electrode placement cannot generally be used in psychophysiological studies. In clinical studies in gastroenterology, this method is often also undesirable. Therefore, other authors have looked for means of becoming independent of the precise anatomical details of abdominal structures. An obvious way of achieving this aim could be a more or less complete mapping of the relevant abdominal area, selecting those positions which give recordings of identifiable physiological source by indirect criteria. These data would also provide an acceptable procedure for electrode positioning by use of skeletal reference, at least in studies with larger groups.

A first step toward such "abdominal potential mapping" was made by Thouvenot et al. (1973). They used an array of 12 unipolar recording sites with leads from epigastric, umbilical, and lumbar regions as shown in Figure 6. Tonković, Penaud, Thouvenot, and Mountafian (1975) employed the same configuration. In addition, they worked with a combination of bipolar and unipolar leads which are redrawn from the original using our anatomical reference system in Figure 7. Six electrode pairs for bipolar recordings (1–6), four single electrodes for unipolar recordings against the left leg (A–D), and a central earth reference (E) are placed on the abdominal surface such that they map the total area between the lower ribs and the pubis.

The authors claim that they were able to identify all the major peaks in the power spectra of their main recordings. Although this is not well supported by the few data presented, their attempt at a more complete electrical mapping of the abdominal surface may be well suited to clarify a few questions on the signal sources of the abdominal potentials. A comparison with Martin's rosette method and Brown's "ladder" configuration might be interesting. Apparently similar mapping attempts have been made in Russian laboratories, but conclusive information on these studies could not be obtained by the present reviewers (Krasil'nikow, 1971, p. 5). Up to 16 channels of EGGs have been recorded simultaneously in those laboratories.

From the psychophysiologist's point of view, sensitivity to various artifacts like movements or large respiratory excursions is very important. Here, too, a variety of recording configurations differ very much. The unipolar recording against the leg, for instance, includes much more respiratory artifacts than the bipolar leads, at least in our experience. We have tested this by instructing people to change their respiratory pattern from thoracic to abdominal breathing, hold their breath, or make gross movements. Bipolar and unipolar recordings were obtained at the same time. Usually larger artifacts were seen in the unipolar recording against a "neutral" electrode at the leg as compared to bipolar rosette

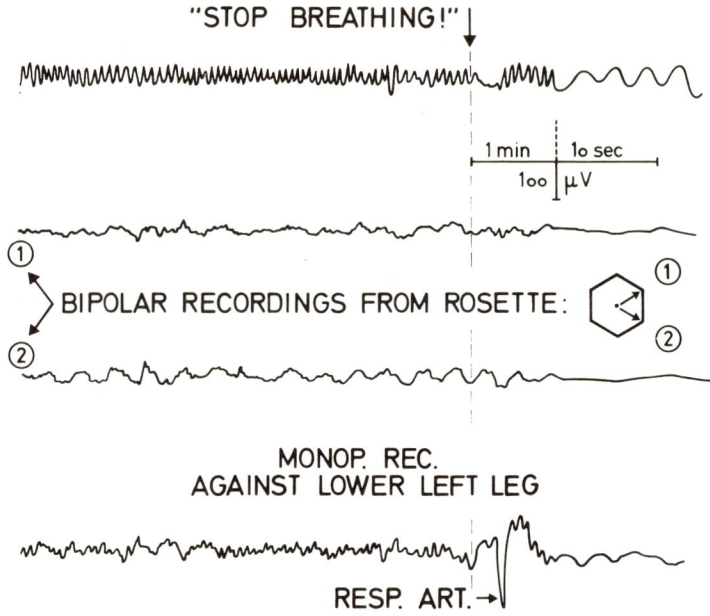

Figure 8. Comparison of "rosette" leads with monopolar recording against left leg. The arrow above the upper record (respiration) indicates voluntary arrest of breathing. This results in a large respiratory artifact in the unipolar, not in the bipolar recordings. Slow waves are clearly visible in both types of EGGs (Hölzl & Brüchle, unpublished data).

leads (Hölzl & Brüchle, 1980). Examples like the one shown in Figure 8, of course, provide only anecdotal information. Systematic comparative studies are needed.

4.3. Signal Analysis

The recording techniques already reviewed cannot be adequately evaluated without relating them to the methods by which the records were analyzed to produce quantitative parameters of the physiological variables assumed to underly the gastrograms. This is especially important with surface electrogastrograms because they are an indirect indicator of electric activity of the gut, the precise source of which is debated. The type of signal analysis used will largely determine whether the parameters obtained are physiologically meaningful. It is equally important when studies of different groups are to be compared. Unfortunately the practice of signal analysis in electrogastrography is as confusing as the many different recording techniques. In defense of the psychophysiologists, it may be stated that gastroenterological specialists have not agreed on techniques of analysis themselves.

4.3.1. Classical Scoring System

In psychophysiology, the best known and most often used system of scoring electrogastrographic records from the abdominal surface was introduced by the Indiana group (Davis et al., 1957) and later systematized by Russell and Stern (1967). In this scoring system the total record is partitioned into half-min (sometimes min) intervals and different parameters are defined for these intervals. Initially a "baseline" is drawn by connecting the points at the beginning and end of each interval as indicated in Figure 9. The other parameters are measured relative to this baseline, but the variations in baseline may itself be analyzed.

4.3.1a. Frequency Measures. Russell and Stern (1967) defined *frequency* as the number of times a tracing crossed the baseline during a standard interval. With 30-sec intervals of analysis, the sum of zero crossings with positive and negative slopes will give the frequency of the basic rhythm in the signal in cycles per min (cpm). With 1-min intervals of analysis, of course, only zero crossings of either positive or negative slope have to be counted. Obviously, measuring peak-to-peak intervals in sec (Russell & Stern, 1967, p. 234; Wenger et al., 1961) results in the reciprocal of the frequency values in cycles per sec (cps or Hz).

It may seem trivial to list these simple relations here, but it can be gathered from the earlier literature that these arbitrary definitions of frequency parameters under certain circumstances produced values which were dependent on the analysis interval and which were often influenced by the relative intensity of the respiratory artifact in the records. For instance, Smith and Hain (1970) also used a zero-crossing measure of frequency. Unlike the dc-recording technique by Davis and co-workers, they used an ac-recording with "a time constant of unusually long duration"; whatever this may mean, let us assume that it is at

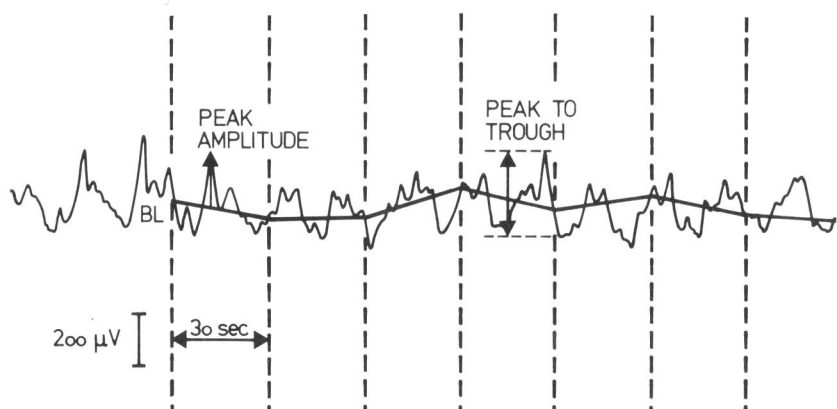

Figure 9. Definition of electrogastrographic signal parameters according to Russell and Stern (1967). BL, baseline; further explanation in text.

least longer than 10-sec, which corresponds to about 1 cpm cutoff frequency (3 db). Under these circumstances, counting the zero-crossings of the tracing in half-min intervals results in correct frequency values in cycles per min under most conditions as long as EKG is filtered out and the respiratory artifact is small compared to the amplitude of the slow waves, which is at least true as long as averages of several analysis intervals of 30 sec are used in the further data analysis. The individual values may become very unstable. Intuitively this may be understood by considering the fact that only about 1½ cycles of slow wave activity may be contained in any one of the intervals of analysis.

This does not necessarily hold for the dc-recording technique by Davis *et al.* (1957, 1959). In this case, slower components of record which have not been eliminated by the highpass filter as in Smith and Hain (1970), interact significantly with the intervals of analysis which are shorter than the period of those slow components. This may result in no zero-crossings at all even though 3 cpm waves may be present, or in too many crossings when a considerable respiratory artifact is present.

These interactions of signal content and analysis interval are quite complicated and often unpredictable. Depending on signal content, period measures may give different frequency estimates from zero-crossing measures. A number of other complications derive from this arbitrary definition of intervals of analysis. To be fair, it must be stated that as long as the polygraph records are scored by hand many of the problems may be avoided (i.e., by drawing a line "through the central positions of all EKG and respiration waves, which may be superimposed upon the EGG"; Russell & Stern, 1967, p. 235). However, this introduces a certain degree of subjectivity.

In any case, the partitioning of the signal into intervals lying in the range of the periods of the signal itself results in adding additional variance not originally present in the signal. For producing stable average signal parameter estimates, the intervals are too short with respect to the slowest components of the signal, and for reliable digitizing of the wave patterns, they are too long with respect to the fastest components (e.g., respiration, assuming that EKG is filtered out with a low-pass filter). In the latter case the well-known sampling theorem, which demands data sampling twice as high as the highest frequency present in the signal, is violated. This is true even for the 3-per-min rhythm and the frequently observed 1-per-min component. For adequate sampling of these rhythms, more than six values per min have to be obtained. With respiration still present in the signal even higher sampling rates (or shorter intervals of analysis) are necessary. With respiration rates ranging from 10 to 40 cpm, for instance, 20–80 values per min must be sampled. (It should perhaps be emphasized here that the sampling theorem does not refer to the highest frequency of interest but to the highest frequency present in the signal, although some people in the field seem to believe the former!) Rigorous low-passing to get rid of the faster components, on the other hand, may seriously distort the signal (Section 4.3.2).

4.3.1b. Amplitude Measures.

The most widely used amplitude measure is *peak amplitude*, the maximum departure (in microvolts) of the signal from the baseline in each standard interval (Russell & Stern, 1967, p. 234). Here again, measures differ depending on whether a dc-recording or an ac-recording with long time constant has been chosen. In ac-recordings (Smith & Hain, 1970), at least as long as appropriate time constants are chosen, peak amplitude will give fairly good estimates of the average amplitude of the underlying rhythm. However, for dc-recordings, the presence of slower components may distort amplitude estimates of the basic electric rhythm even more than its frequency measures. The influence of the respiratory artifact is even stronger, if this is not taken care of in other ways (which may be an unsolvable task). Consider, for instance, the fact that the respiratory artifact may sometimes be present, disappear, and come back again. Then, because of the frequently nonsinusoidal form of the signal, a particular excursion of the pen with certain slope and width cannot be identified as of respiratory or nonrespiratory origin. The complicated result of the superposition of different signal components with varying frequency, amplitude, and phase is discussed in more detail below from the point of Fourier analysis. It should be added that this severe susceptibility of peak amplitude to respiratory artifact is common to dc- and ac-recordings.

Furthermore, the relative content of respiratory artifact may vary with experimental conditions and thus give spurious significance to experimental effect. For instance, when factors like eating or operant responding and their effect on stomach motility are investigated, the respiratory artifact may change in size either by distension of the stomach or change in respiratory style (abdominal or thoracic). This is easily demonstrated by observing the height of the respiratory artifact in examples of generally good gastrograms after feeding and after instruction to change from abdominal to thoracic respiration.

In the original definition of the peak amplitude measure (Davis *et al.*, 1959; Russell & Stern, 1967; Smith & Hain, 1970), the polarity of the deviation from the baseline is disregarded. To give reliable measures of the amplitude of the underlying slow waves, symmetric deviations from the baseline must be assumed. Presumably because this is not always the case, especially with dc-recordings, later authors (e.g., Walker & Sandman, 1977) analyzed positive and negative peak amplitudes separately. The criticisms mentioned above apply to these measures, too, as well as to the peak-to-trough parameter, a third amplitude measure defined by these authors. This measure simply is the distance (in microvolts) from the highest to the lowest point of the EGG recording in the standard interval. An additional problem is associated with this signal parameter. It is not only subject to the artifacts mentioned above, but also contaminates the basic electric rhythm of 3 cpm with slower periodic components (1 cpm) and slow drifts.

In a comparison of gastrographic parameters from classical scoring and spectral analysis from 23 subjects (69 records), Hölzl and Müller (1980) found very low or no correlation of frequency and amplitude measures between the two methods. As spectral analysis produces reliable frequency values for the BER, this lack of correlation is presumably due to the unreliability of classical scoring methods. No preselection of records for "good" BER was applied, however, and the comparison may have been somewhat unfair to the classical method because of little variation in frequency values and other factors.

4.3.1c. Total Motility. Russell and Stern (1967) describe an index of total motility which is essentially the *line* integral of the total gastrographic record within a standard interval of measurement: "It is obtained by running a standard map measurer over the contours of crests and troughs of all waves to be included in the measurement and through the central positions of all EGG and respiration waves . . ." (p. 235). This index is dependent on number *and* amplitude of waves within the interval. With strong respiratory waves present it may be difficult to obtain or it may become subject to observer errors. It is easily shown that this more or less arbitrarily defined parameter has a direct relation to the root mean square value (rms) of the total signal (see Bendat & Piersol, 1971). Both measures are also related to the earlier mentioned "motility index" (MI) by gastroenterologists (see Section 3), which is proportional to the absolute *area* integral of motility records when they deviate little from sinusoidal form.

4.3.1d. "Tonic" Parameters. To account for slow changes in their dc recordings, *displacement* was defined by Russell and Stern (1967) "as the difference . . . between the points at the two ends of the baseline" (cf. Figure 9).

This measure is especially difficult to interpret because with analysis periods of 30 or 60 sec it may either stem from slow potential drifts or from very slow periodic components of about 1 cpm. The definition is in contradiction to the basic sample theorem in signal analysis. Unpredictable interactions with variations of signal contents may be the result. As a measure of "tonic" signal components it may only be used if many periods of analysis are averaged within or across subjects. Even then the interpretation is doubtful.

In the more recent report by Walker and Sandman (1977), another "tonic" parameter, *basal resting level,* has been defined. It is the "amount of dc voltage needed to balance the two EGG electrodes" at the beginning of measurement. So far no gastrointestinal source for this EGG parameter has been identified. Although White (1964a,b) relates it to acid secretion, the empirical basis for doing so is extremely poor (Colcher, Katz, & Goodman, 1957; Goodman, Ginsberg, & Robinson, 1951; Joodman, Colcher, Katz, & Dougler, 1955) and does not stem from surface recordings. Despite careful preparation of nonpolarizable electrodes and skin sites, sizable contact potentials generated at the electrode–skin interface and genuine skin dc potentials are always present. Their relation to the overall dc potential level and the size of the possible gastrointestinal component in it still must be identified.

4.3.1e. Measures of Latency. Russell and Stern (1967) also defined a signal parameter intended to give an estimate of the latency of a response to an external stimulus. This "peak response time" was also used by Walker and Sandman (1977). It is the time from the onset of a stimulus to the point of peak amplitude as defined above. It is easily seen that this latency measure must run into serious difficulties when a small, singular-elicited response is superimposed on a high-amplitude, periodic EGG. In addition, it is easily contaminated with latencies of large excursions of the respiratory artifact which are not easily recognized. The averaged-evoked-response approach is more suitable but requires a computer; it has not been used so far in gastrographic experiments.

4.3.2. Fourier Analysis and Related Signal-Analytic Approaches

Whereas the classical scoring system for gastrograms described in the previous section used more or less arbitrarily defined measures according to the practical demands of hand scoring, some physiological research groups employ a different approach which is based on signal-analytic principles of communication theory and the theory of statistical processes, and which require computer processing of analog signals. The application of this approach to gastrointestinal motility records dates back at least to the early work of Small, Brean, and Farrar (1955), who used autocorrelation methods to describe and analyze the periodic components of intraluminal pressure recordings from the jejunum of rabbits. The autocorrelation function of signals detects distinct periodic components even on a background of high noise levels. The Fourier transform of the autocorrelation function produces the so-called power spectrum which essentially represents the decomposition of the signal into its dominant rhythms (see Chapter 6). Equivalent results are obtained by direct Fourier ("spectral") analyses of gastrograms.

Spectral analyses basically decompose the signal into a series of trigonometric functions (sines and cosines). Their relative amplitudes (or rather, the squared amplitudes) are plotted in the spectra against frequency. When a signal contains only random "noise," all frequencies will be equally strong and the spectrum flat. If, however, dominant rhythms are present, the spectrum will show more or less pronounced peaks at their corresponding frequencies. In this way quantitative evaluation of slow-wave rhythm content in gastrograms is possible. To illustrate the output of this type of analysis an original EGG record, its autocorrelation function, the resulting power spectrum, and corresponding parameters of the analysis are shown in Figure 10. The autocorrelation function is clearly periodic; this periodicity shows in the "frequency domain," that is, in the power spectrum, as a pronounced peak of high relative intensity at about 43.7 MHz or 2.6 cpm. The power at that frequency is proportional to the squared amplitude of the gastrographic "slow wave." (Other spectral and correlational principles and measures are explained in the legend to Figure 10 and in Chapter 6.)

Since the early report by Small *et al.* (1955) a number of research groups have developed further this kind of motility analysis to a point where it may be

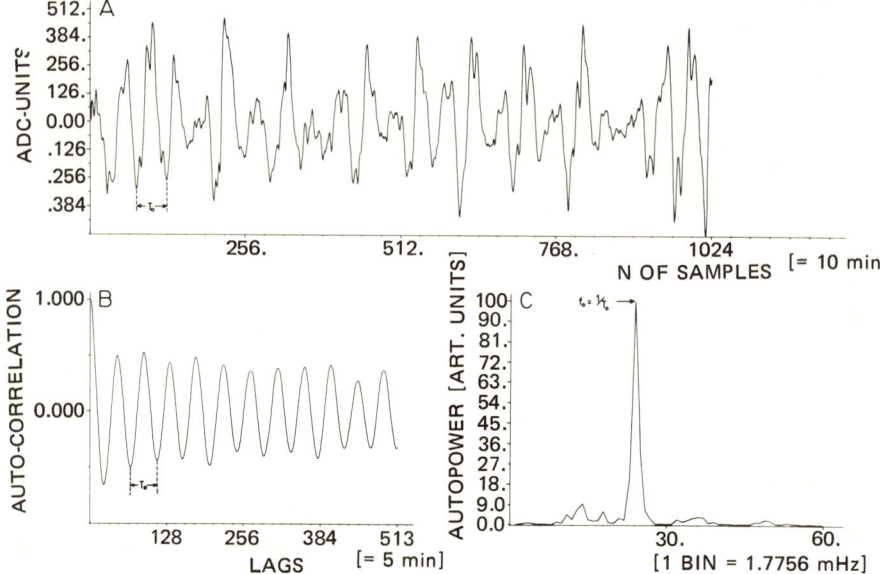

Figure 10. Relation of gastrographic signal, its autocorrelation function, and the corresponding power spectrum. (A) Original gastrogram with respiratory artifact and low-frequency noise as digitized by the analog-to-digital converter. ± 512 ADC units ≅ ± 500 μV. Sampling interval 550 msec, measurement period 1024 samples or circa 10 min. T_0 = period of slow waves (≈ 20 sec). (B) Autocorrelation function (ACF) of record A with "lags" extending up to 5 min. The ACF behaves like a filter accentuating the periodic slow wave component and damping the noise. T_0 = period of slow waves. (C) The power spectrum of record A shows a strong peak at the frequency of the slow wave component, $f_0 = 1/T_0 = 2.6$ cpm, and only minor noise at other frequencies. The absolute or relative height of the slow wave peak gives an estimate of intensity. (Computer plots by G. Müller, based on unpublished data by R. Hölzl & H. Brüchle.)

applied to psychophysiological problems (Brown et al., 1975; Linkens & Cannell, 1974; Nelsen & Kohatsu, 1968; Stevens & Worrall, 1974). Walker and Sandman (1976, 1977) and Hölzl and his co-workers (Hölzl & Scherm, 1975, 1976; Hölzl, Scherm, Schröder, & Kiefer, 1977; and later publications, see Chapter 6) have applied this technique to psychophysiological studies. Because special problems are associated with the use of spectral analysis in this area, a number of technical details have to be considered in order to evaluate the particular use different authors make of this type of analysis. (See Chapter 6 for a more detailed discussion of these problems.)

4.3.2a. Evidence from Physiological Psychology. In their report Stevens and Worrall (1974) compared electrical recordings from the abdominal surface of cats with mechanical recordings from implanted transducers. The position of the electrodes was verified by X-raying. One active electrode was 2 cm caudal to the xiphoid process, and the second was moved about to explore other locations on the abdomen. The reference electrode was always on the skin over the left femoral muscle, similar to the technique used by Davis's group. The authors also applied a more conventional analysis, which was not identical, however, to that used by Davis and his co-workers.

This study was cited later as good evidence for the validity of the EGG and the usefulness of correlational and spectral analyses. A closer look at this evidence reveals, however, that a larger data base is needed. Larger samples of unselected records must be analyzed to evaluate the usefulness of the techniques in psychophysiology on a broader scale. Stevens and Worrall (1974) analyzed only a few hundred periods of slow wave activity (at about 5 cpm, from 3 cats using the conventional hand-scoring method and only one 3-min epoch with auto- and cross-correlation methods). Their results, nevertheless, contain some interesting points for further investigations.

(1) The autocorrelation of one segment of 3 min duration indicates that electrical and mechanical gastrograms show a common periodicity at about 4.2 cpm. But other activity at higher frequencies (9.4 and 11.8 cpm in particular), present in the EGGs, have no counterparts in the mechanical record. Most of the higher-frequency components found by Fourier transformation of the autocorrelation function of this record might also be explained as higher harmonics of the basic rhythm of 4.2 cpm, given the maximal frequency resolution in that study.

(2) Cross-correlations between electrical and mechanical records and the corresponding cross-power spectra indicated a common component at 4.2 cpm as did the comparison of the autopower spectra of the individual records.

A few warnings seem appropriate. Fourier analysis of records with these extremely low-frequency components requires certain precautions to obtain reliable results that can compete with conventional handscoring. With one 3-min segment of a record, frequency resolution is rather limited. With a final Δf of 1.02 cpm ($\sim$ 17 MHz) the possible error of frequency determination of the basic slow-wave rhythm (4.2 cpm or 67 MHz) is as high as 25%. Estimation of amplitude parameters by Fourier analysis is even more unstable than determination of frequency. Transfer of Stevens and Worrall's technique without considering the technical details and their consequences for measurement precision, is therefore not recommended (see also Chapter 6).

4.3.2b. Gastroenterological Research.
Fourier and correlational analyses have also been used by three gastroenterological research groups.

Nelsen and Kohatsu (1968) determined the gastric rate response to feeding in dogs and humans by an autocorrelation technique similar to Small *et al.* (1955), but without using Fourier transformation to obtain power spectra. They used implanted as well as cutaneous and swallowed electrodes. Though promising, to our knowledge, this work was not followed up.

Another attempt to use autocorrelation functions of abdominal potential records and their corresponding power spectra was made by Thouvenot and his associates (Tonković et al., 1975; Thouvenot et al., 1973). In the Thouvenot et al. report, visually identified peaks in the power spectra were assigned to different parts of the gastrointestinal tract according to *a priori* knowledge about typical rhythms from invasive studies, mainly of animals. In Tonković et al., seven frequency classes were defined via histograms of spectral peaks. The latter presumably were identified by visual inspection of the spectra as in the previous report, but this is not clear from the text. The histograms were then divided into arbitrary regions comprising the frequency classes. They were related to different parts of the gut by *a priori* evidence in the Thouvenot et al. report. Whether another record sample would produce the same classification system is rather doubtful, especially because only 32 spectra were used and no systematic variation of experimental conditions was apparently applied.

One of the major problems of the spectral analysis approach is illustrated by Thouvenot's procedure: *How can "significant" components be identified in a complex signal like abdominal surface potentials consisting of several periodic processes plus low- and ultralow-frequency noise?* How can one distinguish higher harmonics and subharmonics of one particular rhythm (from the stomach, for instance) from a genuine contribution of another rhythm generator (e.g., duodenum or colon)? Even to set a statistical criterion of significant peak-height is not easy. A generally accepted solution has not yet been found. The work of the Sheffield group (Duthie and co-workers) provides some relevant information to improve this situation. Starting in the early 1970s, this group has repeatedly and systematically used auto- and cross-correlation functions together with Fourier analysis of internal and external electrical recordings from various segments of the gut, both of humans and animals (Brown, Duthie, Franks, Linkens, & Robertson-Dunn, 1973; Duthie, Kwong, Brown, & Whittaker, 1971; Duthie et al., 1972). Some of these studies bear on the interpretation of the gastrographic power spectra.

Duthie et al. (1971) showed that slow waves of gastric rate (3 cpm) are regularly found in the duodenum of humans. This differs from the results obtained with dogs (Bortoff & Davis, 1968) and casts doubt on Thouvenot's practice of directly ascribing certain peaks of EGG spectra to certain segments of the gut. Brown et al. (1973) appear to have been the first to compare frequency analyses of surface potentials to direct recordings of gastric activity. No actual comparison data were given in this report, however, and only one example of a power spectrum from a surface electrogastrogram was presented.

Later on, Brown et al. (1975) made a more systematic study on the applicability of spectral analysis techniques to human surface gastrograms. Sixteen normal subjects served to produce a total of 128 frequency analyses. The authors found a (statistically) "significant" component at approximately 3 cpm (average 3.02 ± 0.21 cpm) in at least one channel for 88% of the analyzed records. In a careful discussion of the possible sources of this component, Brown et al. (1975)

conclude that of all possible alternatives the stomach is the most likely source. To verify this, simultaneous recordings from internal mucosal suction electrodes (Kwok, 1979) and surface electrodes had been obtained earlier. Frequency analysis revealed a common rhythm of 3 cpm in both types of recordings. This was confirmed by calculating the cross-correlation function between internal and external potentials, although the degree of correlation was not reported. This correlational information was reported for one subject only.

In discussing the possible source of a faster component (between 10 and 12 cpm) Brown *et al.* (1975) raise a number of additional points which must be considered in interpreting gastrographic spectra. From other studies using direct recordings it was concluded that the small and large intestines are most likely the origin of the 12 cpm component. Because this was obtained mainly in the fasting state, and not after the meal, dislocation of stomach and/or intestines by filling was suspected to be the cause. (This also led to the increase in amplitude of the BER detected from the surface.) The authors correctly state that there is a need for cutaneous recordings from many electrode sites before a firm conclusion can be reached. For instance, differences in higher harmonic signal content between fasting and postprandial states may well account for this finding, which could be due to a higher incidence of contraction-correlated spike potentials after the meal. This presumably would be reflected in a change of EGG wave from sinusoidal to rectangular forms. Rectangular waves contain harmonic components of the base rhythm. Those are normally not distinguishable from genuine fast rhythms. Kwok (1979) claims to have been able to relate fast activity in the surface record (9–10 cpm) to spike activity in the serosal signal using a Fourier and autoregression approach simultaneously (see Section 4.3.3). Only *direct* cross-correlational studies and coherence function analysis (see Chapter 6) of *simultaneous* recordings on a larger scale can settle the issue.

In general, the problem of correlating certain aspects of the gastrographic spectra, other than the well-known fundamental of the 3 cpm rhythm, with physiological events has not been solved. This is as true for Fourier approaches as it is for classical scoring. However, a number of improvements have been added.

Linkens and Cannell (1974) described an interactive graphics program for this type of analysis, capable of performing fast Fourier transforms (FFT, with suitable windowing and calibration) and calculating auto- and cross-correlograms (via inverse FFT) as well as digital filtering in the frequency domain. While these options are now standard in any good computer software package for spectral analysis, the possibility of calculating (and displaying) the 95% confidence limits and bandwidth as derived by Durrani and Nightingale (1973) deserves special attention. It might provide one way of defining "significant component," which is the major problem with this type of analysis. This technique has been used with some success in later studies of the Sheffield group (Smallwood, Brown, & Duthie, 1976) on direct recordings from the gastric muscle, but was said not to be useful with colonic records (Stoddard, Duthie, Smallwood, & Linkens, 1979). This limitation presumably applied to surface gastrograms as well. Therefore, according to Stoddard *et al.* ". . . visual detection of peaks is mandatory" (p. 477). This reintroduces a subjective element into the analysis (Smallwood, Linkens, & Stoddard, 1980). If one wants to avoid this by automatic significance testing one has to use long epochs of recording, thus sacrificing detection of short-term changes in the signal. In addition weak and/or inconstant activity will not often lead to a significant peak, and it may result in more than one peak or in flat peaks (cf. Stoddard *et al.,* 1979, for a quantitative analysis): "Waxing-and-waning" and similar activity patterns violate the stationarity assumption of Fourier analysis and may lead to spurious spectral components not present in the original signal. These and related problems eventually led that group to use a totally different approach (Smallwood, Linkens, Kowk, & Stoddard, 1980; Smallwood, Linkens, & Stoddard, 1980), which is briefly discussed in Section 4.3.3b.

Despite the problem discussed, spectral analysis seems at present to be the best type of signal analysis in surface gastrography, both in empirical and theoretical respects. This has been questioned by some psychophysiological researchers comparing the classical scoring system with Fourier techniques (Lilie, 1974; Walker & Sandman, 1977). Unfortunately, the particular procedures used by those authors do not provide for a *fair* comparison, because some of the requirements necessary for interpretable power spectra were either not met or procedural parameters necessary to evaluate the authors' analyses were not specified. For example, the precise bandpass characteristics of the recording system, dc removal prior to Fourier analysis, "windowing" (see Chapter 6), and parameter definition in spectrum, may decide whether the outcome of the analysis is of value or not. Quite unfavorable conditions for spectral analysis of gastrograms were typically defined.

This is the case, too, for the study by Walker and Sandman (1977). They came to the conclusion that spectral analyses had no advantage over the classical scoring system, and even produced fewer significant differences between experimental conditions. A quick look at the original report shows that with their rather short period of measurement (3 min) frequency resolution becomes quite low. In that case the procedure becomes sensitive to low-frequency noise and insensitive to subtle signal changes, thus increasing error variance. It is not astonishing that there is little more to be won by a crude spectral analysis than a crude traditional scoring system.

4.3.3. Filter Techniques

4.3.3a. Fixed Bandpasses. Common Fourier techniques have the serious disadvantage of obscuring short-term changes in signal parameters by their inherent averaging logic. To obtain suitable frequency resolution of 1 to 2 MHz (~ 0.1 cpm) at least 10-min epochs of recording are needed (see Chapter 6 for an alternative solution). That makes it difficult to follow minute-to-minute changes of slow wave frequency or amplitude after feeding, a pharmacological treatment, or during biofeedback training of motility.

One obvious way of isolating a well-known frequency band such as the 3 cpm slow wave activity is filtering the noisy original signal by suitable electronic filters or equivalent digital filter algorithms. The problem is that the frequency of slow waves may be quite inconstant or change systematically with experimental manipulations such as feeding (cf. Nelsen & Kohatsu, 1968). With a bandpass filter which is narrow enough to reject low-frequency noise near the signal band and set at a fixed midfrequency at the beginning of measurement, those frequency changes would be misinterpreted as amplitude changes when the slow wave runs out of the passband of the filter. Movement artifacts are difficult or impossible to reject by bandpassing. The ever-present respiratory component in surface gastrograms is also not easily filtered out. Higher harmonic components of a nonsinusoidal EGG may partially overlap with the respiration band. Filtering it out would result in severe distortion of the EGG signal. In particular, it may reject the most relevant contraction-related fast activity. For special applications, such as biofeedback experiments, however, this simple filter approach may be useful as long as the broader original signal band (e.g., 0.01 to 200 MHz) is secured and analyzed by conventional or Fourier techniques for control purposes and as long as frequency changes are negligible within experimental periods. When this is not the case, one of the following methods must be applied.

4.3.3b. Tracking Filters. Quite early gastroenterological research groups tried to devise filter methods capable of adequately dealing with changing frequencies of slow waves. Such a filter or algorithm has to readjust its midfrequency to "track" the wandering basal signal frequency, and is, therefore, called a "tracking filter."

Various types of tracking filters exist. One of the best known is the so-called phase-locked loop filter (PLL). It has been widely used in FM- and AM-demodulation as well as in the tracking filters for telemetric receivers (cf. MacKay, 1968). The first to introduce this principle into electrogastrography was Nelsen (1967). This technique basically uses a voltage-controlled, sine-wave oscillator (VCO), the frequency of which is readjusted in a feedback control loop until the phase difference between input signal and output of VCO is zero. In that way the VCO signal "locks" into the input signal and "tracks" its basal rhythm over wide frequency ranges. In the original report surface gastrograms of 15 patients and volunteers were filtered with an analog computer, and promising results were obtained. Later a digital computer program with a number of practical improvements was written for a laboratory computer (PDP 8), but seemingly no systematic large-scale studies followed the initial attempts. Smallwood

(1978a,b) constructed a practical PLL circuit with modern integrated components and presented test data which merit further study.

From the point of view of the psychophysiologist, the above-mentioned PLL versions have some serious limitations. The first is that they do not readily supply wave-to-wave amplitude estimates. Although there are possibilities, for example, by complex multiplication of the input signal with the VCO output, at present no empirical information on the value of this manipulation seems available. Another difficulty of these circuits is their problematic low-frequency behavior. It tends to make the response of the filter to changes very slow, or even unreliable. Therefore, Smallwood, for instance, stored his gastrogram on analog tape and played it back at a speed 60 times as high as the recording speed, thus working in a higher-frequency range. For biofeedback procedures and similar experiments, where real-time processing is essential, Smallwood's technique is not applicable.

Finally, the problem of identification of signal source applies to these filter methods as well as to others. If the technical problems mentioned above can be solved—which seems very probable—and physiologically meaningful signal bands can be identified for subsequent filtering, the filter approach might become extremely useful in clinical investigations where cumbersome signal processing must be avoided.

In closing, it should be mentioned that more advanced filter techniques which take into account signals with nonsinusoidal form (like slow waves with spikes on top) have been available for some time from communication engineering but have not been utilized for processing of gastrograms. The methods of "matched" and "optimal" filtering are quite involved technically and require close cooperation with specialists in biomedical engineering to ensure proper application. Where this is provided, however, unexpected progress in application studies are the result as research in the cardiovascular area has shown (e.g., Stemmler & Thom, 1979).

4.3.3c. Autoregressive Filter Methods.

Smallwood and his co-workers in Sheffield (Smallwood, Linkens, Kwok, & Stoddard, 1980; Smallwood, Linkens, & Stoddard, 1980) have introduced a type of digital filters into the field of electrical gut recordings which originally stem from econometric time series analysis (Box & Jenkins, 1970), and these have also proved to be valuable in biosignal, in particular EEG analysis (e.g., Lopes da Silva, Dijk, & Smits, 1975; Rösler, 1980): These are the so-called autoregressive or AR filters.

In contrast to Fourier techniques AR methods model the signal not as a series of trigonometric functions in the frequency domain but as a series of linearly dependent values in the time domain. Each signal value (x_t) at a particular point in time (t) is predicted by a linear combination of previous values (x_{t-i}) with weights (a_i [$i = 1, 2, \ldots, p$]):

$$x_t = a_1 x_{t-1} + a_2 x_{t-2} + \cdots + a_p x_{t-p} + z_t$$

The number of terms (p) and the weights or coefficients (a_i) are determined by linear regression techniques so that the error term (z_t) has minimal variance, hence the term "autoregression." The resulting vector of coefficients, roughly speaking, describes the signal composition analogous to the Fourier coefficients in spectral analysis (see Chapter 6). In fact, equivalent spectra may be calculated from AR analyses (Linkens, 1978; Rappelsberger & Petsche, 1975; Rösler, 1980).

AR methods have several advantages over conventional Fourier analysis. One of them is that the resulting spectra are smoother because the error term does not reappear in the spectra. Fourier-type spectra, on the other hand, contain all signal components included in the analysis and have to be smoothed, for example, by averaging of several spectra.

AR methods model the signal explicity as a sum of AR components plus a (Gaussian) error term. They are, therefore, called "structural" approaches whereas Fourier decomposition is "descriptive" in the sense that it does *not* imply that the signal is "really" made out of superimposed sine waves (Box & Jenkins, 1970). Therefore, some of the interpretation problems associated with power spectra of gastrograms, which were discussed in Section 4.3.2, can be avoided with AR analysis. In addition, *significance testing* of periodic components becomes clear (Linkens, 1978).

Furthermore AR models also may be constructed as on-line filters to detect significant *deviations* from previous signal composition, such as single contractions on top of ongoing periodic slow-wave activity. This approach has been as successfully used in detection of "transient nonstationarities" in the EEG as spike-and-wave complexes in epileptics (Lommen, 1976; Praetorius, Bodenstein, & Creutzfeldt, 1977). This approach may well open a new line of EGG processing with particular value in psychophysiological studies where single gastrointestinal events are the target of research (such as in studies on visceral perception, biofeedback, and elicited gastrointestinal responses to external stimuli; cf. Chapters by Stern, Walker, and Whitehead, in this volume).

4.4. Validity of Electrogastrograms—Critical Evaluation

4.4.1. Psychophysiological Studies

Much of the available information on the physiological source of surface EGG was dealt with in previous sections. It should have become clear by now that, despite some progress since the earlier reports by Davis and his co-workers, the question of validity of EGG is still debatable. The past evidence is comprehensively reviewed by Russell and Stern (1967) and Brown (1972).

Those studies tried to relate EGG measures directly to Code's Wave Types I–III by which *manometric* recordings of gastric motility had been characterized (Hightower, 1962). This attempt has generally *not* been successful except for the

BER which has the same frequency as rhythmically appearing Type-II waves. Brown (1972) did not seem to be aware of this problem when citing Hightower's (1962) monograph on manometric studies of gastric motility as if it dealt with types of EGG waves. The latter are much more complex (cf. Section 2.3). The older attempts to correlate features of the EGG with those of manometric records suffer from the additional weakness that the latter are debated measures of motility themselves (cf. Texter et al., 1957; Truelove, 1968; and Section 2.1).

In general the "validation philosophy" of the earlier studies has been rather weak. Very seldom have direct correlative studies with simultaneous invasive and surface recordings and adequate analysis of their correlation been attempted. When this has been done, only a few sample records were compared in a qualitative way. Moreover, mechanical and electrical recordings are treated interchangeably giving rise to misunderstandings.

More direct evidence on the validity of the EGG stems from the study of Stevens and Worrall (1974), which was mentioned earlier. Its basic results (apart from those discussed previously) may be summarized as follows: (1) By using conventional frequency analysis (number of baseline crossings; Davis et al., 1957), the authors found good correlations of frequency parameters of the slow wave component in electrical and mechanical records (3.76–4.54 cpm) but no corresponding fast activity in the mechanical record (12.9–16.5 cpm). It has to be kept in mind, however, that these data stem from three animals only and that the tracings had been visually selected for the minimum number of movement artifacts "having good activity." In our experience this procedure would lead to the loss of one-third to two-thirds of records in human gastrography under usual conditions of psychophysiological experiments. Also the observed correlations (.84, .86, and .85) are not too impressive under these rather favorable conditions. The coefficients indicate that 28% of the frequency variance is still not accounted for. (2) No attempt has been made to secure validation data on conventional amplitude measures. (3) No correlations of amplitude measures derived from power spectra were obtained in the study. Power spectra and cross-power spectra from many records would be necessary to accomplish this task.

Summing up, only *frequency parameters* of the surface electrogastrograms have been validated against mechanical records with partial success. This conclusion had been drawn already by Kohatsu (1970) in his review of gastroenterological studies on the electrogastrogram. Although fairly good correlations of frequency parameters indicate "that the EGG is at the very least correlated with gastric motility" (Stevens & Worrall, 1974, p. 179), the direct gastric counterparts of amplitude measures of the gastrogram, whether defined by conventional analysis or by Fourier analysis, have not been identified so far.

Obviously separate validation of different signal parameters such as frequency and amplitude of slow waves and incidence of single contractions is mandatory because validity of one measure may not imply validity of another.

4.4.2. Gastroenterological Studies

Further validation data were obtained by gastroenterological groups in Sheffield, England (Brown *et al.*, 1975), and Tours, France (Thouvenot *et al.*, 1973; cf. Section 4.3.2).

The direct cross-correlation study by Brown *et al.* (1975) is of particular interest. It shows that implanted serosal and abdominal surface electrodes measure the same basic physiological process—mass action potentials of gastric smooth muscles. With the more primitive method of contact electrodes on an intragastric balloon and somewhat qualitative data handling, Davis *et al.* (1959) had earlier shown a similar correspondence with surface recordings.

In general, these groups using Fourier and cross-correlational analysis to evaluate surface gastrograms in relation to internal motility records have found good correspondence of basic slow wave rhythms from both sites, but only frequency terms were compared. Data on the validity of amplitude estimates are still lacking. Amplitude changes in surface recordings may be brought about in several ways. An increase at the surface can stem simply from an increase in slow waves at the level of smooth muscle layers of the stomach, which may or may not be correlated with contraction. It could also reflect increased spiking activity on top of slow waves which also shows only as an increase in 3 cpm amplitude of surface EGG, which again would be correlated with contraction. Furthermore, identification of wave types other than rhythmic 3 cpm activity has not been achieved by these groups. The reason for this lies in the kind of spectral analysis they used. It obscures "waxing-and-waning" patterns in the record and other transient features characteristic of electromotor behavior of the stomach found by direct investigation. The related question of interpretation of different peaks in the spectrum of a gastrogram as distinct components rather than harmonics of one and the same nonsinusoidal periodic process has been discussed earlier at some length. It is a serious problem for straightforward validation studies, and is still unsolved.

The work by Brown *et al.* (1975) and Thouvenot *et al.* (1973) also deals with the question of the physiological source of abdominal potentials. Even when their gastrointestinal origin is taken for granted other parts of the gut than the stomach could contribute. For a long time the colon, especially its transverse part, was considered to be a possible candidate. It shows frequency bands near gastric base rhythms (50 MHz or 3 cpm; Konturek & Rösch, 1976; Taylor, 1973; and Taylor, Duthie, Smallwood, & Linkens, 1975). Whether the colon can be excluded as a source of slow waves in surface gastrograms, as readily as Brown *et al.* (1975) seem to believe, remains to be verified by cutaneous recordings from many electrode sites at the same time (Brown *et al.*, 1975).

Recently a critical monograph on "Myoelectrical Activity of the Stomach" by Smout (1980) appeared which deals with surface electrogastrography in dogs and humans. In contrast to previous work, Smout presented a more thorough empirical and theoretical analysis of the main problems in gastrography. The relation of simultaneous recordings from serosal and surface electrodes in the postprandial and the interdigestive interval was studied. A rosette configuration was used. Signals were analyzed visually and by Fourier analysis. In general, the results corroborated earlier findings by providing a better empirical basis. While details of Smout's data cannot be presented here, some of his conclusions are important in respect to further research and future clinical applications (Smout, 1980, pp. 95–99):

1. Both electrical control activity (ECA) and electrical response activity (ERA), that is contraction-related potentials, are reflected in the electrogastrogram.
2. The sinusoidal form of EGG waves and the ERA-related amplitude changes can be explained by a dipole model of gastric action.
3. Low-frequency components (i.e., below 3 cpm) of yet unknown origin occur (cf. Chapter 6 and Hölzl, Heltzel, Brückner, Eder, Müller, Skambraks, & Kleinschmidt, 1981).
4. After a test meal, the main frequency of the EGG falls and subsequently rises above fasting levels. The amplitude increases. Probably also the position of the antrum relative to the cutaneous electrodes changes. This results in a shift of optimal lead so that maximal 3 cpm activity is recorded from a different electrode after a meal.
5. Tachygastria may be detected noninvasively by the EGG. This phenomenon was previously reported to be associated with gastric retention in clinical cases (cf. Smout, 1980, p. 99). In this way the EGG may lead to a better understanding of motor disorders of the stomach.

The author of the present report does not fully agree with Smout's somewhat pessimistic view on the use of surface gastrography in the analysis and diagnosis of more classic stomach disorders like peptic ulcers. But it is certainly true that much research has still to be done to develop electrogastrography to the point of being a clinical diagnostic tool.

Composition of abdominal potentials may very well vary with anatomical variations, body position, filling state, and a number of other experimental conditions, so that presently available data from a few small-scale studies may not apply to psychophysiology settings with different conditions. For instance, low-frequency noise may increase in periods where subjects have to be active. This produces a nonspecific increase in total signal energy including 3 cpm bands without any gastric change. Misinterpretation of spectral parameters of EGG would result. Similar systematic experimental effects on signal composition are easily constructed (see Sections 2.1 and 3).

Not only, then, is there a need for separate validation of each signal parameter but also the validation question must be asked anew for each experimental setting.

5. Magnetogastrography

Magnetogastrograms (MGG) are obtained when small magnets, iron rods, or other magnetically active objects are introduced into the stomach, and resulting magnetic field changes during stomach contractions are detected by magnetometers.

5.1. Classical Methods

Wenger *et al.* (1955, 1957) were apparently the first to use this method for noninvasively recording stomach wall movements. The subject, usually while sitting, swallows a small polystyrene-coated magnetic rod (Alnico V, 5 mm diam, 12 mm long, weight 2.5 g) together with approximately 100 ml water. The procedure is said to be sensitive to magnet movements less than 1° with a commercial magnetometer (Waugh Type W-2, Irwin Laboratory, L. A.). Precise flux sensitivity of the device was not given nor was the typical field strength of the magnetic rod.

In a later publication (Wenger *et al.*, 1961), this research group discussed the method further. They concluded that their "magnetometer method" gave only crude measures of contraction amplitudes but reliable indications of time and frequency of contractions.

Only partial correspondence was found with intragastric balloon recordings. The authors related their findings to the wave-type classification well known from manometric studies (see Section 2.2 , and Code *et al.*, 1952). They stated that mostly Type I waves, but no Types II and III were found 2–4 hr after eating. It has been discussed at some length in earlier sections of this chapter how problematic it is to use the nomenclature of manometric events for other types of motility recordings. Localized stomach wall movements as detected by the magnetometer method are not the same as intragastric pressure changes when the stomach lumen contracts.

Even less information on the correlation with pressure recordings is available for the MGG than for the EGG. Engel and McFall (1959) contributed to this problem. Despite the scarcity of data presented in the original report, it is interesting for its technical ingenuity. The authors used dogs as subjects. The magnets were either implanted in the stomach wall together with strain gauges or magnets fastened with surgical thread onto a balloon probe for pressure recordings. In that way they were able to compare magnetic changes with stomach wall movements directly measured with strain gauges and manometry. Again, only partial correspondence in terms of traditional wave types was found.

Unfortunately, no larger-scale studies on further development of these promising methods have been published. There is one anecdotal report of a similar technique by Davis et al. (1957), who measured the MGG to validate their EGG records. They used an iron rod instead of a magnet, and a minedetecting device which responds to metal in general and not only to magnets. Hölzl et al. (1977) picked up movements of a small magnet via the voltage changes induced in a two-coil system. This system was not very sensitive, however, and was later abandoned.

Edwards, Hill, and Treadwill (1967) improved the original method by extra shielding of the magnetic probe against extraneous fields. They enclosed the magnetometer in a hollow cylinder of magnetic insulating material open only at the frontside toward the magnet to be sensed. This improved the signal-to-noise ratio but no quantitative test data were presented. Edwards et al. (1967) drew attention to the problem of reliable positioning of the probe. Since the signal strength of changes in magnetic flux is inversely proportional to the cube of the distance between the magnet and the probe, unreliable positioning may present a major source of variance in MGG recording. The authors constructed a mounting support for the probe which allowed reproducible positioning over the subject, who was lying on his back.

Edwards et al. (1967) also tried to solve the problem that the ingested magnet moves downstream with time, and records can only be interpreted if information on magnet location is available. They tied the magnet to a tooth with digestable surgical thread and defined antral position by the presence of 3 cpm activity. This was confirmed by letting the magnet pass on until duodenal 12 cpm rhythm appeared, and then drawing it back until 3 cpm waves reappeared. The investigators report that they never had any problems with gagging due to the thread being in the esophagus. This is somewhat astonishing in the light of observations made by researchers who used telemetering capsules tied to a tooth (e.g., Horowitz & Farrar, 1962). It may be that a small magnet does not produce such forceful tightening of fastening threads as are produced by much bigger telemetering capsules.

5.2. Three-Axes Magnetogastrogram with Freely Moving Magnet

The author of the present review and his co-workers have adapted the classical magnetometer method to a clinical psychophysiological laboratory and used it in conjunction with electrogastrography (Hölzl, 1979). Teflon-coated standard stirring magnets 5 mm in diameter and 14 mm long were used. They were not fastened by a thread. To overcome the problem of undefined magnetic axis because of unknown orientation of the magnet in the stomach, a three-axes miniature magnetometer (3 × 4 × 12 cm) with built-in transducing and amplifying circuity was used (Develco). Position is defined relative to fixed skeletal points but the problem of the variable abdominal anatomy relative to these points remains unsolved. (Details of the method are discussed in Chapter 6.)

5.3. Magnetogastrographies with Ferromagnetic Tracer Material

Frei, Gunders, Pajewsky, Alkan, and Eshchar (1968) reported on the use of ferrites as an alternative to barium sulfate as contrast material for X-ray investigation of the gastrointestinal tract. The magnetic properties of the material allowed for manipulation from the outside by a magnet so that particular parts of the gastrointestinal tract could be displayed in more detail.

Later, gastric emptying was studied by this research group with the same substance (Benmair, 1975; Benmair, Dreyfuss, Fischel, Frei, & Gilat, 1977; Frei, Benmair, Yerushalmi, & Dreyfuss, 1970). They used a special differential probe to measure the effective magnetic susceptibility in the gastric area after ingestion of a test meal containing 20% of magnesium ferrite. The gradual decline in susceptibility due to gastric emptying is plotted against time. The exponential emptying curves obtained seem to correspond very well with those seen with radioactive tracer techniques.

This noninvasive method of continuous measurement of gastrointestinal "transit" has given promising results in over 60 patients and is equally applicable in lower parts of the gastrointestinal tract (Benmair, Fischel, Frei, & Gilat, 1977). Because of the radio-opaqueness of the material additional X-ray control in specified intervals is possible. The technique requires an external energizing ac field. This may be a disadvantage in psychophysiological applications. If this could be overcome and also contractile activity mirrored in the fine grain of the activity, a convenient method for psychophysiological motility and emptying studies would be available.

First attempts in this direction were made in the Hölzl's laboratory. A recording example from an unpublished pilot study by Hölzl, Bolsinger, and Brüchle is shown in Figure 11.

The magnetic field changes induced by movement of the ingested ferrite (test meal prescription according to Benmair, 1975) before the background (earth-)dc-field were measured by a highly sensitive differential three-axes magnetometer system ("Förster probe"; cf. Chapter 6), which allowed for dc-field compensation. No additional energizing field was used. (The system is described in more detail in Chapter 6.) Bipolar EGGs were simultaneously recorded from the abdomen according to the rosette method. Visual and computer analysis shows good correspondence of 3 cpm activity in EGGs and ferrite MGGs. Also,

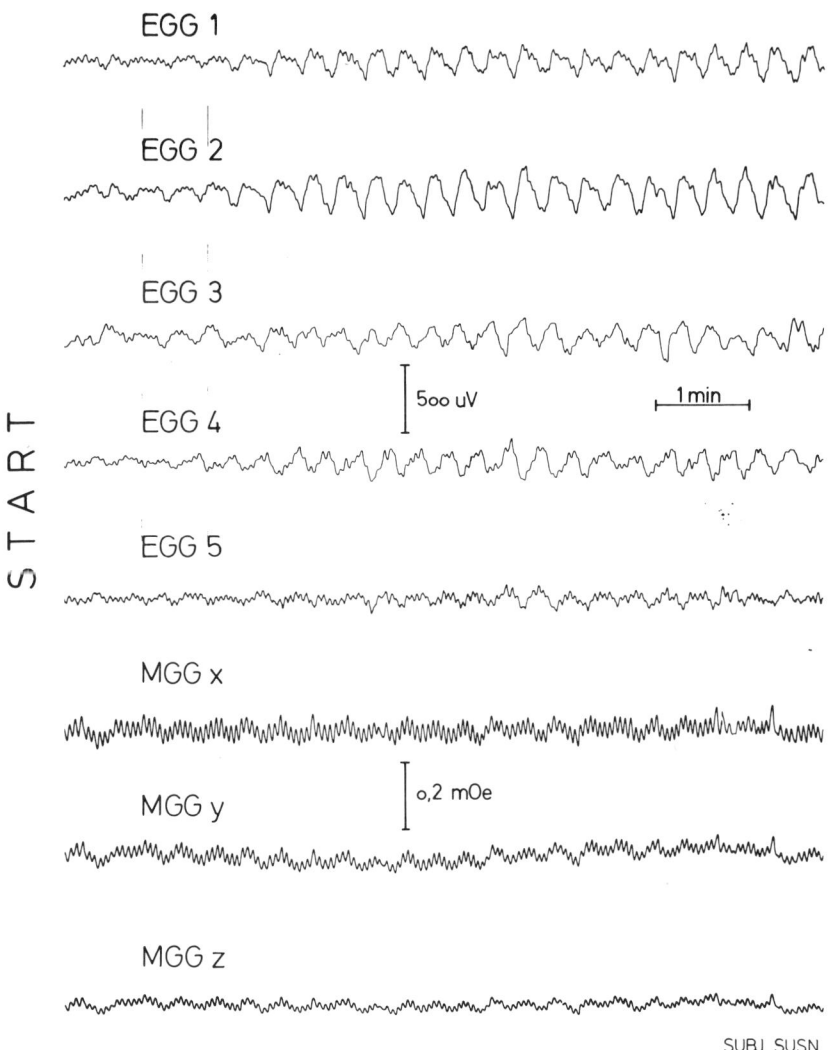

Figure 11. Sample records of simultaneous electrogastrograms from the rosette configuration (numbers as indicated in Figure 5D), and magnetogastrograms with Benmair's ferrite technique. Only the ac components of the three axes in space are shown. The ferrite meal was taken immediately before the "START" point = begin of records in figure (Hölzl & Brüchle, unpublished data).

a strong respiratory component is superimposed on the rather weak magnetic records, and wave amplitudes gradually decline with the evacuation of stomach content. This is much stronger in the dc component, which is not shown on the record. After 20 min a first readjustment of dc-field compensation was needed.

In other subjects, this readjustment was sometimes quicker. Therefore, separate amplification of ac and dc components of ferrite MGGs is necessary. Then, high amplification of the ac component for detection of 3 cpm activity and moderate amplification of the dc or slowly changing component for measurement of emptying is possible. It should be mentioned that calibration of the system is difficult, and the method is not yet ready for routine use. Some subjects also have problems with the test meal because of pulverulence produced by the ferrite granules on chewing. This was already mentioned by Benmair, Dreyfuss, Fischel, Frei, and Gilat (1977). In addition diarrhea was produced in one of our cases, presumably by residual HCl-soluble magnesium oxide in the ferrite preparation.

5.4. Signal Analysis

Nothing much, unfortunately, can be reported on signal analysis. Workers in the field did not pay attention to the problem, presumably because frequency was considered to be the only reliable parameter (of the MGG) which is easily obtained by visual counting of waves as long as they are relatively undisturbed. Unfortunately, this is not the case in the majority of recordings with the possible exception of those using implanted magnets.

Respiration is always a strong source of artifacts, but also quite minute body movements, change in position, and tonus of abdominal muscles cause sizable responses (the latter by dislocation of the stomach). These artifacts are much more pronounced in the MGGs than in the EGGs, and not easily dealt with by conventional methods. Until recently, therefore, amplitude measures of the MGG were difficult to interpret.

On the other hand, the MGG has the big advantage of actually indicating mechanical movement of stomach walls. It is, therefore, not subject to the possible criticisms which have been raised against the EGG. Further development of the MGG techniques including signal analysis by more advanced methods, as in the case of EGGs, seems to be worthwhile.

6. Conclusion

From the literature available, one may conclude that surface gastrograms, in general, provide highly valuable measures of gastrointestinal electromotor activity, especially for basic and clinical psychophysiology. These measures have unnecessarily been overlooked by psychophysiologists and most gastroenterologists without good grounds, as Walker and Sandman (1977) rightly criticized. The conviction that gastrograms are cumbersome to record, difficult to analyze, and impossible to interpret is certainly an irrational one. There are, however, real problems of calibration and correlation with the physiological source for which routine solutions are not readily available. With the advent of better and flexible electronic equipment, advanced signal processing techniques on the basis of the fast Fourier transform, and also more direct correlation studies, these problems have become manageable.

In addition, the evidence on the clinical usefulness of the surface gastrogram is accumulating slowly but steadily. Some of it is not well known in the English-language literature but still deserves attention. Russian gastroenterologists, for instance, have done extensive work on the diagnostic use of the electrogastrogram for routine ulcer screening (Androsov, Firsova, & Tolstych, 1973; Levin & Belousov, 1963). It is difficult to evaluate these studies because the methodology and statistical design are not well documented in the literature which is easily accessible to Western readers (cf. Krasil'nikow, 1971; Sobakin *et al.*, 1962). Similar work has been done by French and East German researchers (Martin *et al.*, 1971; Schulz, Reitzig, Koblitz, Lisewski, & Schulze, 1975).

The effects of surgical interventions such as highly selective vagotomy and pharmacological treatment by spasmolytic substances have successfully been demonstrated (Eder, 1981; Heltzel, Hölzl, & Brückner, 1978; Heltzel *et al.*, 1980; Hölzl *et al.*, 1981; Winhaiter, 1981). From these studies it also became clear that clinical studies often present technical and methodological difficulties quite different from those in laboratory studies with healthy subjects, and methods may not always be transferred to clinical settings or groups without modification (e.g., Hölzl *et al.*, 1981).

ACKNOWLEDGMENTS

Preparation of this chapter would not have been possible without the assistance of Alexandra Solder, who did the drawings, and Silvia Pattay, who typed various versions of the manuscript. Their help is gratefully acknowledged. The diligence and patience of Silvia deserves special mentioning. Bill Whitehead and Stefan Lautenbacher read an earlier version of the paper and made valuable suggestions, but are not responsible for the remaining deficiencies.

7. References

Aeberhard, P. Der gastrointestinale myoelektrische Komplex. *Zeitschrift für Gastroenterologie,* 1977, *15,* 202–208.

Adler, H. F., Atkinson, A. J., & Ivy, A. C. The study of motility of the human colon: An explanation of dyssynergia of the colon, or the "unstable colon." *American Journal of Digestive Diseases,* 1941, *8,* 197.

Alvarez, W. C. The electrogastrogram and what it shows. *Journal of the American Medical Association,* 1922, *78,* 1116–1119.

Alvarez, W. C., & Mahoney, I. J. Action currents in stomach and intestine. *American Journal of Physiology,* 1922, *58,* 476–493.

Androsov, N. S., Firsova, P. P., & Tolstych, P. I. The value of electrogastrogram in estimation of the gastric motor function in cancer. *Voprosy Onkologii*, 1973, *19*, 39–43.

Beaumont, W. *Experiments and observations of the gastric juices and physiology of digestion.* Plattsburg, Pennsylvania: F. P. Allen, 1833.

Bendat, J. S., & Piersol, A. G. *Random data: Analysis and measurement procedures.* New York: Wiley, 1971.

Benmair, Y. *Use of a ferromagnetic tracer for measurement of gastric emptying and some other medical physics purposes.* Unpublished Ph.D. thesis, Weizmann Institute of Science, Feinberg Graduate School, 1975.

Benmair, Y., Dreyfuss, F., Fischel, B., Frei, E. H., & Gilat, T. Study of gastric emptying using a ferromagnetic tracer. *Gastroenterology*, 1977, *73*, 1041–1045.

Benmair, Y., Fischel, B., Frei, E. H., & Gilat, T. Evaluation of a magnetic method for the measurement of small intestinal transit time. *American Journal of Gastroenterology*, 1977, *68*, 470–475.

Bortoff, A., & Davis, R. S. Myogenic transmission of control slow waves across the gastroduodenal junction in situ. *American Journal of Physiology*, 1968, *222*, 1295–1298.

Box, G. E. P., & Jenkins, G. M. *Time series analysis.* San Francisco: Holden-Day, 1970.

Brown, B. H., Duthie, H. L., Franks, C. I., Linkens, D. A., & Robertson-Dunn, B. Correlation and spectral techniques applied to the analysis and modeling of gastrointestinal electrical signals. *International Symposium on Measurement and Process Identification by Correlation and Spectral Techniques*, Bradford, 1973.

Brown, B. H., Smallwood, R. H., Duthie, H. L., & Stoddard, C. J. Intestinal smooth muscle electrical potentials recorded from surface electrodes. *Medical and Biological Engineering*, 1975, *13*, 97–103.

Brown, C. C. Instruments in psychophysiology. In N. S. Greenfield & R. A. Sternbach (Eds.), *Handbook of psychophysiology.* New York: Holt, Rinehart & Winston, 1972.

Bruch, H. *Eating disorders: obesity, anorexia nervosa, and the person within.* New York: Basic Books, 1973.

Burnstock, G., Holman, M. E., & Prosser, C. L. Electrophysiology of smooth muscle. *Physiological Review*, 1963, *43*, 482–527.

Cannon, W. B. The influence of emotional states on the functions of the alimentary canal. *American Journal of the Medical Sciences*, 1909, *137*, 480–487.

Cannon, W. B. *The wisdom of the body* (Rev. ed.). London: Routledge & Kegan Paul, 1939.

Cannon, W. B., & Lieb, C. W. The receptive relaxation of the stomach. *American Journal of Physiology*, 1911, *29*, 267–273.

Cannon, W. B., & Washburn, A. L. An explanation of hunger. *American Journal of Physiology*, 1912, *31*, 436–454.

Carlson, A. J. Contributions to the physiology of the stomach. I. The character of the movements of the empty stomach in man. *American Journal of Physiology*, 1912, *31*, 151. (a)

Carlson, A. J. The relation between the contractions of the empty stomach and the sensation of hunger. *American Journal of Physiology*, 1912, *31*, 175–192. (b)

Code, C. F., & Carlson, H. C. Motor activity of the stomach. In C. F. Code (Ed.), *Handbook of physiology* (Vol. 4, Sec. 6). Baltimore: Williams & Wilkins, 1968.

Code, C. F., Hightower, N. C. Jr., & Morlock, C. G. Motility of the alimentary canal of man: Review of recent studies. *American Journal of Medicine*, 1952, *13*, 328.

Colcher, H., Katz, G. M., & Goodman, E. N. Simultaneous multirecording of gastric potential. *Clinical Research Procedures*, 1957, *5*, 195.

Cooke, A., & Christensen, J. Motor functions of the stomach. In M. H. Sleisinger & J. S. Fordtrau (Eds.), *Gastrointestinal disease.* Philadelphia: Lippincott, 1973.

Cragg, B. G., & Evans, D. H. L. Some reflexes mediated by afferent fibres of the abdominal vagus in the rabbit and cat. *Experimental Neurology*, 1960, *2*, 1–12.

Daniel, E. E. Nerves and motor activity of the gut. In F. Brooks & P. Evers (Eds.), *Nerves and the gut*. Thorofare: Slack, 1977.
Daniel, E. E., & Irvin, J. Electrical activity of gastric musculature. In C. F. Code (Ed.), *Handbook of physiology* (Vol. 4, Sec. 6). Baltimore: Williams & Wilkins, 1968.
Davenport, H. W. *Physiology of the digestive tract*. Chicago: Year Book Medical Publishers, Inc., 1971.
Davis, R. C., & Berry, F. Gastrointestinal reactions during a noise avoidance task. *Psychological Reports*, 1963, *12*, 135–137.
Davis, R. C., Garafolo, L., & Gault, F. P. An exploration of abdominal potentials. *Journal of Comparative and Physiological Psychology*, 1957, *50*, 519–523.
Davis, R. C., Garafolo, L., & Kveim, K. Conditions associated with gastrointestinal activity. *Journal of Comparative and Physiological Psychology*, 1959, *52*, 466–475.
Deckner, C. W., Hill, J. T., & Bourne, J. R. Shaping of gastric motility in humans. *Proceedings of the 80th Annual Convention of the American Psychological Association*, 1972, *7*(2), 759–760.
Deller, D. J., & Wangel, A. G. Intestinal motility in man. I. A study combining the use of intraluminal pressure recording and cineradiography. *Gastroenterology*, 1965, *48*, 45–57.
Duret, R. L., & Arguello, M. Electromanometric studies of the effects of metoclopramide in man (title translated). *Semaine des Hôpitaux*, 1969, *45*, 1678–1691.
Durrani, T. S., & Nightingale, J. M. Probability distributions for discrete Fourier spectra. *Proceedings of the Institute of Electrical Engineering*, 1973, *120*, 299–311.
Duthie, H. L. Electrical activity of gastrointestinal smooth muscle. *Gut*, 1974, *15*, 669–681.
Duthie, H. L., Kwong, N. K., Brown, B. H., & Whittaker, G. E. Pacesetter potential of the human gastroduodenal junction. *Gut*, 1971, *12*, 250–256.
Duthie, H. L., Brown, B. H., Robertson-Dunn, B., Kwong, N. K., & Whittaker, G. E. Electrical activity in the gastroduodenal area—Slow waves in the proximal duodenum. *American Journal of Digestive Diseases*, 1972, *17*, 344–350.
Eder, R. *Die Magenmotilität bei Patienten mit Ulcus duodeni vor und nach selektiver proximaler Vagotomie im Vergleich mit unbehandelten Kontrollen*. Unpublished doctoral dissertation, Universität München, 1981.
Edwards, A. E., Hill, R. A., & Treadwill, T. Improvements in the magnetometer technique of measuring gastric motility. *Psychophysiology*, 1967, *4*, 116–118.
Engel, B. T., & McFall, R. A. The magnetometer method for recording localized movement of the stomach wall. *Journal of Applied Physiology*, 1959, *14*, 1069–1070.
Fedor, J. H., & Russell, R. W. Gastrointestinal reactions to response-contigent stimulation. *Psychological Reports*, 1965, *16*, 95–113.
Fink, G., & Stacher, G. Eine neue Endoradiosonde zur Messung intraluminaler Drucke im Magen-Darm-Trakt. *Acta Chirurgica Austriaca*, 1972, *4*, 1–6.
Frei, E. H., Gunders, E., Pajewsky, M., Alkan, W. J., & Eshchar, J. Ferrites as contrast material for medical X-ray diagnosis. *Journal of Applied Physics*, 1968, *39*, 990–1001.
Frei, E. H., Benmair, Y., Yersuhalmi, S., & Dreyfuss, F. Measurements of the emptying of the stomach with a magnetic tracer material. *IEEE Transactions Magnetics*, 1970, *MAG-6*, 348–349.
Furman, S. Intestinal biofeedback in functional diarrhea: A preliminary report. *Journal of Behavior Therapy and Experimental Psychiatry*, 1973, *4*, 317–321.
Ganong, W. F. *Medizinische Psychologie*. Berlin: Springer, 1972.
George, J. D. Gastric acidity and motility. *American Journal of Digestive Diseases*, 1968, *13*, 376–383.
Goodman, E. N., Ginsberg, I. A., & Robinson, M. A. An improved apparatus for measuring the electrogastrogram. *Science*, 1951, *113*, 682.
Goodman, E. N., Colcher, H., Katz, G. M., & Dangler, C. L. The clinical significance of the electrogastrogram. *Gastroenterology*, 1955, *29*, 598–608.

Griggs, R. C., & Stunkard, A. The interpretation of gastric motility: Sensitivity and bias in the perception of gastric motility. *Archives of General Psychiatry*, 1964, *11*, 82–89.
Heltzel, W., Hölzl, R., & Brückner, W. L. Noninvasive measurement of gastric motility after selective proximal vagotomy. *Proceedings of the 5th World Congress of the Collegium Internationale Chirurgiae Digestivae*, Sao Paulo, 1978, 2 (No. 235).
Heltzel, W., Hölzl, R., Eder, R., Kleinschmidt, J., & Brückner, W. L. Kombinationsgrastrographie: Beurteilung der Magenmotilität bei Ulcus duodeni-Patienten vor und nach selektiver proximaler Vagotomie mit Pyloroplastik. *Proceedings of the 21st Meeting of the Österreichische Gesellschaft für Chirurgie*, Wien, 1980.
Hightower, N. C. Motility of the alimentary canal of man. In J. A. Rider & H. C. Möller (Eds.), *Disturbances in gastrointestinal motility*. Springfield, Ill.: Charles C Thomas, 1962.
Hoagland, H., Rubin, M. A., & Cameron, D. E. The electroencephalogram of schizophrenics during insulin hypoglycemia and recovery. *American Journal of Physiology*, 1937, *120*, 559–570.
Hölzl, R. Noninvasive measurement of gastrointestinal motility in experimental psychosomatics. In W. H. G. Wolters & G. Sinnema (Eds.), *Psychosomatics and biofeedback*. Utrecht: Bohn, Nijhoff, 1979.
Hölzl, W., & Brüchle, H. Unpublished data, 1980.
Hölzl, W., & Müller, M. Unpublished data, 1980.
Hölzl, R., & Scherm, R. *Indirekte Messung der Magenmotilität durch Kombination von EGG und MGG*. Paper read at the 5th Arbeitstagung Psychophysiologische Methodik, Wien, June 1975.
Hölzl, R., & Scherm, R. The use of indirect measures of motility in behavioral analysis and treatment of psychosomatic disorders of the gastrointestinal tract. Paper read at the 6th Annual Convention of the European Association for Behavior Therapy, Spetsae, Greece, September 1976.
Hölzl, R., Scherm, R., Schröder, G., & Kiefer, H. Die indirekte Messung der Magenmotilität und ihre Veränderung unter verschiedenen Belastungsbedingungen. In W. H. Tack (Ed.), *Bericht über den 30. Kongreß der DGfP*. Göttingen: Hogrefe, 1977.
Hölzl, R., Schröder, G., & Kiefer, H. Indirect gastrointestinal motility measurement for use in experimental psychosomatics: A new method and some data. *Behavior Analysis and Modification*, 1979, *3*, 77–97.
Hölzl, R., Heltzel, W., Brückner, W. L., Eder, R., Müller, G., Skambraks, M., & Kleinschmidt, J. Noninvasive measurement of gastric motility in humans by combination of electrogastrogram and magnetogastrogram. *European Surgical Research*, 1981, *13*, 108.
Horowitz, L., & Farrar, J. T. Intraluminal small intestine pressures in normals and in patients with functional gastrointestinal disorders. *Gastroenterology*, 1962, *42*, 455–464.
Hubel, K. A. Voluntary control of gastrointestinal function: Operant conditioning and biofeedback. *Gastroenterology*, 1974, *66*, 1085–1088.
Jansson, G. Vago-vagal reflex relaxation of the stomach in the cat. *Acta Physiologica Scandinavica*, 1969, *75*, 245–252.
Kohatsu, S. A study of the human electrogastrogram using cutaneous electrodes. *Japanese Journal of Smooth Muscle Research*, 1968, *4*, 148.
Kohatsu, S. The current status of electrogastrography. *Klinische Wochenschrift*, 1970, *48*, 1315–1319.
Konturek, S. J., & Rösch, W. Gastrointestinale Motilität. In S. J. Konturek & M. Classen (Eds.), *Gastrointestinale Physiologie*. Baden-Baden: Witzstrock, 1976.
Kramer, K. Physiologie der Verdauung. In G. F. Domagk, J. Eisenburg, & K. Kramer (Eds.), *Ernährung, Verdauung, Intermediärstoffwechsel (Physiologie des Menschen*, Vol. 8), München: Urban und Schwarzenberg, 1972.
Krasil'nikov, L. G. Koinicheskoye znacheniye elektrogastrografii (Clinical importance of electrogastrography). *Sovietica Meditsina*, 1960, *3*, 107.
Krasil'nikov, L. G. *Electrogastrography*. Moskow: BME, Ezegodnik III, 1971.

Kwok, H. H. L. Autoregressive analysis applied to surface and serosal measurements of the human stomach. *IEEE Transactions on Biomedical Engineering*, 1979, *BME-26* (7), 405–409.

Levin, G. L., & Belousov, A. S. Electrogastrographic studies in gastric and duodenal stenosis. *Klinicheskaya Meditsina*, 1963, *41*(7), 51.

Lilie, D. The electrogastrogram. In R. F. Thompson & M. M. Patterson (Eds.), *Bioelectric recording techniques. Part C: Receptor and effector processes*. New York: Academic Press, 1974.

Linkens, D. A. Methods of analyzing rhythmic electrical potentials in the gastrointestinal tract. In H. L. Duthie (Ed.), *Gastrointestinal motility in health and disease*. Lancaster: MTP Press, 1978.

Linkens, D. A., & Cannell, A. E. Interactive graphics analysis of gastrointestinal electrical signals. *IEEE Transactions on Biomedical Engineering*, 1974, *BME-2*, 335–339.

Lommen, J. G. Automatic computation of autoregressive model's order in the detection of transient nonstationarities in EEGs using a recursive algorithm. In B. van Eijnsbergen & F. H. Lopes da Silva (Eds.), *Progress Report No. 5*. Utrecht: Medish Fysisch Instituut TNO, 1976.

Lopes da Silva, F. H., Dijk, A., & Smits, H. Detection of non-stationarities in EEGs using the autoregressive model—An application to EEGs of epileptics. In B. van Eijnsbergen & F. H. Lopes da Silva (Eds.), *Progress Report No. 4*. Utrecht: Institute for Medical Physiological (TNO), 1974.

MacKay, R. S. *Bio-medical telemetry*. New York: Wiley, 1968.

Martin, A., & Thillier, J. L. L'électro-gastroentéro-graphie (E.GE.G). *La Presse Médicale*, 1971, *79*, 1235–1237.

Martin, A., & Thillier, J. L. Le vectogastrogramme. *La Nouvelle Presse Médicale*, 1972, *1*, 452–456.

Martin, A., Thouvenot, J., & Touron, P. Varations périodiques de potentiels cutanées abdominaux en relation avec l'activité digestive. *Comptes Rendus des Séances de la Sociétée Biologique*, 1967, *161*, 2595–2600.

Martin, A., Moline, J., & Murat, J. Apport de l'électrosplanchnographie (E.S.G.) au diagnostique préopératoire d'une ulcération gastrique. *La Presse Médicale*, 1971, *70*, 1277–1278.

Martin, H., & Saller, K. *Lehrbuch der Anthropologie* (Vol. 3). Stuttgart: G. Fischer, 1962.

Nelsen, T. S. Use of phaselock techniques for retrieval of the electrogastrogram from cutaneous and swallowed electrodes. *Digest of the 7th International Conference on Medical Electronics and Biological Engineering*, Stockholm, 1967.

Nelsen, T. S. A theory of integrated gastrointestinal motor activity based on the chain oscillator model. *American Journal of Digestive Diseases*, 1971, *16* (new series), 543–547.

Nelsen, T. S., & Kohatsu, S. Clinical electrogastrography and its relationship to gastric surgery. *American Journal of Surgery*, 1968, *116*, 215–222.

Nelsen, T. S., & Kohatsu, S. The stomach as a pump. *Rendic. Rendiconti di Gastro Enterologia*, 1971, *3*, 65–71.

Praetorius, H. M., Bodenstein, G., & Creutzfeld, O. D. A new approach to automatic EEG analysis. *Electroencephalography and Clinical Neurophysiology*, 1977, *42*, 84–94.

Quigley, J. P., & Brody, D. A. A physiologic and clinical consideration of the pressures developed in the digestive tract. *American Journal of Medicine*, 1952, *13*, 73–81.

Rappelsberger, P., & Petsche, H. Spectral analysis of EEG by means of autoregression. In G. Dolce & H. Künkel (Eds.), *CEAN: Computerized EEG analysis*. Stuttgart: Fischer, 1975.

Rhodes, J., Bernando, D. E., Phillips, S. F., Rovelstad, R. A., & Hofmann, A. F. Increased reflux of bile into the stomach in patients with gastric ulcer. *Gastroenterology*, 1969, *57*, 241–252.

Rösler, F. Statistische Verarbeitung von Biosignalen: Die Quantifizierung hirnelektrischer Signale. In U. Baumann, H. Berbalk, & G. Seidenstücker (Eds.), *Klinische Pyschologie—Trends in Forschung und Praxis* (Vol. 3). Bern: Huber, 1980.

Rudick, J., & Janowitz, H. D. Gastric physiology. In H. L. Bockus (Ed.), *Gastroenterology*. Philadelphia: Lippincott, 1974.

Russell, R. W., & Stern, R. M. Gastric motility: The electrogastrogram. In P. H. Venables & I. Martin (Eds.), *A manual of psychophysiological methods*. Amsterdam: North-Holland, 1967.
Sarna, S. K., Daniel, E. E., & Kingma, Y. J. Simulation of electrical activity of small intestine. *Gastroenterology*, 1970, *58*, 1050.
Schröder, G. *Indirekte Messung der Magenmotilität unter verschiedenen Belastungsbedingungen.* Unpublished thesis, Universität Marburg and Max Planck Institute of Psychiatry, Munich, 1977.
Schulz, J., Reitzig, P., Schulze, E., Bärsch, J., Etzold, H., & Lisewski, G. Über die Aussagemöglichkeiten der Elektrogastroenterographie. *Deutsche Zeitschrift für Gesundheitswesen*, 1973, *28*, 2485–2488.
Schulz, J., Reitzig, P., Koblitz, F., Lisewski, G., & Schulze, E. Elektrogastrographische Untersuchungen bei akuten gastroenterologischen Erkrankungen. *Deutsches Gesundheitswesen*, 1975, *30*, 956–958.
Schütze, U., Wiedemann, K., Hanf, K., Lorenzen, F., & Emmonegger, H. Wirkung von Dihydroergovalin und Methylergometrin auf die Darmmotilität. *Medizinische Welt*, 1979, *30*, 1166–1168.
Small, M. D., Brean, J. W., & Farrar, J. T. An application of autocorrelation methods to the interpretation of intestinal motility records. *Journal of General Physiology*, 1955, *38*, 695–707.
Smallwood, R. H. Analysis of gastric electrical signals from surface electrodes using phaselock techniques: Part 1—system design. *Medical and Biological Engineering and Computing*, 1978, *16*, 507–512. (a)
Smallwood, R. H. Analysis of gastric electrical signals from surface electrodes using phaselock techniques: Part 2—system performance with gastric signals. *Medical and Biological Engineering and Computing*, 1978, *16*, 513–518. (b)
Smallwood, R. H., Brown, B. H., & Duthie, H. L. An approach to the objective analysis of intestinal smooth muscle electrical potentials recorded from surface electrodes. In G. Vantrappen (Ed.), *Proceedings of the 5th International Symposium on Gastrointestinal Motility*. Herentals: Typoff Press, 1976.
Smallwood, R. H., Linkens, D. A., Kwok, H. L., & Stoddard, C. J. The use of autoregressive modelling techniques for the analysis of colonic myoelectrical activity in man. *Medical and Biological Engineering and Computing*, 1980, *18*, 591–600.
Smallwood, R. H., Linkens, D. A., & Stoddard, C. J. Analysis and modelling of amplitude changes in human duodenal slow waves. *Clinical Physics and Physiological Measurement*, 1980, *1*, 47–58.
Smith, J. M. Changes in gastrointestinal motility during conditioned suppression. *Proceedings of the 80th Annual Convention of the American Psychological Association*. 1972, *7*, 650–652.
Smith, J. M., Renault, P. F., & Schuster, C. R. Operant schedule control of differential changes in gastrointestinal motility. *Proceedings of the 81st Annual Convention of the American Psychological Association*, 1973, *8*(2), 849–850.
Smith, R. M., & Hain, J. D. Relationship between somatization and effects of stress on electrogastric waveform in humans. *Psychological Reports*, 1970, *27*, 755–765.
Smout, A. J. P. *Myoelectric activity of the stomach (gastroelectromyography and electrogastrography)*. Delft, Holland: University Press, 1980.
Sobakin, M. A., Smirnow, J. P., & Mishin, L. N. Electrogastrography. *IRE Transaction on Biological and Medical Electronics*, 1962, *9*, 129–132.
Stacher, G., & Fink, G. Schlaf und Motilität der Speiseröhre. *Zeitschrift für Gastroenterologie*, 1974, *12*, 251–256.
Stemmler, G., & Thom, E. Ein Programm für die interaktive Auswertung des Herzschlagabstandes aus stark artefaktbehafteten EKG-Aufzeichnungen. *EDV in Medizin und Biologie*, 1979, *10*(4), 122–127.

Stern, R. M. Effects of variation in visual and auditory stimulation on gastrointestinal motility. *Psychological Reports*, 1964, *14*, 799–802.

Stern, R. M. Effects of contrasts in stimulation on gastrointestinal motility. *Psychological Reports*, 1965, *16*, 156–158. (a)

Stern, R. M. A re-examination of the effects of response-contingent aversive stimulation on gastrointestinal activity. *Psychophysiology*, 1965, 2, 217–223. (b)

Stevens, J. K., & Worrall, N. External recording of gastric activity: The electrogastrogram. *Physiological Psychology*, 1974, *2*, 175–180.

Stoddard, C. J., Duthie, H. L., Smallwood, R. H., & Linkens, D. A. Colonic myoelectrical activity in man: Comparison of recording techniques and methods of analysis. *Gut*, 1979, *20*, 476–483.

Stunkard, A. J., & Koch, C. The interpretation of gastric motility: Apparent bias in the report of hunger by obese persons. *Archives of General Psychiatry*, 1964, *11*, 74–82.

Stunkard, A. J., & Fox, S. The relationship of gastric motility and hunger. *Psychosomatic Medicine*, 1971, *33*, 123–134.

Taylor, I. Myoelectric activity in the rectosigmoid in man. In E. E. Daniel, K. Bowes, J. A. L. Gilbert, B. Schofield, T. K. Smitka, & G. Scott (Eds.), *4th International Symposium on Gastrointestinal Motility*. Vancouver: Mitchell Press, 1973.

Taylor, I., Duthie, H. L., Smallwood, R., & Linkens, D. Large bowel myoelectrical activity in man. *Gut*, 1975, *16*, 808–814.

Texter, E. G., Smith, H. W., Moeller, H. C., & Borborka, G. J. Intraluminal pressures from the upper gastrointestinal tract I. Correlations with motor activity in normal subjects and patients with esophagal disorders. *Gastroenterology*, 1957, *32*, 1013–1024.

Thouvenot, J., & Martin, A. Possibilité d'étude de l'activité globale du tube digestif par dérivation cutanée abdominale. *Procédés du 1er Congrès Français d'Electronique Médical*. Tours, 1967.

Thouvenot, J., Tonković, S., & Penaud, J. Electrosplanchnography—Method for the electrophysiological exploration of the digestive tract. *Acta Medica Jugoslavica*, 1973, *27*, 227–247.

Tiemann, F., & Reichertz, P. Über das intestinale Elektrogastrogramm (E.I.G.) und seine Bedeutung für die Klinik. *Medizinische Klinik*, 1959, *54*, 654–668. (a)

Tiemann, F., & Reichertz, P. Experimentelle Grundlagen des Elektro-Intestinogramms. *Medicina Experimentalis*, 1959, *1*, 17–26. (b)

Tonković, S., Penaud, J., Thouvenot, J., & Mountafian, J. P. Une application de l'analyse spectrale dans le traitement des signaux électrosplanchnographiques. *Medical and Biological Engineering and Computing*, 1975, *13*, 226–271.

Torgersen, S. Developmental anatomy of pyloric canal and etiology of infantile pyloric stenosis. *Acta Radiologica Scandinavica*, 1942, *32*, 935.

Truelove, S. C. The place of motility studies in the management of motor disorders of the large bowel. *American Journal of Digestive Diseases*, 1968, *13*, 484–487.

Venables, P. H., & Martin, I. (Eds.). *A manual of psychophysiological methods*. Amsterdam: North-Holland, 1967.

Walker, B. B., & Sandman, C. A. The bidimensionality of the electrogastrogram. *Psychophysiology*, 1976, *14*, 81.

Walker, B. B., & Sandman, C. A. Physiological response patterns in ulcer patients: Phasic and tonic components of the electrogastrogram. *Psychophysiology*, 1977, *14*, 393–400.

Walker, B. B., Lawton, C. A., & Sandman, C. A. Voluntary control of electrogastric activity. *Psychosomatic Medicine*, 1978, *40*, 610–619.

Weber, J., & Kohatsu, S. Pacemaker localization and electrical conduction patterns in the canine stomach. *Gastroenterology*, 1970, *59*, 717–727.

Weisbrodt, N. W. *Gastrointestinal physiology*. London: Butterworths, 1974.

Weltz, G. A. *Magenphysiologie für Röntgenzwecke*. Leipzig: Thieme, 1940.

Wenger, M. A., Engel, B. T., & Clemens, T. L. Initial results with the magnetometer method of recording stomach motility. *American Psychologist,* 1955, *10,* 452.
Wenger, M. A., Henderson, E. B., & Dinning, J. S. Magnetometer method for recording gastric motility. *Science,* 1957, *125,* 910.
Wenger, M. A., Engel, B. T., Clemens, T. L., & Cullen, T. D. Stomach motility in man as recorded by the magnetometer method. *Gastroenterology,* 1961, *41,* 479–485.
White, E. H. Surface recording of gastrointestinal motility. *Psychological Reports,* 1964, *14,* 321–322. (a)
White, E. H. Additional notes on gastrointestinal activity during avoidance behavior. *Psychological Reports,* 1964, *14,* 343–347. (b)
Whitehead, W. E., & Drescher, V. M. Perception of gastric contractions and self-control of gastric motility. *Psychophysiology,* 1980, *17,* 552–558.
Wirnharter, A. *Der Einfluss von intravenös verabreichtem Buscopan auf nicht-invasive Motilitätsindizes im Einfach-Blindversuch.* Unpublished doctoral dissertation, Universität München, 1981.
Wolf, S., & Welsh, J. D. The gastrointestinal tract as a responsive system. In N. S. Greenfield & R. A. Sternbach (Eds.), *Handbook of psychophysiology.* New York: Holt, Rinehart & Winston, 1972.
Wolf, S., & Wolff, H. G. Studies on a subject with a large gastric fistula. *Transactions of the American Physiology Society,* 1942, *57,* 115–137.
Wolf, S., & Wolff, H. G. *Human gastric function.* New York: Oxford University Press, 1943.
Zander, W. Beitrag zur Verifizierung der spezifischen Konfliktverarbeitung bei psychosomatischen Krankheitsbildern: Untersuchungen an Patienten mit Ulcus duodeni. *Médicine et Hygiène,* 1976, *32,* 152–154.
Zander, W. *Psychosomatische Forschungsergebnisse beim Ulcus duodeni.* Göttingen: Vandenhoeck and Ruprecht, 1977.

6

CONJOINT GASTROGRAPHY
Principles and Techniques
GERHARD M. MÜLLER, RUPERT HÖLZL, and
HEINRICH A. BRÜCHLE

1. Introduction

The last chapter discussed some of the problems involved in the psychophysiological use of surface gastrograms as noninvasive measures of gastrointestinal motility. No general solution to these problems has yet been found, but it is possible to define practical solutions for special applications. The following paragraphs will deal with methods developed in our laboratory during the last few years to produce sensitive and specific measures of the periodic components of gastric electromotor activity. These are the well-known basic electrical rhythm (BER) in the electrical records and the periodic Types I and II waves in the mechanical records, both occurring at a frequency of about 3 cpm. We assume that changes in the frequency and amplitude of these components will suffice as indicators of gastrointestinal responses to "stress," in clinical studies with patients suffering from functional gastrointestinal disorders.

Hölzl and Scherm (1975, 1976) and Hölzl, Scherm, Schröder, and Kiefer (1977) tried to circumvent the difficulties both electrogastrograms (EGG) and magnetogastrograms (MGG) have in reliably recording identifiable components of gastric motor activity by combining both types of recording and rejecting nonoverlapping noise bands in both signals. They have termed this method

---

GERHARD M. MÜLLER, RUPERT HÖLZL, and HEINRICH A. BRÜCHLE • Department of Psychology, Max Planck Institute of Psychiatry, Munich, The Federal Republic of Germany.

conjoint gastrography (CGG) (see also Hölzl, 1979; and Hölzl, Schröder, & Kiefer, 1979).

There are many possible ways of combining EGGs and MGGs. A simple way would be to look for concurrent excursions on the record which are not due to respiration. Davis, Garafolo, and Kveim (1959) apparently did this in an attempt to validate their recordings of surface potentials. In this way, one would be able to exclude EGG waves with no apparent contraction correlates on the one hand and low-frequency artifact from the MGG having no gastric counterpart. While not every EGG wave leads to contraction, a stomach contraction must have an electrical correlate, that is, a spike potential on top of a slow wave. This correlate appears on the surface somewhat distorted, with respiration and other artifacts superimposed, so that isolation from the EGG record alone is difficult or impossible.

Although it is possible to visually identify areas of agreement and areas of disagreement between two physiological recordings by looking for concurrent excursions, it is technically very difficult to do this reliably because the waveforms are very complex. This chapter describes some of the details of an alternative, more reliable method of conducting conjoint gastrographic analyses.

2. Rationale of Conjoint Gastrography

For routine application in the psychophysiological laboratory or in clinical studies some automatic way of using EGG and MGG information in conjunction must be found. The promising results of spectral analyses of electrogastrograms have led to the attempt to combine EGG and MGG by way of their spectral parameters. This method was called *conjoint spectral gastrography* (CSG; Hölzl, 1979; Hölzl *et al.*, 1979).

Several EGGs and MGGs are Fourier-analyzed as described in the previous chapter. Significant peaks in the gastrographic spectra are evaluated in respect to frequency and amplitude (or power). Peaks are identified as of *gastric* origin when they lie within a certain frequency range, for example, 1–4 cpm, *and* the "parliament" of electro- and magnetogastrograms "agreed" on them, that is, the peaks in EGGs and MGGs are correlated according to some criterion. Furthermore, peaks must not stem from respiration. To ensure this, the latter is recorded concomitantly and spectrally analyzed, too.

The type of CGG is determined by how EGGs and MGGs are combined, how correlated activity is specified, and how criteria of correlation are defined. Answers to these questions differ for every application. A special version employed in the authors' laboratory and their particular kinds of EGG and MGG recordings are described below.

3. Electrogastrograms

3.1. Recording Sites

Bipolar recordings from a modified Martin rosette against the middle electrode are employed. (This configuration was shown in Figure 5D of the preceding chapter.) In some studies a unipolar EGG is obtained from the second rosette electrode (Electrode 1 in Figure 1) against a reference site on the left tibia, at a relatively muscle-free point, halfway between the ankle and the head of the tibia. This "peripheral" EGG corresponds closely to the original site used by Davis, Garafolo, and Gault (1957; cf. Chapter 5). The grounding electrode is placed on either the hip bone or the middle of the sternum. The latter is preferred when the EKG from the chest and other biopotentials are recorded in addition to gastrograms, because it provides for a ground lead from a point which is nearer the center of the electrode configuration. This ensures optimal common mode rejection for differential amplifiers. Simultaneous multichannel recording from those leads is routinely used in this laboratory. A minimum of four channels of abdominal mapping, that is EGG 1–4 in Figure 1, should be obtained.

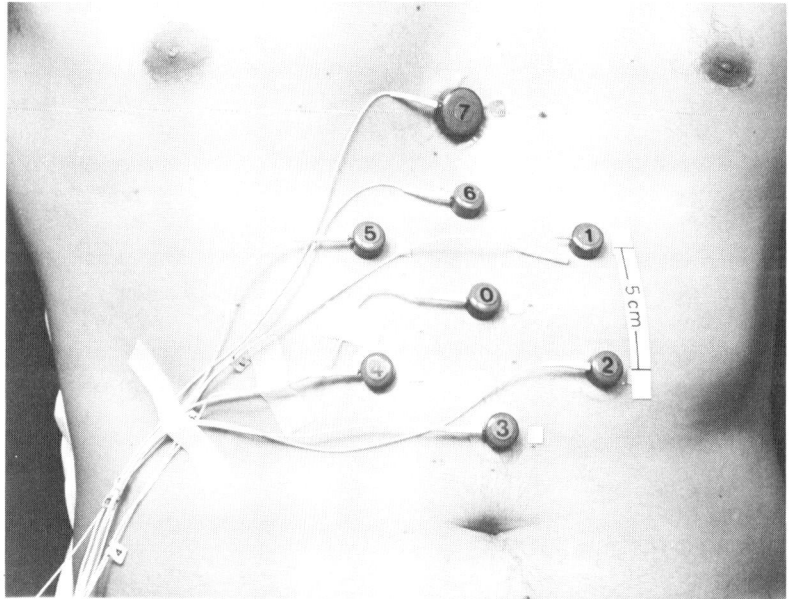

Figure 1. Electrode field *in situ*. The configuration is a modified Martin rosette. Fixation tapes partially removed. (0) Middle electrode; (1)–(6) electrodes for EGG 1 through EGG 6; (7) ground electrode. The correct fastening of electrode wires is shown at electrode (0). Wires are detachable (1). (IVM, E 221.)

3.2. Electrodes and Skin Preparation

In principle any nonpolarizable silver–silver-chloride electrode is sufficient, but mechanical properties and geometric dimensions of electrodes have also to be considered. Ideally electrodes of minimal size with short, highly flexible connection wires should be used. This minimizes movement artifacts. We have tested several electrode types in the laboratory and in clinical settings. The best EGGs with minimum polarization, drift, low-frequency noise, and movement artifacts were recorded with Beckmann skin electrodes (active diameter = 8mm). Their only drawbacks lie in the outer diameter (16 mm) and the fact that the wires are firmly attached to tbe body of the electrode. With multichannel recordings the electrode field may become too dense and the wires a source of mechanical interference. The present procedure therefore uses Type E 221 IVM silver–silver-chloride electrodes (active diameter = 8 mm). They are smaller, with an outer diameter of 12.5 mm, and have detachable wires. Thus the subject can easily be prepared in another room and the electrodes connected to the detachable leads with the subject already sitting in the chair in the final position. With ac recordings with a lower cutoff frequency of 0.01 Hz (3 dB), the IVM electrodes show performance equal to the Beckmann electrodes. The electrodes are applied to the skin with closely fitting standard stick-on rings. The active area of these electrodes is recessed in the housing. This reduces movement artifact.

Double fixation of electrode wires is essential with all types of electrodes, and a small loop between fixation tapes is recommended. It allows small movements in the abdominal area without pull on the electrode.

Figure 1 shows a typical electrode field *in situ* with fixations tapes removed for the middle electrode (Electrode 0 in Figure 1) and the final bundle of wires leading to the preamplifiers at the back of the chair.

Various disposable electrodes from EKG suppliers have also been used. Most of them turned out to be unreliable, too large for abdominal mappings, and very sensitive to movement, even coming off frequently during a positional change of the subject. The stick-on part of those electrodes is normally made from polystyrene foam, which is not flexible enough for the soft, moving abdominal area. However, for clinical measurement over a short time disposable EKG electrodes for infants manufactured by Hewlett-Packard (Type 14389A) perform well, although the stiffness of the original clip-on cables still presents a problem. Movement artifacts stemming from minor dislocations of the electrode area relative to the skin are not easily avoided whenever the subject has to be active during measurement. This disadvantage was found to be compensated for by the quickness of application, which may be a major requirement in clinical studies on a large scale.

Careful skin preparation has been considered important for good EGGs by all workers in the field. The present authors found this problem less serious provided that a good grounding site (< 3 kΩ) was achieved in optimal position together with a good differential amplifier. The following procedure is applied in our laboratory: Marked skin sites are thoroughly cleaned with surgical spirit (benzine) instead of alcohol. The latter may dehydrate the skin and thereby increase its resistance. Then standard electrode jelly (e.g., Beckmann paste) is rubbed in gently but thoroughly until no more jelly is absorbed. After a few seconds the excess of jelly is wiped off with cotton. When the skin appears dry again, prepared electrodes are applied with stick-on rings and cautiously checked for adherence. Only the grounding site is abraded cautiously just before the jelly treatment. Two to three gentle strokes with sandpaper (finest grade) will suffice. The electrode impedance, especially that of the grounding lead, is checked with a low-current (< 20 μA), low-frequency (10 Hz) ac ohmmeter.[1] The procedure is repeated if one electrode shows a resistance above 10 kΩ.

The subject is then seated in the chair and actual measurement is begun not earlier than half-an-hour after application.

3.3. Amplifiers and Filters

Any standard polygraph with differential dc amplifiers and suitable low-pass filters and time constants may be used. In the earlier studies from our group, EGGs were recorded with a Beckmann Dynograph R whose input couplers (9806 C) had been changed to provide time constants up to 20 sec. The limited number of channels and limited dynamic range of the amplifiers, however, led us to develop the special gastrographic amplifier system[2] described in Figure 2. It provides up to 32 channels of EGGs in groups of 4.

Two requirements must be met by the amplifier system: It should be insensitive to extraneous noise, especially to low-frequency interference; it should be applicable in electrically adverse environments; and it should allow true dc recordings *and* high amplification ($K = 100,000$) of ac components in the EGG in the presence of large standing (dc) potentials. This exceeds the dynamic range of most amplifiers and recording systems.

To meet the first condition, we place separate differential preamplifiers of moderately high input impedance (1 MΩ) near the subject. Low-level signals have to travel only the short distance (< 1 m) from the subject to the input plugs of a preamplifier. There the signal is amplified by a factor of 1000 and connected with low-output impedance to the final amplification stage ($k_{max} = 100$) in the

---

[1] Built by R. Rink and K. Mair, Electronic Workshop of the MPIP, Munich. Their assistance is gratefully acknowledged.
[2] This was done in close cooperation with H. J. Langer, Eching (by Munich). The system may be purchased from his company.

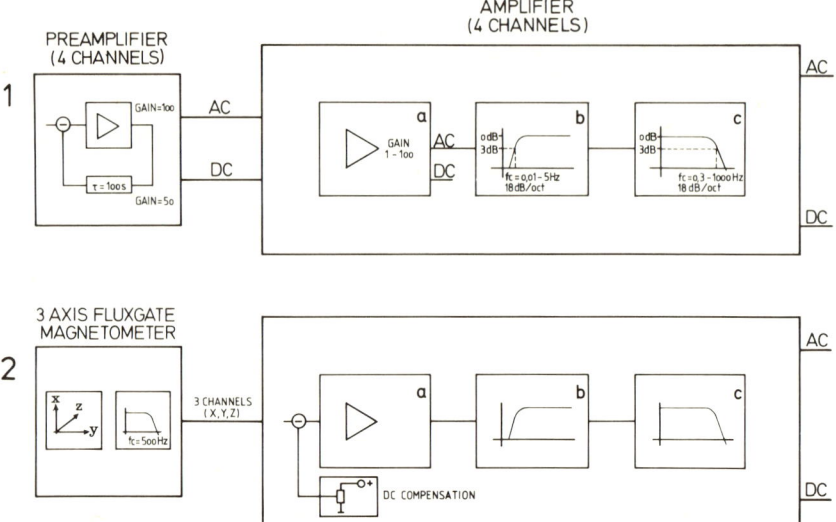

Figure 2. Block diagram of amplifier system. (1) Electrogastrographic amplifiers (left to right). Eight preamplifiers with four channels each: dc compensation for offsets up to ± 100 mV; f_c = 0.00159 Hz; time Constant τ = 100 sec; gain: 50 for dc–0.01 Hz, 1000 for 0.01–1000 Hz; input impedance = 1 MΩ. Eight main amplifiers with four channels each: (a) Gain: 1, 2, 5, 10, . . . 100; (b) high pass: dc, 0.01, 0.02, 0.05, 01, . . . 5 Hz, cutoff frequency, f_c; (c) low pass: 0.3, 2, 5, 10, 20, . . . 100 Hz, cutoff frequency, f_c; filter rolloff: 18 dB/octave. (2) Magnetogastrographic amplifiers (left to right): three-axis fluxgate magnetometer; main amplifier: identical to EGG amplifier, but only three channels in use; additional manual dc compensation for each channel. (From H. Langer, Eching by Munich, 1978; see Footnote 2.)

control room. Inpute impedance of the preamplifier has been reduced in favor of low noise amplification which is 3 μV_{pp} from dc to 100 Hz.

Incorporated in the final-stage amplifier module are the controls for amplification ranging from 1000 to 10 μV full scale (i.e., - 1 V) and high- and low-pass filters with 18 dB/octave rolloff. The 3-dB cutoff frequencies of the high-pass filter lie at 0.01–5Hz, that of the low-pass filter at 0.3–1000 Hz. The high-pass control has an additional "dc" position which selects true dc recording if so desired. Corresponding standing potentials may be monitored by miniature galvanometers in the front panel of the final amplification module.

The second requirement (sensitive dc recording) is met by separate ac and dc amplification in the preamplifier module. But instead of using a resistance–capacitance (RC) network, a negative feedback loop provides for automatic compensation of dc offsets at the input stage up ±100 mV, thus simulating a time constant of 100 sec without the disadvantages of conventional circuits, which often have difficulties with very low frequencies in signals with large dynamic ranges. The amplification ratio for the "ac" component in the pre-amplifier is 1000; for the "dc" component, which actually is the compensation voltage, amplification is reduced to 50. For each of the four channels in one amplification group, the two components may be connected to separate main amplifier modules permitting simultaneous dc and ac recording. For the latter a frequency band from 0.01 to 0.3 Hz (0.6–18 cpm) is selected by the filter controls. This is the standard gastrogram setting in our laboratory.

4. Magnetogastrograms

4.1. Magnetometers and Magnetic Capsules

Two types of magnetic capsules have been used by our group. The simplest ones are magnetic stirring rods 12 mm long and 5 mm in diameter. They have an inert Teflon coating and can be swallowed without hazard by the subjects. A spherical version (10 mm in diameter) was also tested, but no systematic differences in signal amplitude or quality were found (Hölzl, 1979; Schröder, 1977). Stirring rods are much cheaper than the spheres and need not be retrieved by subjects. They seem well suited for routine usage. However, they vary strongly in magnetic strength, and some calibration procedure or the use of relative measurements are recommended to reduce error variance. In our earlier studies, movement of the magnets in the stomach were detected by two coils (4000 windings each) connected in series with the differential inputs of a Beckman Dynograph R with altered time constants as described above. However, because of insensitivity and spatial nonselectivity of the method, a three-axis flux-gate magnetometer (Develco 9200 C) has been applied since then. The probe is quite small (10.2 × 3.5 × 3.2 cm) and contains complete integrated electronic circuitry to give three channels of low-impedance output voltages proportional to magnetic flux in the three axes of space when supplied with a suitable low dc voltage source (±12 V). Sensitivity is 2.5 V/600 mOe with a measurement range of ±600 mOe.[3] Output ripple lies at 5 mV$_{pp}$. This amounts to a resolution of 2% of full range. The probe has a frequency range from dc to 500 Hz (3 dB). Without suitable amplifiers and filters, very sensitive records of MGGs including dc field measurements indicative of magnet position can thus be made. Other magnetometers with similar specifications may be used as well.

For MGGs made with the ferrite powder technique developed by Benmair (1975; cf. previous chapter) this type of magnetic probe, however, is not sufficient. For that purpose a Förster probe (Förster Reutlingen, Type 1.107) is employed which increases sensitivity by several orders of magnitude (down to 1 mOe full-scale).[4] The system has two additional features which make it particu-

---

[3]"mOe" = one thousandth of an oersted, the unit of magnetic field strength.
[4]The measurement system was lent to us by Dr. Hertz, IABG, Munich, whom we want to thank for

larly suited for the ferrite technique. First, dc field compensation is easily possible over a wide range. High amplification of the ac field components in the presence of relatively strong dc fields presents no problem. Second, extraneous magnetic field interference can be excluded by true difference measurement between two probes in a line for each axis. Thus the extraneous field component with a flat gradient may be subtracted from the field stemming from the swallowed magnetic substance and producing a steep gradient. Despite its expensiveness and the somewhat bulky electronic circuitry, the single probe is extremely small (6 × 1 × 1 cm). The two probes of a pair representing one axis are mounted on a polyvinylchloride bar at 34-cm distance.

4.2. Amplifiers and Filters

Compatible with the electrogastrographic amplifier system described earlier, a magnetogastrographic module has been constructed which plugs into the system case instead of an EGG output amplifier module. This MGG module accepts signals from conventional three-axis flux-gate magnetometers such as Develco 9200C and Helatronic MAG 030 and provides suitable dc supply voltages (± 12 V). The dc field component from the magnetometers may be compensated manually in the final amplifier stage but not at the probe itself as in the Förster system. This limits measurement range but is sufficient for measurements with magnetic rods. Compensation voltage is available at an output port. Amplification ratios and filter choice are identical to the final stages of the electrogastrographic amplifiers. Any other system could be used, of course, as long as it provides for suitable amplification of output signals of magnetic probes, high- and low-pass filters as specified, and, most important of all, dc field compensation. The latter is a necessary requirement for high amplification of ac field components.

4.3. Procedure

In MGG recording, reliable probe positioning and some control over magnet location in the gut are essential. Both problems are difficult to solve, but practical answers and be found. In our laboratory the following routine is adhered to.

Subject sits in an adjustable laboratory chair in a slightly reclining position (see Figure 3). The magnetometer probe is positioned directly over the middle electrode of the EGG rosette 5 cm distant from the front plane of the probe. Its y

---

his generous assistance. The help of P. Bolsinger (MPIP), who did the first tests, is also acknowledged.

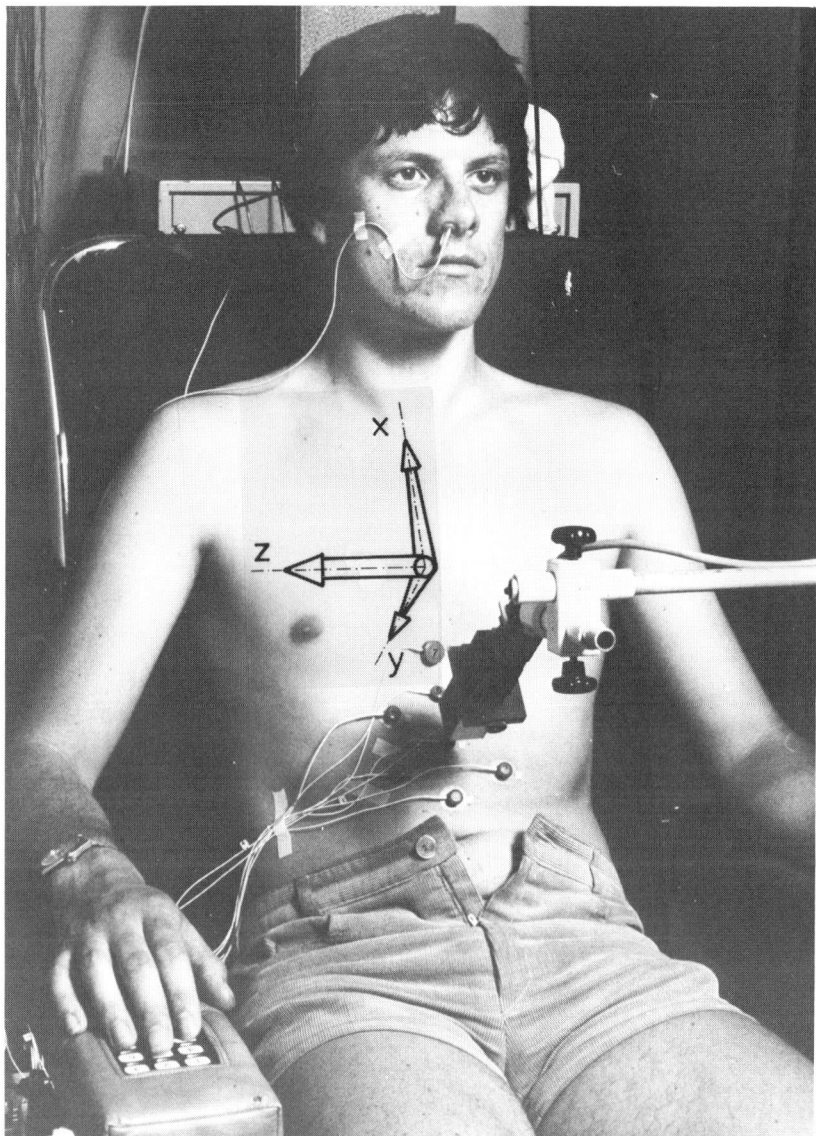

Figure 3. Subject *in situ*. The Develco magnetometer for standard measurements is mounted. The *y* axis is orthogonal to the abdominal plane in 5-cm distance direct over the middle electrode. Nasal thermistor with adapter is also shown (see Section 5 and Figure 4).

axis is orthogonal to the abdominal plane defined by the lower end of the sternum and the hip bones. The magnetometer mounting allows adjustments in all directions. Fairly good reproduction of probe positions is possible in this way. For certain research purposes, however, only relative rather than absolute field strength should be used.

Magnet location is controlled only indirectly in most of our studies: By careful control of sitting position, and by having the subject eat a small standard meal (see p. 133) before swallowing the magnet, the magnet will stay in the stomach in most cases for periods of 1–2 hr because of its high specific weight. This can be checked in the MGG record itself which shows clear 3 cpm activity after some minutes when the magnet is in the stomach. The latter disappears when the magnet moves through the pylorus, and is replaced by fast activity after large erratic excursions indicating pyloric passage. Cross-correlation functions between EGGs and MGGs also change in a characteristic way (see Section 7.4.4) when the magnet leaves the stomach. In our experience, tying the magnet to a tooth with surgical thread causes too much gagging, so the procedure by Edwards, Hill, and Treadwell (1967) was not adopted even though it may produce more reliable control of location.

Three axes of MGG are always recorded simultaneously and analyzed separately because orientation of the magnet remains undefined. Figure 3 indicates the relation of magnetic axes to the abdomen.

4.4. Procedure with Ferrite Test Meal

When using Benmair's (1975) ferrite technique with the Förster probe, a different procedure must be followed. A test meal consisting of 50 g magnesium ferrite powder, 140 cm^3 of milk, and 60 g instant chocolate pudding is prepared according to Benmair's recipe (Benmair, 1975, p. 22). Immediately before measurement, the subject is asked to eat the mixture quickly with a plastic spoon or to use a thick straw. Compensation of the dc field is adjusted and measurement commenced.

Some of the problems inherent in MGG recording with rods, such as uncontrolled tumbling movements of the magnet or early loss through the pylorus are avoided here. On the other hand, there is continuous transit of magnetic substance from the stomach into the duodenum and, in consequence, strong drifts of the dc field take place all the time. Frequent readjustments are necessary. For longer recording periods repeated test meals must be given. Unless one also wishes to measure gastric emptying, this method is not recommended for general use. These comments do not bear on the original ferrite method with active susceptibility measurement using an external excitation field (see Chapter 5). Probe positioning is as essential here as with conventional magnetometers. The same procedure as above is followed.

5. General Procedure and Control Measurements

Subject preparation includes a standard test meal of 200 g of yogurt and control of food intake prior to measurement. Routinely, no less than 14 hr but no more than 18 hr of fasting is required. Test sessions are scheduled between 8 and 11 A.M. Subjects are asked to avoid heavy meals, certain foods, and alcohol the day before the experiment. Time and content of the last meal is recorded. The main variance of gastrointestinal activity stems from eating. It must be controlled if gastrographic data from psychophysiological experiments are to be interpretable.

The subject takes the test meal while sitting in the chair and after all adjustments have been made. Then he brings the magnet near his mouth, dc compensation is readjusted, and the subject is asked to swallow the magnet together with some water (25 ml). Thus the effects of meal and magnet on EGG and MGG, respectively, can be monitored. Intervals between the start and end of eating and the beginning of actual measurements are held within certain limits (10–30 min), but usually not absolutely constant because of necessary readjustments. These intervals are therefore recorded and taken into account in the analysis.

Other important concomitant variables of gastrographic measures are body build and respiratory activity. The latter is a major source of artifact in EGG *and* MGG and is recorded routinely together with them. Despite the nonlinearity inherent in the transduction process, this laboratory uses an improved version of the thermistor method for respiration recording. A miniature thermistor (Valvo NTC) with a thermal time constant of 9 sec and 2.2 kΩ resistance is used. Filter settings are at 0.05 Hz (HP) and 1.0 Hz (LP). Alternatively a Beckman Thermistor Coupler 9858 may serve. The thermistor is fastened to the right nostril by a special adapter shown in schematic drawing in Figure 4 and *in situ* in Figure 3. The nasal adapter (cf. Hölzl, 1976) ensures a more constant stream of the respiratory air around the thermistor and prevents heating of the thermistor by adventitious contact with the inner nostril wall. Thus not only frequency but also amplitude values of the thermistor become interpretable as long as respiratory frequency does not vary too much, and summation measures of amplitude over longer recording periods such as spectral power can be used. Conventional belt techniques interfere with the electrode field of multichannel EGGs.

Various body measures are taken. Body height and weight, circumference, medial and horizontal diameters at the height of the middle electrode of the rosette, and the thickness of fat layer near the rosette are routinely registered. They serve as important covariates of gastrographic amplitudes and can be used to reduce between-subject variance. Abdominal diameters are measured with calipers for large objects (GPM No. 108). A *Lange* skinfold caliper (Cambridge Scientific Industry) serves to evaluate the fat layer.

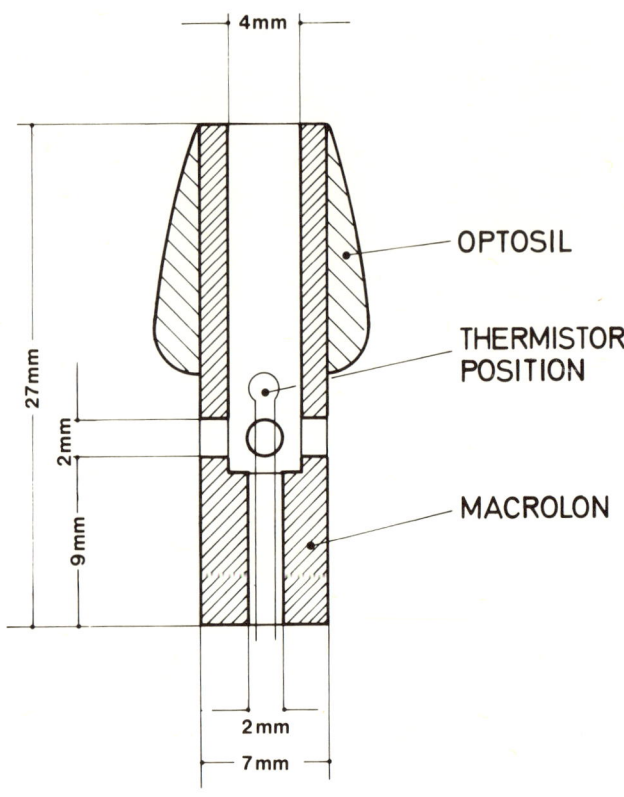

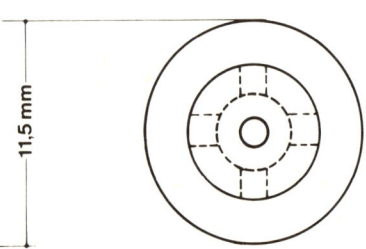

Figure 4. Nasal adapter (schematic drawing). The thermistor is inserted in a Macrolone® tube with small outlets for the respiratory air. Dental cement (aptosil) was used to adapt the form of the probe to the nostril (see Figure 3).

6. Data Acquisition

6.1. Laboratory Configuration

Gastrograms and other physiological variables are transduced and amplified with either the gastrography system described or any standard physiological recorder. Data are digitized by a laboratory computer with a sampling frequency of 1.82 Hz after low-passing at 0.3 Hz (3 dB). The data stream is divided in 10-min epochs (1024 data points, one every 550 msec, that is, 563.2 sec). These epochs are stored on disk or digital tape and enter further processing such as Fourier analysis. Their length has been chosen with respect to spectral analysis to produce sufficient frequency resolution for gastrogram analysis (see Section 7.2). Data acquisition programs[5] include on-line calculation and display of power spectra together with incoming digitized raw gastrograms for data monitoring during measurement, and suitable calibration routines. Stored digitized data are analyzed off-line after completion of the experiment. This can be done on the lab-computer itself (a PDP 8/e in our case) with a FORTRAN II package including programs for spectral analyses, coherent averaging, cross-correlation, and output routines for line-printer and plotter (see Section 7). This package is used for small-scale experiments only. For clinical studies with larger data bases, off-line analysis using a midicomputer (DEC 2060 at the authors' institution) with a more elaborated FORTRAN IV package is preferred. The system is not specific to this particular kind of environment. This applies also to the following paragraphs. The set of equipment described should be viewed as *one* realistic example.

6.2. Portable Data Logging

In clinical studies portable data acquisition and storage may be necessary because patients awaiting operation cannot be moved or for other practical reasons. For these applications several kinds of portable data logging are available. The simplest method is direct storage of analog data on FM or PCM tape recorders (Philips Analog 7 and Johne & Reilhofer PCM System TM 8K13, respectively), fast replay (32-fold) with digitization on the laboratory computer, and off-line analysis as described above. Stimuli and instructions are presented from a commercial tape recorder which also defines trigger signals on the data recorder, so that the clinic personnel can be fully in charge of the procedure, and no specialist is required except in the final analysis.

Recently a microcomputer-based 32-channel data logger for clinical gastrography was constructed which stores EGG data directly on magnetic cassettes

---

[5]The present programs are based on a package of SABR routines by Dr. Ben Dawson, M.I.T. (Cambridge, Massachusetts), who implemented the system during his visit at the MPIP in 1977. Current main programs (FORTRAN II) are by H. Brüchle, MPIP, Munich.

in digitized form. This circumvents time-consuming replay of analog data because the digital cassette data may be fed directly into the midicomputer (DEC 2060).[6] This technique is especially valuable when large amounts of data from screening studies have to be dealt with.

7. Signal Analysis

7.1. Overview

As indicated above gastrograms are acquired at a rate of one value every 550 msec (.1.82 Hz). Epochs of 1024 values (9.39 min) are the units of analysis. In the off-line analysis initially data are multiplied by calibration constants to produce physically interpretable values comparable over different studies using different equipment. Mean and standard deviation (rms value) are calculated and printed, and finally the mean is subtracted to get a vector with zero mean. This vector is multiplied by a suitable weight function ("windowing"). This improves performance of the following stage, the fast Fourier transform (FFT) of signals. After Fourier transformation, autopower spectra of all channels and cross-power spectra between EGGs and MGGs are calculated. These terms will be explained further in the following paragraphs. (For a general understanding see the previous chapter, by Hölzl.) Critical relative maxima ("peaks") of auto- and cross-power spectra are defined by a peak detection routine, and concordant peaks in defined regions of the autospectra of EGG and MGG identified by use of combined and weighted peak vectors from cross-spectra. Frequency and amplitude (root power) of these concordant peaks are printed and stored as spectral parameters of identified periodic gastrogram components. In particular, one component around the well-known 3 cpm activity is evaluated like that. In addition, a slower component is invariably found. It is treated likewise. Furthermore the absolute maximum power of frequencies below the respiratory peak is stored. These spectral parameters (calculated for each channel over 1 epoch of approximately 10 min) or simple scalar transformations of them enter the usual statistical group analyses like analysis of variance, etc.

Before going into details of the techniques described a short digression on some basic principles of Fourier analysis and explanation of spectral analytic terms seems in order. Violation of underlying assumptions may lead to erroneous conclusions from spectral data.

7.2. Principles of Fourier Analysis in Gastrography

Fourier techniques are based on the work of the famous French mathematician after whom they were named. These techniques were originally designed for

---

[6]The data logger was constructed and built by P. Bolsinger, MPIP, Munich.

the mathematical analysis and description of periodic physical phenomena. The spectrum and related types of analysis have also been called "spectral analysis" because they basically decompose these signals into a series of pure sine or cosine waves much as an optical prism decomposes white light into a series of pure "spectral" colors. Fourier techniques in general, however, have a much wider scope. To understand their basics, consideration of the Fourier series expansion may be helpful. It expresses any nonsinusoidal periodic function (or time signal) as a series of sine (or cosine) functions of different frequencies and amplitudes. The first element of the series is a sine (or cosine) function with the same frequency as the frequency of the original periodic signal. It is called the base frequency. The other sine wave components in the series lie at integer multiplies of the base frequency. They are called "higher harmonics." Different periodic signals like square waves or triangular waves differ in the relative amplitude and also the phase relationships of the component sine waves in which they can be expanded. Plotting these amplitudes or their squares as a function of frequency results in an "amplitude" or "power spectrum" with values at discrete frequencies. It is therefore called a "line spectrum" (cf. Figure 5). The term "power" is derived from the equivalent term in electrical engineering, where power dissipated across a resistor R equals U^2/R, with U the voltage drop across R. In an ac circuit in particular U^2 is the mean square value of the line voltage. U is the "root mean square" (rms) voltage. Correspondingly the values of the "amplitude spectrum" in Figure 5 may be interpreted as the rms values of the particular sine waves of which the periodic signal is composed. Generalization of the Fourier expansion to nonperiodic signals like transients or random signals leads to the spectral representation of time-varying signals in general.

The Fourier series in that case changes into the Fourier integral or Fourier transformation (see Section 7.3.1), and the "spectrum" becomes a continuous rather than a discrete function of frequency. That means that the signal "contains" all frequencies in a given interval, and not just certain "lines." A signal varying completely at random ("white noise") contains these frequencies to equal extents. Its spectrum is flat. If some frequencies predominate in an otherwise random signal the spectrum will have "peaks" in that frequency range. This typically is the case with physiological signals like the α-EEG or the EGG with 3 cpm activity plus noise. The periodic components in these noisy records may be detected therefore by spectral analysis. The "spectra" discussed so far are called "autopower" (or autoamplitude) spectra because they refer only to one signal and its periodic content. Pairs of signals (like EGGs and MGGs) may also be analyzed to detect their *common* periodic content. These spectra are called "cross-power spectra."

The original formulations of Fourier dealt with *continuous* signals of *infinite* length. Realistic physical signals, however, are of *limited* length and usually have to be sampled at *discrete* intervals.

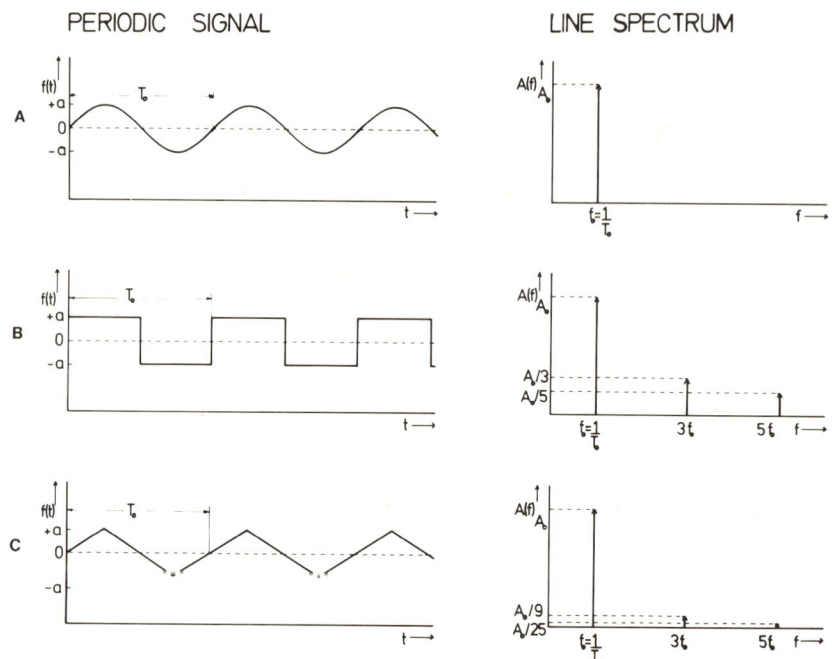

Figure 5. Harmonic analysis of simple periodic signals. (A) Pure sine wave with amplitude A_0 and frequency $f_0 = 1/T_0$, where T_0 is the period length of the wave. The "power" or mean square in the spectral representation is given by $\frac{1}{2}a^2$; the "root mean square" by $a/\sqrt{2}$. This value corresponds to the height of the single "line" of the spectrum $A_0 = a/\sqrt{2}$ (right half of figure). A well-known example is given by the relation of the "effective voltage" of an ac network (110 or 220 V_{rms}) to the peak voltage in the power line (156 or 311 V_{0P}). (B) Symmetric square wave; terms as in (A). Intensity of harmonics at $(2k + 1) \cdot f_0$ (with $k = 0,1,2, \ldots$) falls off with a diminishing factor of $1/(2k + 1)$: $A_1 = \frac{1}{3}A_0$, $A_2 = \frac{1}{5}A_0$, ...; notice that A_0 has a value different from the one in (A); $A_0 = a/\pi\sqrt{2}$. (C) Symmetric triangular wave; terms as in (A). Intensity of harmonics falls off with a diminishing factor of $1/(2k + 1)^2$: $A_1 = \frac{1}{9}A_0$, $A_2 = \frac{1}{25}A_0$, ... $A_0 = 2a/\pi^2\sqrt{2}$ (From I. N. Bronstein & K. A. Semendjajew, *Taschenbuch der Mathematik* [18th ed.]. Thun: Harri Deutsch, 1979.)

Spectral analysis of such signals requires some preconditions, the most important of which is defined by the so-called sampling theorem of Shannon (cf. Randall, 1977, p. 19). It states that frequencies contained in the sampled signal and lying above one half of the sampling frequency f_s (the Nyquist frequency) are misinterpreted as slow signals very much as the stroboscope reduces wheel rotation by "sampling" flashes. Sometimes the erroneous statement may be heard that the sampling theorem simply requires that f_s *doubles the highest frequency of interest*. It must be emphasized that in contrast to this conviction f_s has to be the double of the *highest frequency actually contained* in the signal. Figure 6 illustrates the situation. When sampling gastrograms with 3 cpm or 50 MHz as the highest frequency of interest, sampling with $f_s = 100$ MHz (or 6 values per minute) would not be sufficient as long as higher-frequency components such as respiration artifact (250 MHz or 15 cpm) or higher harmonics of the gastrogram itself (6, 9, 12, . . . cpm) are present. For these components the sampling theorem would be violated and slower components *in* the area of interest added to the 3 cpm rhythm (cf. Figure 6D and caption). Only low-passing the signal just above the highest frequency of interest allows reduction in sampling frequency to double of the highest frequency of interest. Low-pass cutoff frequencies must be reported if signal acquisition is to be evaluated.

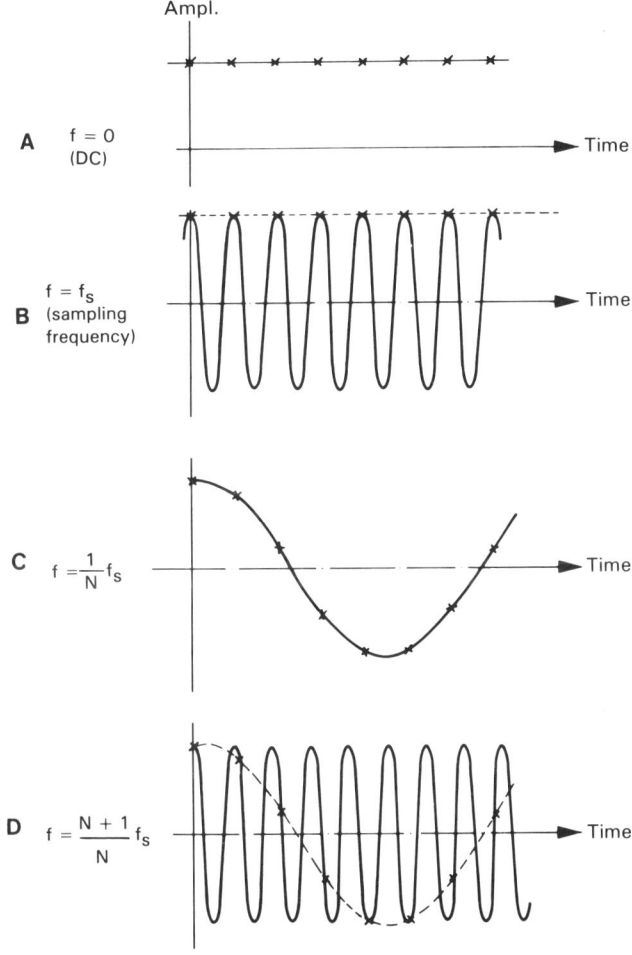

Figure 6. Illustration of "aliasing." (A) Zero-frequency or dc component. (B) Component at sampling frequency f_s interpreted as dc. (C) Frequency component at $(1/N)f_s$. (D) Frequency component at $(N + 1)/Nf_s$ interpreted as $(1/N)f_s$; this artifactual frequency, usually in the range of interest, even with the original f above it, will be added to the spectrum. (Adapted from Randall, 1977, p. 21. Reproduced with permission.)

The fact that instead of infinite signal lengths, time-limited epochs of measurement are used has two important implications. The first is limitation of frequency resolution, Δf. This is the distance of two adjacent spectral lines which can just be distinguished in the spectrum. Smaller frequency changes of a "peak" (representing a significant periodic component like the 3 cpm activity) cannot be detected. Δf is given by $1/T$, where T is the epoch length. For sufficient resolution in 3 cpm detection, for instance, 10-min records are therefore necessary ($\sim$ 3% resolution). The second effect of limited measuring time results from the fact that Fourier transforms used to calculate the spectra assume periodic continuations of the record segment. Usually discontinuities at its start and end points will arise. This adds components to the signal spectrum which were not present in the original. To minimize these unwanted effects the operation of "windowing" is employed. It consists of multiplying the input with a mathematical function, usually bell-shaped, before transforming. Deeper understanding of the effects of windowing on the resulting spectra requires reference to the "*convolution theorem*" (see p. 143). "Windowing" on the other hand reduces frequency resolution (typically by a factor of 2). This also has to be kept in mind by the investigator employing these techniques to a practical problem. Relevant information should always be reported.

The next section discusses some basic mathematical relationships which justify the requirements stated above for the interested reader. The particular operations used in CGG follow in Section 7.4.

7.3. Basic Fourier Mathematics[7]

7.3.1. *Fourier Expansion and Transformation Formulas*

If $g(t)$ is a periodic function, that is

$$g(t) = g(t + n \cdot T) \quad (1)$$

which is piecewise monotonic and continuous, $g(t)$ may be expressed definitely by a sum of sine waves at equally spaced frequencies $f_k = k \cdot f_1$ with $f_1 = 1/T$ and $k \in N$:

$$g(t) = \sum_{k=-\infty}^{+\infty} G(f_k) \exp(j2\pi f_k t) \quad (2)$$

with

$$G(f_k) = \frac{1}{T} \int_{-T/2}^{+T/2} g(t) \exp(-j2\pi f_k t) dt \quad (3)$$

---

[7]This section is based on Randall (1977, pp. 5–48).

$G(f_k)$ is a sequence of complex coefficients $(a + i \cdot b)$. They are called "Fourier coefficients" or "spectral components of $g(t)$." Their absolute values $(a^2 + b^2)^{1/2}$ represent the amplitudes, the angle arctan $(b/a) = \phi$ the phase of the sine waves the signal is thought to be made of. The exponential functions with imaginary argument are only another way of expressing trigometric functions like sine waves (Euler's equation). The formulas 2 and 3 for periodic functions may be generalized for nonperiodic signals by lettering $T \to \infty$. This implies that $f_1 = 1/T \to 0$ and $G(f)$ becomes a continuous function of f and, therefore, the summation in (2) an integration:

$$g(t) = \int_{-\infty}^{+\infty} G(f) \exp(j2\pi ft) df \qquad (4)$$

with

$$G(f) = \int_{-\infty}^{+\infty} g(f) \exp(-j2\pi ft) dt \qquad (5)$$

and the limiting condition

$$\int_{-\infty}^{+\infty} g(t) dt < \infty \qquad (6)$$

Equation 5 is called "forward Fourier transform," 4 the "inverse Fourier transform," and both together represent a "Fourier transform pair." It is the representation of a continuous time-varying signal in the "frequency domain" and vice versa. When the time signal is not continuous but sampled at discrete intervals Δt, as in digitizing physiological signals with a laboratory computer, the formulas of the transform pair take slightly different forms:

$$g(t_n) = \frac{1}{f_s} \int_{-f_{s/2}}^{+f_{s/2}} G(f) \exp(j2\pi ft_n) df \qquad (7)$$

and

$$G(f) = \sum_{n-\infty}^{+\infty} g(t_n) \exp(-j2\pi ft_n) \qquad (8)$$

where $t_n = n \cdot \Delta t$, Δt is the sampling interval, and $f_s = 1/\Delta t$ the sampling frequency.

When the sampled time series stems from a periodic function, the transform pair takes the simpler form:

$$g(n) = \sum_{k=0}^{N-1} G(k) \exp(j2\pi kn/N) \qquad (9)$$

and

$$G(k) = \frac{1}{N} \sum_{n=0}^{N=1} g(n) \exp(-j2\pi kn/N) \qquad (10)$$

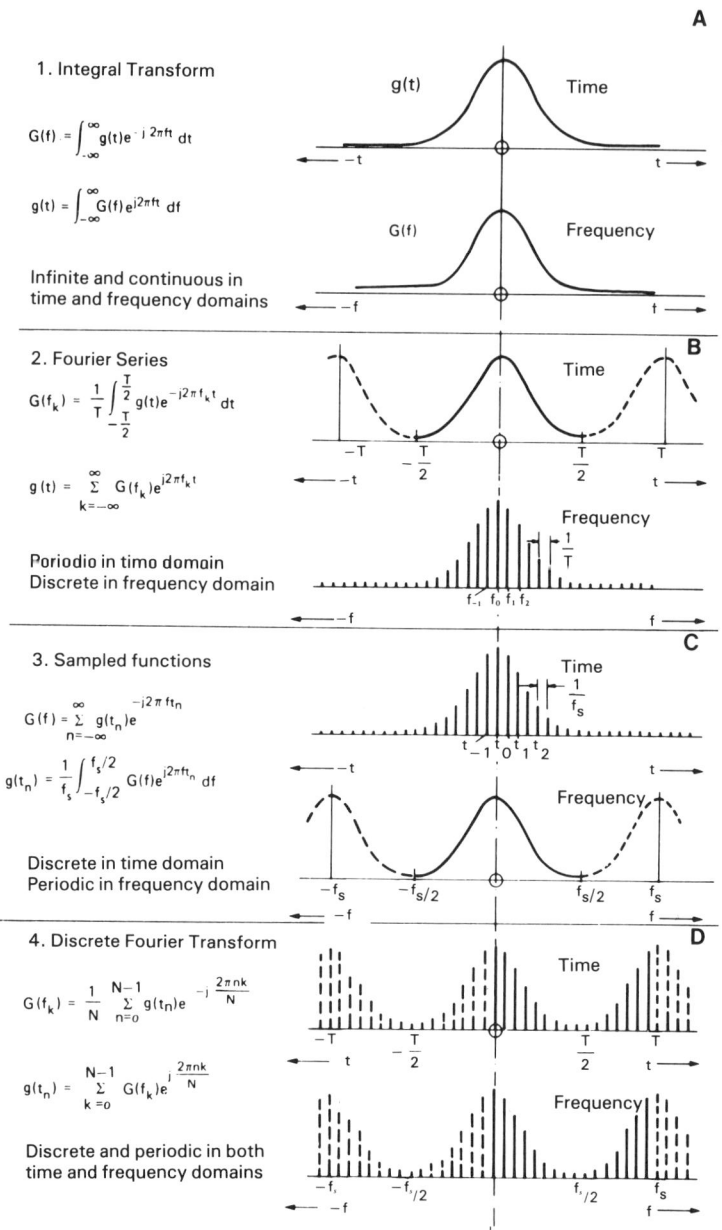

Figure 7. Various forms of the Fourier transform. (Adapted from Randall, 1977, p. 16. Reproduced with permission.)

This transform pair is better known as the "discrete Fourier transform" or DFT.

Figure 7A–D illustrates these different types of Fourier transforms and their implications.

As shown in Figure 7D, the DFT implies periodic continuation of the time signal outside the measurement interval T, with period $T = N \cdot \Delta t$. This has important consequences when the DFT or its famous algorithmic realization, the "fast Fourier transform" (FFT), is applied to spectral decompensation of sampled time signals of finite length (see Section 7.2 and below).

The DFT of a periodic time signal has a spectrum which is discrete and has only components at integer multiples of the fundamental frequency $f_1 = 1/T$ (cf. Equations 1 and 2, and Figure 7B and D).

The Fourier transform has some useful properties. One of them is symmetry, i.e., if $g(t)$ is a real-valued function, as generally will be the case, then the transform $G(f)$ is conjugate even:

$$G(f_k) = G^*(-f_k) \tag{11}$$

Where G^* is the complex conjugate of G:

$$G(f_k) := a + i \cdot b \Rightarrow G^*(-f_k) = a - i \cdot b \tag{11a}$$

One of the consequences is that, because of the antisymmetry of imaginary parts, the zeroth frequency or dc component is always real. Another one is that only one half of the complex vector of coefficients need to be stored, because the other half can be calculated according to equation 11a (see Oppenheim & Schafer, 1975, Chapter 3).

7.3.2. The Concept of Convolution

Basic to some further operations in spectral analysis is the operation of "convolving" (convolution of) two signals.

Convolution of two time functions $f(t)$ and $h(t)$ is defined mathematically as

$$g(t) = \int_{-\infty}^{+\infty} f(\tau) h(t-\tau) d\tau, \tag{12}$$

and often symbolically represented with an asterisk:

$$g(t) = f(t) * h(t) \tag{13}$$

When $f(t)$ is the input to a physical system, say a filter, and $h(t)$ is the response of the filter to an impulse, the convolution $g(t)$ of input and the impulse response will give the output of the filter. This is the most commonly known application of the convolution integral.

When $f(t)$ and $h(t)$ are represented by discrete periodic series, $f(n)$ and $h(n)$, with period N, the N-point DFT of their periodic convolution $g(n)$ will be

$$G(k) = F(k) \cdot H(k) \tag{14}$$

with

$$g(n) = \sum_{l=0}^{N-1} f(l)h(n-l) \tag{15}$$

$$F(k) = \sum_{n=0}^{N-1} f(n)\exp(-j2\pi kn/N) \tag{16}$$

and

$$H(k) = \sum_{n=0}^{N-1} h(n)\exp(-j2\pi kn/N) \tag{17}$$

Relations 14 and 15 are known as the "convolution theorem," which means that "convolving" two signals in the time domain corresponds to multiplication in the frequency domain. Vice versa, multiplication in the time domain corresponds to convolution in the frequency domain. This is often symbolized in the following way:

$$f(t) * h(t) \circ\!\!-\!\!\bullet F(k) \cdot H(k) \tag{17a–18a}$$

$$f(t) \cdot h(t) \circ\!\!-\!\!\bullet F(k) * H(k) \tag{17b–18b}$$

7.3.3. Estimation of Spectra

Whereas an input sequence $f_x(t)$ generally is real, it follows from equation (3) that the corresponding frequency components $X(k)$ will be complex valued and may thus be written as $X(k) = a_k + j \cdot b_k$. The values of the so-called "power spectrum" are given by the squared absolute values of these complex components multiplied by 2 for the antisymmetric parts (cf. Equation 11):

$$X_{\text{pow}}(k) = 2|X(k)|^2 = 2(a_k^2 + b_k^2) \tag{19}$$

or as "root mean square" (rms) or amplitude spectrum

$$X_{\text{rms}}(k) = [X_{\text{pow}}(k)]^{1/2} \tag{19a}$$

To simplify notation let the Fourier transform of $f_x(t)$ (cf. Equation 3) now be represented as

$$\mathcal{F}\{f_x(t)\} := F_x(k) \tag{20}$$

Then the autopower spectrum may be written as

$$|F_x(k)|^2 = F_{xx}(k) \tag{21}$$

where $F_x(k)$ is a complex spectral component, and $F_{xx}(k)$ is the real-valued "power" of the component with frequency k. $F_{xx}(k)$ may also be calculated from the autocovariance or autocorrelation functions of the time signal $f_x(t)$.

The autocovariance function $\text{Cov}_{xx}(\tau)$ of a function $f_x(t)$ is defined as

$$\text{Cov}_{xx}(\tau) = \lim_{T\to\infty} \frac{1}{T} \int_{-T/2}^{T/2} f_x(t) \cdot f(t+\tau) dt \tag{22}$$

The autocorrelation function $R_{xx}(\tau)$ is obtained by normalizing $\text{Cov}_{xx}(\tau)$ to a maximum value of 1:

$$R_{xx}(\tau) = \text{Cov}_{xx}(\tau) / \text{Cov}_{xx}(0) \tag{23}$$

Fourier transformation of $\text{Cov}_{xx}(\tau)$ leads to the autopower spectrum:

Comparison with Equation 12 shows that Equation 22 can be regarded as the convolution of $f_x(t)$ with $f_x(-t)$ and thus be represented as multiplication in the frequency domain

$$\mathcal{F}\{f_x(t)\} = F_x(k) \tag{24a}$$

$$\mathcal{F}\{f_x(-t)\} = F_x(-k) = F_x^*(k) \tag{24b}$$

[cf. Equation 11]

$$\{f_x(t) * f_x(-t)\} = F_x(k) \cdot F_x^*(k) = |F_x(k)|^2 \tag{25}$$

Therefore, autopower spectrum and autocovariance function make up another Fourier transform pair. This is the so-called Wiener–Khinchine relation.

The power spectrum may thus be obtained in two ways: (a) direct forward Fourier transform of the signal and squaring (Equations 10 and 19), (b) forward Fourier transform of the autocovariance function.

On the other hand the autocovariance function may be obtained by forward transformation of the time signal calculating the power spectrum and inverse transformation instead of using Formulas 22 and 23. Especially when using the FFT algorithm, this results in a great reduction of computer time.

Other applications which will be used later are *cross-power spectra* and *coherence spectra*.

In the convention above, the cross-power spectrum of two signals is given by

$$F_{xy}(k) = F_x^*(k) \cdot F_y(k) \tag{26}$$

where $F_x^*(k)$ represents the complex conjugate (cf. Equation 11a) of the Fourier transform $F_x(k)$ of signal $f_x(t)$.

In contrast to the real-valued autopower spectrum $F_{xx}(k)$ (Equation 21), the cross-power spectrum usually is complex. The real part of $F_{xy}(k)$ is known as the "co-spectrum," the imaginary part as "quad-spectrum."

When $F_y(k) = F_x(k)$, $F_{xy}(k)$ reduces to $F_{xx}(k)$, because of Equation 16 and Equation 21.

Coherence spectra give a measure of the extent to which $f_y(t)$ is determined by $f_x(t)$ as a function of frequency k:

$$\gamma_{xy}^2(k) = \frac{|\bar{F}_{xy}(k)|^2}{\bar{F}_{xx}(k) \cdot \bar{F}_{yy}(k)} \tag{27}$$

where $\bar{F}_{xy}(k)$ is a cross-spectrum obtained by averaging over cross-power spectra of a number of records (co- and quad-spectra averaged separately). $\bar{F}_{xx}(k)$ and $\bar{F}_{yy}(k)$ are averaged autopower spectra from the same set of records.

7.3.4. Effects of Time Windows on Spectra

Practical application of the DFT in spectral analysis of real time signals works with data segments of finite length (see Section 7.2). A finite data set can be viewed as the result of a multiplication of an infinite time signal with a rectangular window with values of 1 in the recording interval, and 0 elsewhere. The DFT of the finite data segment consequently will give the spectral composition of that product.

"Windowing" a time signal corresponds to a convolution in the frequency domain:

When a discrete signal $f(n)$ is truncated to a finite record length N, the resulting signal $\tilde{f}(n)$ may be represented as the product of $f(n)$ and the rectangular window $w_{\text{rect}}(n)$:

$$w_{\text{rect}}(n) := \begin{cases} 1 & \text{for } 0 \leq n \leq N - 1 \\ 0 & \text{otherwise} \end{cases} \quad (28)$$

$$\tilde{f}(n) = f(n) \cdot w_{\text{rect}}(n) \quad (29a)$$

or

$$\tilde{f}(n) = \begin{cases} f(n) & \text{for } 0 \leq n \leq N - 1 \\ 0 & \text{otherwise} \end{cases} \quad (29b)$$

The convolution theorem states that the complex spectrum of the truncated signal $\tilde{f}(n)$ is obtained by convolving the spectrum of the original signal $f(n)$ with the spectrum of the window:

$$\tilde{F}(k) = F(k) * W(k) \quad (30)$$

The result is a "smeared" version of $F(k)$. The effect is sometimes called "leakage" because it can be viewed as if energy from spectral lines in the original "leaked" through to other, adjacent frequencies.

Figure 8 shows the effects in time and frequency domain of multiplying a pure sine wave with a rectangular window (i.e., truncating it to finite length). From the spectrum of the rectangular window the reason for distortion of spectra by addition of frequency components can be understood: "side lobes" have considerable power which falls off relatively slowly with increasing distance from "main lobe." The rationale for additional windowing with nonrectangular (bell-shaped) windows is reduction of these side lobes and nullification of discontinuities at the limits of the truncation interval. The rectangular window has the narrowest main lobe, but the highest side lobes, whereas spectra of the other windows tapering off smoothly to zero in the time domains show greatly reduced side lobes. On the other hand their main lobe is much wider and frequency resolution diminished.

7.4. Auto- and Cross-spectral Analyses of Conjoint Gastrograms

As described above gastrographic input data for spectral analyses consist of data vectors containing $1024 = 2^{10}$ points sampled at a rate of 550 msec per point giving a record length of 563.2 sec ~ 10 min. With up to 16 channels this amounts to an input matrix of 1024×16, 12-bit numbers entering off-line

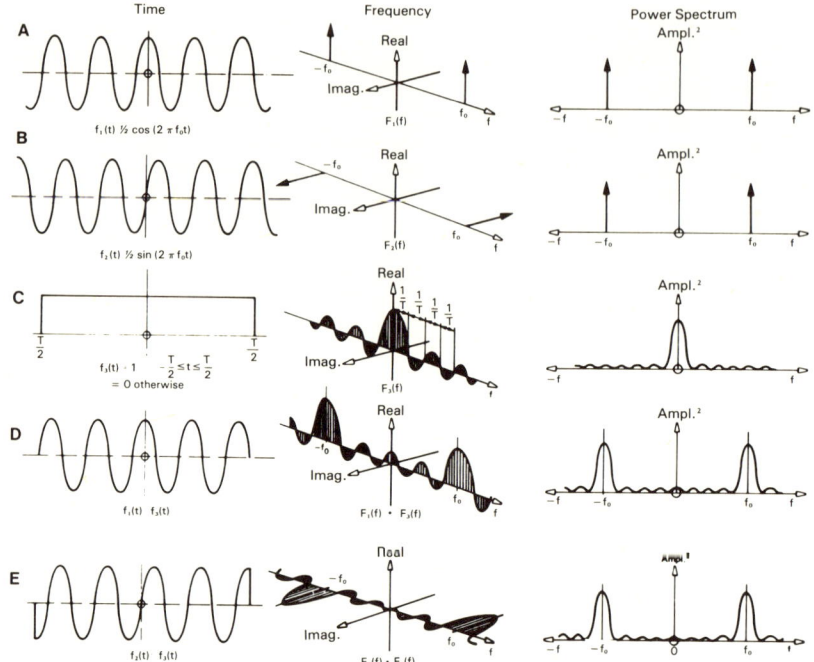

Figure 8. Effect of truncating a signal to finite length. (A) Cosine wave (sine wave + 90°) and its Fourier transform. (B) Sine wave and its Fourier transform. (C) Rectangular window and its Fourier transform. (D) Truncated cosine wave and its Fourier transform. (E) Truncated sine wave and its Fourier transform. (Adapted from Randall, 1977, p. 46. Reproduced with permission.)

analysis programs.[8] The input matrix is analyzed in three steps: preconditioning, Fourier transformation with calculation of spectra, and evaluation of spectra. Record length has been chosen for optimal performance of transforms which work faster with record lengths equal to powers of 2.

7.4.1. Preconditioning

Initially input data are rescaled by multiplication of a vector of scaling factors defined to give numbers with real physical dimensions such as μV (×100) for the EGGs mOe (millioersted) for the MGGs, etc. These seemingly trivial transformations turned out to be essential for comparison across experi-

---

[8]The package was written by G. M. Müller, MPIP, Munich, using subroutines from the IEEE-package (Weinstein & Digital Signal Processing Committee, 1979), Calcomp Graphics Software, Benson Graphics Software and from the Computer Center of the MPIP. Programs are in FORTRAN Version 05A, which is running under the Operating System Tops-20V4 of the Digital Equipment Corporation on a DEC 2060. They will run without major changes on other installations as well.

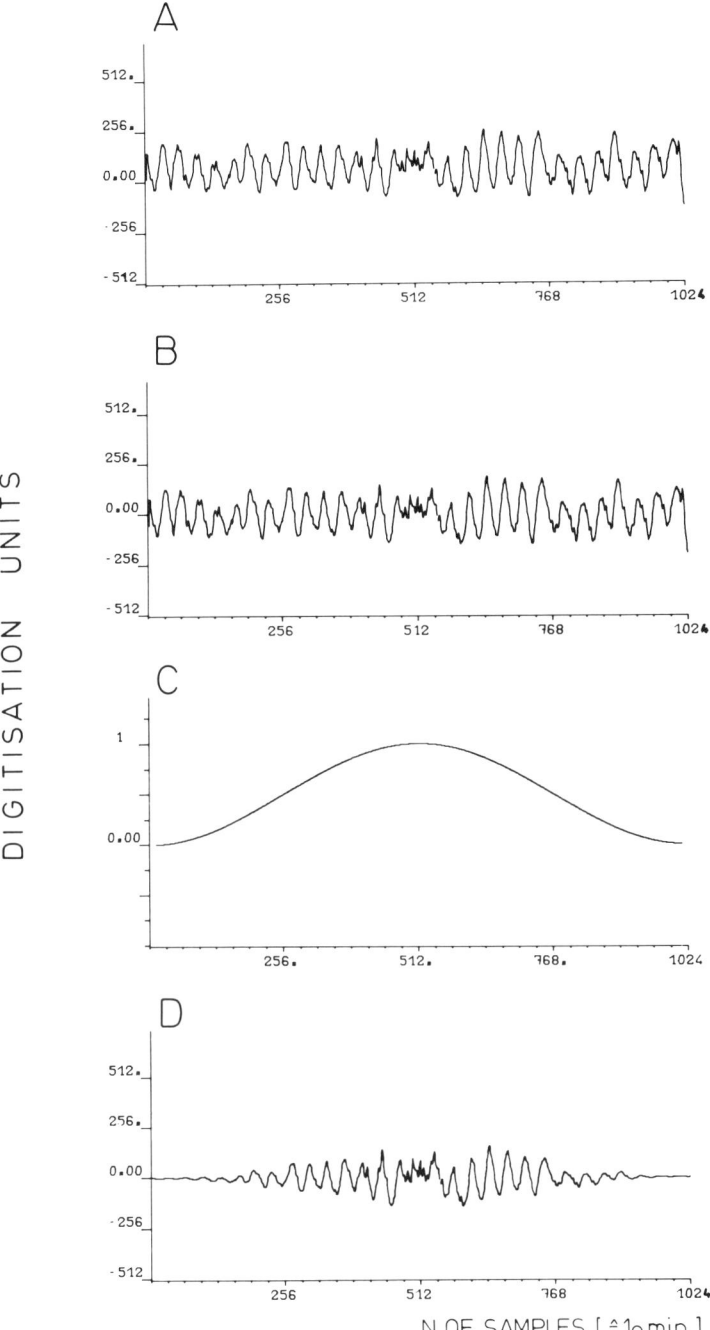

Figure 9. Illustration of preconditioning. (A) Original signal. (B) Signal after dc removal. (C) Windowing function (Hanning). (D) Signal after dc removal and multiplication by the Hanning function ("windowing").

ments with different equipment or calibration. After rescaling, dc offsets in the signal are eliminated by subtraction of the *mean* from raw values. At the same time the overall "root mean square" (rms or standard deviation) is calculated, stored, and printed. It is an overall index of intensity, and can be used to control calibration and to calculate normalized spectral parameters. In particular estimation of signal-to-noise ratio is achieved by comparing rms with amplitudes of specific components.

The next step in preconditioning, that is, "windowing" the input data field, is especially important. Its rational basis was discussed in Section 7.3.3. In our case data points are multiplied by the Hanning function. Figure 9A–D illustrate the effect of the preconditioning procedure. Because the preconditioned records begin and end with zero values periodic continuation implicit in the DFT will not produce discontinuities.

7.4.2. Fourier Transform

The final preconditioned input array shown in Figure 9D is transformed by the FFT routine SFTF (IBM Scientific Subroutine Package). It produces a complex output vector of length $(N/2 + 1)$, that is 513 real and imaginary Fourier coefficients ($N = 1024$) as a function of integer multiples of the fundamental frequency $\Delta f = 1/T = 1.7756$ mHz for $T = 563.2$ sec. Δf represents the "resolution" of the spectrum. The Fourier coefficients, roughly speaking, contain amplitude and phase information in respect to the different sine and cosine wave components the signal is thought to be made of (see Section 7.3).

Calculating the absolute values ($a^2 + b^2$) of the complex values ($a + i \cdot b$) for each frequency results in the autopower spectrum of the signal. It is shown in Figure 10 without (A) and with (B) windowing.

The graphs represent the "intensity" with which different frequency components are contained in the original signal irrespective of their phase relationships. This loss of phase information is the reason why no simple one-to-one correspondence between the form of the original signal and its power spectrum is to be found. The stabilizing effect of the window is clearly seen in the lower left of Figure 10. It must be paid for, however, with a reduction in frequency resolution. The power of a particular component is smeared over adjacent bins (see previous section). This has to be kept in mind when we advance to the next step in the analysis.

Similarly to the calculation of the autopower spectra from single channels cross-power spectra of EGG–MGG pairs are computed. Basically they indicate common periodic components in both channels of a pair.

In Figure 10D the absolute values of a cross-power spectrum between the EGG record of Figure 10B and the one MGG channel (MGGY, Figure 10C) of the same subject are plotted as a function of frequency. A clear peak in the 3 cpm

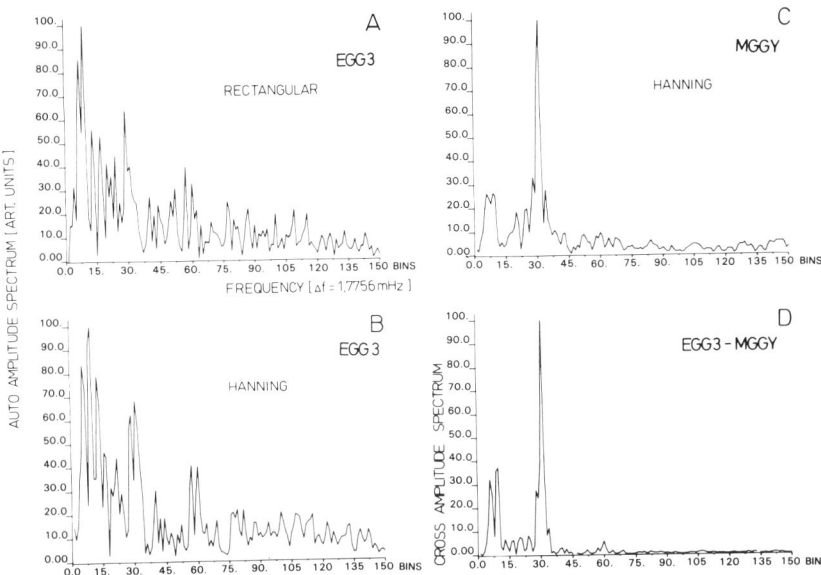

Figure 10. Auto- and cross-power spectra of gastrograms. (A), (B) Effects of windowing on autopower spectra of electrogastrogram record from Figure 9 (EGG3); rectangular (i.e., no additional) window—(A); Hanning window—(B). (C) Autopower spectrum of corresponding MGGY (with Hanning window). (D) Cross-power spectrum of EGG3 (Figure 9) and MGGY. (Spectra were normalized in respect to greatest component ≐ 100 units.)

region is to be seen indicating concordant periodicity of that frequency in EGG and MGG. The increase in selectivity for that component is demonstrated by further damping of other frequencies in Figure 10B.

Results of auto- and cross-power computation enter the next step in the analysis, that is, the calculation of single frequency and amplitude parameters of significant and concordant peaks. In practice only the complex spectra are stored and power vectors recalculated in the initial part of the peak detection routine described below. The reason for this is to be found in the particular hardware environments of our programs where enough CPU-time is readily available but disk memory is limited. This is easily changed for other installations.

7.5. Evaluation of Spectra

Evaluation of a spectrum means defining "significant" frequency components with respect to frequency and amplitude. This could be done by statistical testing of peaks in an autopower spectrum, for instance, against deviation from white noise, that is, flat spectrum. Because of the instability of FFT power estimates this would be a very insensitive procedure, accepting only very large and distant peaks (e.g., Smallwood, Linkens, & Stoddard, 1980).

In conjoint gastrography a different approach has been used: More or less empirically defined, very sensitive, but unselective peak finding routines determine a vector of relative maxima (frequency and amplitude) in the autopower spectrum of a signal. Some of the peaks in this list of "admissible candidates" will simply stem from instability ("ripple") because thresholds are set very low. By combining EGGs and MGGs, however, in a suitable manner selectivity is increased again. Peaks are accepted only when they represent common activity in EGGs and MGGs. In that way peaks from uncorrelated spectral noise and peaks not representing electrical as well as mechanical activity will not be selected as significant. To increase selectivity further in most applications only those spectral peaks are included in the final output step which in addition can be related to the well-known 3 cpm band of ECA or Type II waves (see previous chapter) or a repeatedly found 1 cpm component (see below, Section 8).

7.5.1. Peak Detection

In a first step, the number of points f_i with amplitude a_i of the autopower spectrum are reduced to the vector of extrema, that is, points of relative maxima or minima. At the same time the absolute maximum (f_{abs}, a_{abs}) is determined and stored (Figure 11). f_{abs} in the example is f_{31}.

The array of extrema is then examined for clear relative maxima, which have rising *and* falling slopes steeper than a preset criterion tanα *or* rise higher in amplitude over preceding and succeeding minima than a preset percentage p of the absolute maximum (a_{abs}) of the amplitude spectrum. Criteria were set lower

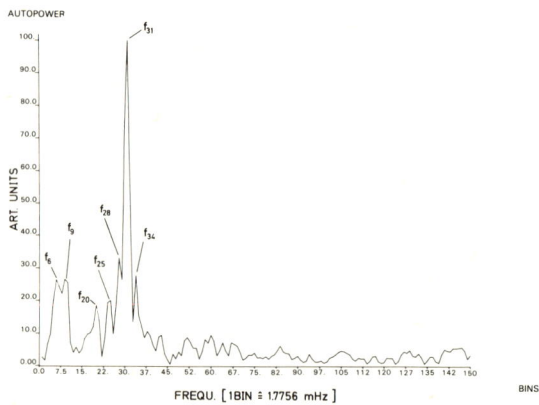

Figure 11. Peak detection routine. Peaks found according to preset criteria are marked with arrows, normalized spectrum; see text for further details.

for autopower spectra than for cross-power spectra. The reason for this is to have low selectivity for finding "admissible candidates," but high selectivity in their identification by concordance for EGGs and MGGs (see Section 7.5.2). By considering rising *and* falling slopes the routine is capable of rejecting double or multiple peaks with no significant trough in between (e.g., f_6 and f_9 in Figure 11). Then the midpoint of the double peak is chosen as its corresponding midfrequency "bin" $[f_7 = \frac{1}{2}(f_6 + f_9)$ in the example]. The amplitude value of the double peak is defined as the mean of its constituents $[a_7 = \frac{1}{2}(a_6 + a_9)$ in the example]. Small peaks on top of rising or falling slopes of a bigger peak are ignored (f_{28} in Figure 11). In Figure 11 f_7 (double), f_{20}, f_{25}, f_{31}, and f_{34} have been found to be "significant" peaks. The vector of their frequencies (in spectral "bins"), f_j, and the vector of their amplitudes, $\bar{a}_j$, are the output of the peak routine.

7.5.2. Peak Identification

For identification of a significant autopower peaks common to EGG and MGG absolute cross-power spectra between them are evaluated with the peak detection routine described above after normalization in respect to their absolute maxima. Normalized amplitudes of peaks detected are summed up for each "bin" over all cross-power spectra, that is, over 21 EGG–MGG combinations in the standard channel configuration of 7 EGGs and 3 MGGs. Absolute maxima are searched in the resulting summation vector within two specified frequency regions from 8 to 32 MHz and from 32 to 70 MHz. They represent the main components at 1 cpm and 3 cpm (about 17 and 50 MHz, respectively). These maxima define the points of highest probability of common peaks in autopower spectra. They therefore constitute the midpoints of very narrow search intervals for the autospectra. Highest peaks in this intervals are identified as the slow (3 cpm) and ultraslow (1 cpm) wave components. Their frequencies (f_0, f_u) and amplitudes (a_0, a_u) are stored as final spectral parameters together with the point of absolute maximum (f_{abs}, a_{abs}) left to the peak of the respiratory artifact. Earlier verions of peak identification used combination of autospectra alone, and calculation of cross-correlograms between EGGs and MGGs to specify common components.

8. Selected Results

During the past few years a number of methodological studies were completed investigating signal content, statistical properties, various covariates (including body measures) of CSG parameters, and their correlation with invasive manometric measurements (e.g., Eder, 1981; Hölzl, Müller, Skambraks, & Brüchle, 1981; Skambraks, 1981). A limited selection of these data will be presented here.

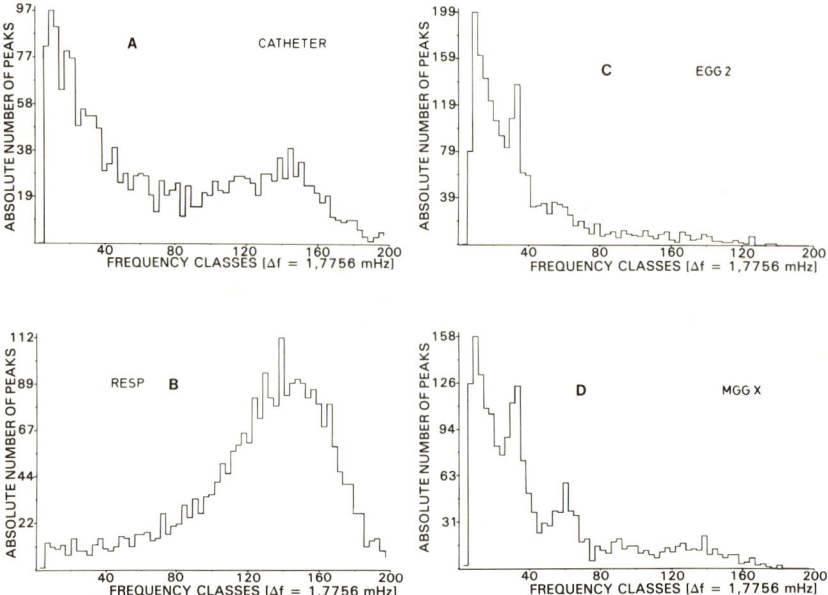

Figure 12. Peak distributions of autopower spectra. (A) Peak distribution of catheter. (B) Peak distribution of respiration (for comparison). (C) Peak distribution of EGG2. (D) Peak distribution of MGGX. Based on 150 records and about 1000 peaks. (Reanalyzed data from Eder, 1981).

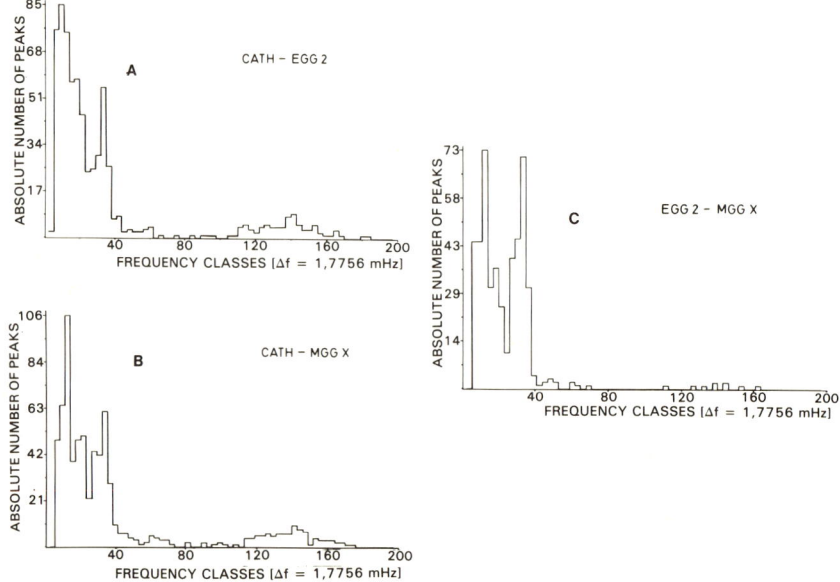

Figure 13. Peak distributions of cross-power spectra. (A) Peak distribution of Catheter and EGG2. (B) Peak distribution of Catheter and MGGX. (C) Peak distribution of EGG 2 and MGGX. (Data base: cf. caption to Figure 12.)

8.1. Peak Histograms

Frequency distributions of spectral peaks of many auto- and cross-power spectra have been calculated. They invariably show a two-component structure with modal values at about 1 cpm and 3 cpm. Figure 12 illustrates this with data from one study in which intraluminal pressure recordings were also obtained. Quite similar frequency distributions are shown in different channels. These bimodal peak distributions have been replicated in three other studies with new subjects under different conditions. The total data base encompasses now more than 10,000 spectra and 50,000 peaks. The general form of distributions is retained when only *absolute* maxima of spectra are included with the exception of our type of catheter measurement in which power of ultraslow components normally exceed that of the slow component.

Peak histograms of cross-power spectra also exhibit the bimodal form. This is shown in Figure 13 for the same study as in Figure 12.

8.2. Cross-Correlograms

The two components mentioned above also appear in cross-correlation functions between EGGs and MGGs on the one hand, and catheter recordings and gastrograms on the other hand. Usually only a clear common 3 cpm component is shown, but sometimes a 1 cpm wave is superimposed (Figure 14A and B). This signal structure may change contingent upon experimental conditions as is demonstrated in Figure 14B and C.

This poses the interesting question whether validation of noninvasive motility measures is dependent upon experimental conditions (see Chapter 5).

8.3. Coherence Functions

While comparison of autospectra, cross-spectra and cross-correlation functions so far give good evidence on the validity of surface recordings in certain respects and for single subjects, they are no real proof of causal relationship. This is different for coherence functions (see Section 7.3.3). They show the general degree to which one variable (e.g., the EGG) is determined by another variable (e.g., intraluminal pressure recordings) as a function of frequency of periodic components, and averaged over many records within and/or between subjects. For one study (Eder, 1981) coherences of catheter, EGG, and MGG recordings were computed, and medium to good correspondences found. Absolute peak values of the coherence functions are not very high, probably due to heterogeneity of conditions averaged. Relative size of coherence specific to 3 cpm activity, however, is impressive (Figure 15).

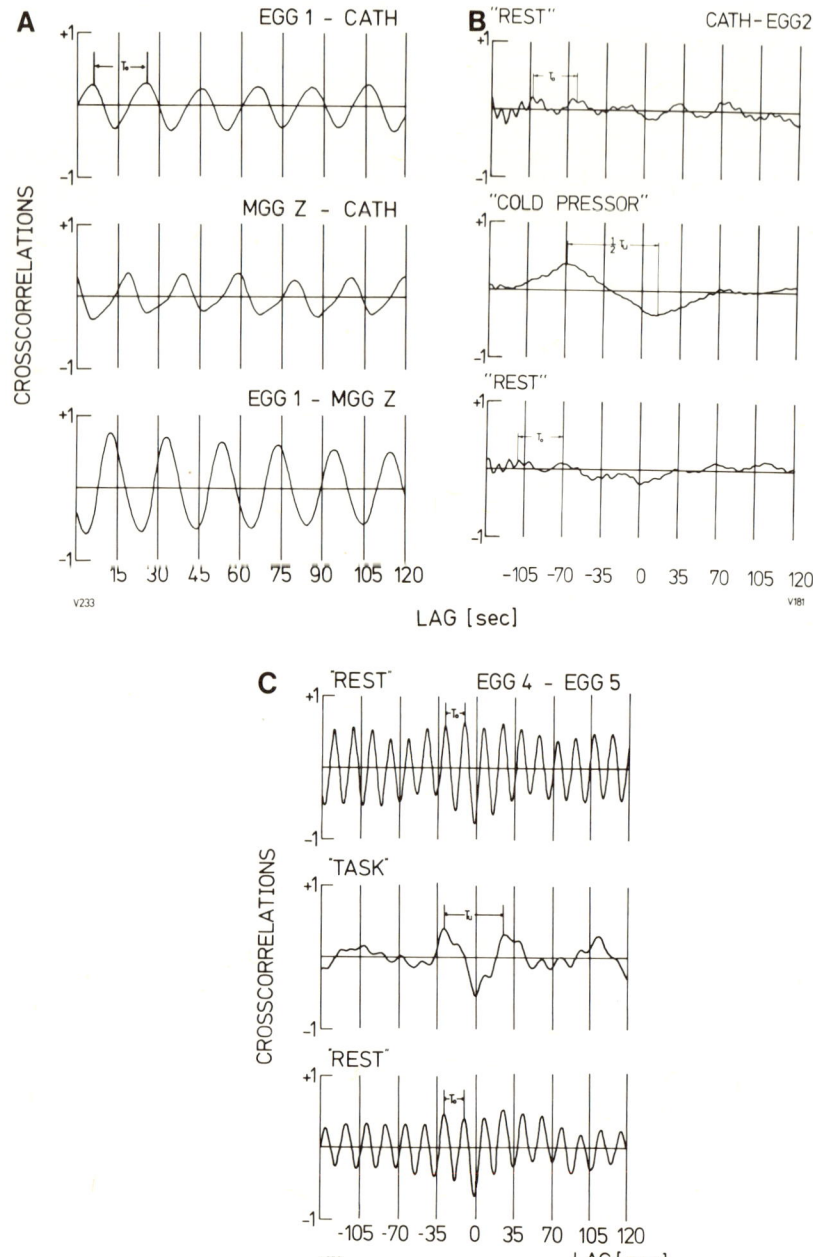

Figure 14. Cross-correlograms of surface gastrograms and intraluminal pressure recordings under different conditions. (A) Cross-correlograms of surface gastrograms and intraluminal pressure re-

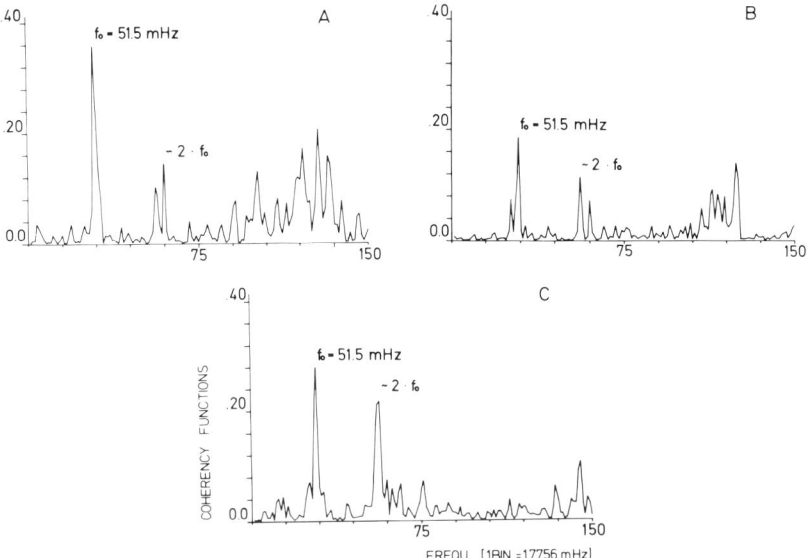

Figure 15. Coherency functions of surface gastrograms and intraluminal pressure recordings. (A) Coherency function of catheter and EGG 2, (B) coherency function of catheter and MGGX, and (C) coherency function of EGG 2 and MGGX. f_0 corresponds to 3 cpm activity and $2f_0$ to its first harmonic. Based on 150 records of 10 min each (reanalyzed data from Eder, 1981).

Further studies on direct correspondence of parameters of surface recordings and invasive measures of electromotor activity of stomach are needed, of course, but data available today obviously justify extension of this type of research.

ACKNOWLEDGMENTS

The work reported in this chapter has developed out of early research of Rupert Hölzl with the late R. Scherm, G. Schröder, and H. Kiefer. Without the results of their dedicated work the present studies would not have been undertaken. Their contributions are gratefully acknowledged. A number of other people assisted in preparation of this paper. Among them, Hildegard Koch (manuscript), Alexandra Solder, and Constanze Dahmes (drawings) deserve special

cording (Eder, 1981); 10-min sample from a single subject (No. V233); T_0 = period of 3 cpm component. (B) Change of correlated component during cold pressor test (source: Eder, 1981, subject no. V181); T_0 as above, T_u = period of ultraslow (1 cpm) component. (C) Change of correlated component between two EGGs during a difficult perceptual discrimination task (cf. Hölzl et al., 1979; unpublished data by Lautenbacher & Hölzl, 1981).

mention for their endurance. The valuable assistance of the MPIPs electronics and mechanic workshops and photolab is also acknowledged.

9. References

Benmair, Y. *Use of a ferromagnetic tracer for measurement of gastric emptying and some other medical physics purposes.* Unpublished doctoral dissertation, Weizmann Institute of Science, Feinberg Graduate School, 1975.

Davis, R. C., Garafolo, L., & Gault, F. P. An exploration of abdominal potentials. *Journal of Comparative and Physiological Psychology,* 1957, *50,* 519–523.

Davis, R. C., Garafolo, L., & Kveim, K. Conditions associated with gastrointestinal activity. *Journal of Comparative and Physiological Psychology,* 1959, *52,* 466–475.

Eder, R. *Die Magenmotilität bei Patienten mit Ulcus duodeni vor und nach selektiver proximaler Vagotomie im Vergleich mit unbehandelten Kontrollen.* Unpublished doctoral dissertation, Universität München, 1981.

Edwards, A. E., Hill, R. A., & Treadwell, T. Improvements in the magnetometer technique of measuring gastric motility. *Psychophysiology,* 1967, *4,* 116–118.

Hölzl, R. *Eine einfache Verbesserung der Atmungsaufzeichnung mit der Thermistormethode.* Unpublished manuscript, Munich, Max Plank Institute of Psychiatry, 1976.

Hölzl, R. Noninvasive measurement of gastrointestinal motility in experimental psychosomatics. In W. H. G. Wolters & G. Sinnema (Eds.), *Psychosomatics and biofeedback.* Boston: Bohn, Nyhoff, 1979.

Hölzl, R., & Scherm, R. *Indirekte Messung der Magenmotilität durch Kombination von EGG und MGG.* Paper presented at the 5th "Arbeitstagung Psychophysiologische Methodik," Wien, June 1975.

Hölzl, R., & Scherm, R. *The use of indirect measures of mobility in behavioral analysis and treatment of psychosomatic disorders of the gastrointestinal trait.* Paper presented at the 6th Annual Convention of the European Association for Behaviour Therapy, Spretsae (Greece), September 1976.

Hölzl, R., Scherm, R., Schröder, G., & Kiefer, H. Die indirekte Messung der Magenmotilität und ihre Veränderung unter verschiedenen Belastungsbedingungen. In W. H. Tack (Ed.), *Bericht über den 30.Kongress der DGfP.* Göttingen: Hogrefe, 1977.

Hölzl, R., Schröder, G., & Kiefer, H. Indirect gastrointestinal motility measurement for use in experimental psychosomatics: A new method and some data. *Behavioural Analysis and Modification,* 1979, *3,* 77–97.

Hölzl, R., Müller, G., Skambraks, M., & Brüchle, H. Die klinische Validierung einer nichtinvasiven Methode zur Messung der Magenmotilität. *Zeitschrift für Psychosomatik,* 1981, *27,* 50–58.

Oppenheim, A. V., & Schafer, R. W. *Digital signal processing.* Englewood Cliffs, New Jersey: Prentice Hall, 1975.

Randall, R. B. *Application of B & K equipment to frequency analysis.* Naerum (Denmark): Brüel & Kjaer, 1977.

Schröder, G. *Indirekte Messung der Magenmotilität unter verschiedenen Belastungsbedingungen.* Unpublished Master's thesis, University of Marburg and Max Planck Institute of Psychiatry, Munich, 1977.

Skambraks, M. *Psychophysiologische und psychologische Unterschiede zwischen Patienten mit Ulcus ventriculi aut duodeni, Personen mit vegetativen Magenbeschwerden und normalen Kontrollpersonen.* Unpublished thesis for diploma, University of Munich and Max Planck Institute of Psychiatry, Munich, 1981.

Smallwood, R. H., Linkens, D. A., & Stoddard, C. F. Analysis and modelling of amplitude changes in human duodenal slow waves. *Clinical Physics and Physiological Measurement*, 1980, *1*, 47–58.

Weinstein, C. J. (Chairman),& Digital Signal Processing Committee (Eds.). *Programs for digital signal processing*. New York: IEEE Press, 1979.

7

MEASUREMENT OF GASTRIC ACID SECRETION

PETER R. WELGAN

1. Introduction

Scientific interest in the psychophysiology of the stomach originated with the studies of Beaumont (1833), who directly observed the effects of mood changes on the gastric mucosa of a patient with a gastric fistula. In a similar manner, other fistulous patients have been examined as a source of information about emotional influences on the acid secretory and motor activity of the stomach (e.g., Gordon & Chernya, 1940; Richet, 1878; Wolf & Wolff, 1943; Wolf, 1965). With the advent of modern electronic monitoring systems, such as the Beckman pH electrode and titration methods, researchers have expanded the scope of their investigations of the psychological influences on the gut beyond the visual inspection methods used with fistulous patients. Wolf and Welsh (1972) have reviewed the research on the effects of psychological variables on gastric function for the reader interested in a detailed analysis of this aspect of the subject.

Gastric acid secretions are of primary importance in the study of psychological influences on the stomach, because changes in gastric activity have been shown to be closely associated with specific emotional reactions and to an extent, they are learned.

Increased interest in the psychophysiology of gastric acid secretions has created a need for standardized approaches to research in this field. This chapter reviews the current acid measurement procedures in medicine and psycho-

---

PETER R. WELGAN • Department of Psychiatry and Human Behavior, University of California at Irvine and 1001 Dove Street, Suite 280, Newport Beach, California 92660.

physiology and analyzes their merit in human psychological research. In addition, the chapter reviews the specific procedures for subject preparation and acid monitoring techniques.

2. Measurement of Gastric Acid

Hydrochloric acid is secreted into the stomach by the parietal or oxyntic cells in a concentration three million times greater than that found in the blood and tissues. Grossman (1978) indicates that the formation of hydrogen ions occurs in the parietal cells through aerobic metabolism, a process which eventually produces very-high-energy phosphate bonds. For each hydrogen ion secreted by the parietal cells, a molecule of carbon dioxide from the arterial blood or mucosal metabolism is converted into bicarbonate. The bicarbonate eventually enters the interstitial fluids, and the resulting levels of alkalinity in the blood, known as alkaline tide, provide an indicator of hydrochloric acid production in the stomach.

Parietal cells contain high concentrations of the enzyme, carbonic anhydrase, which acts as a catalyst in the formation of hydrochloric acid. Acid is secreted at a constant concentration of 165 mEq/L (Cummins, 1963). The acid concentration of the stomach contents changes as the hydrogen ions combine with various contents present (e.g., mucus, saliva, protein). A detailed analysis of the process of acid formation may be found in Grossman (1978).

The current methods of acid measurement in psychophysiology are modifications of standard gastroenterological test procedures. A review of these procedures is necessary for an understanding of the transition to psychological research. There are three methods of gastric acid measurement in gastroenterology: (1) the pH method, (2) the pH meter–titration method, and (3) the indicator titration method.

2.1. The pH Method

Hydrochloric acid is commonly measured in terms of its pH value and concentration in the gastric juice. As originally defined pH is the potential of hydrogen in a solution. It is the symbol for the logarithm of the reciprocal of the hydrogen ion concentration expressed in gram atoms per liter of a solution. A solution with a pH 7, such as water, has 0.0000001 gram atom of hydrogen ion per liter and is considered neutral. Values of pH from 7 to 0 indicate increasing acidity while pH values from 7 to 14 indicate increasing alkalinity. When determined with the glass electrode, however, pH represents the negative logarithm of the hydrogen ion activity and not concentration since electrode potentials are generated at the glass solution interface by differences in ionic activities. For example, in infinitely dilute or ideal solutions ionic activity and concentration are equivalent. However, at hydrogen ion levels encountered in gastric juice of pH 3 or less, a considerable departure from the ideal occurs. Using traditional methods of determining hydrogen ion concentration under these conditions, such as titration to a fixed pH value, systematic and nonlinear errors result. The errors arise from the difficulty in measuring the total acid present in gastric juice because pH is a measure of only the free or dissociated hydrogen ions present. It does not reflect the bound or undissociated hydrogen ions in solution. Free hydrogen ions are distinguished from bound or combined hydrogen ions because saliva and mucus in the stomach act as buffers which bind many hydrogen ions so long as the pH of the stomach is below 7.2. These bound hydrogen ions are a part of the total hydrogen ions secreted by the stomach, but they cannot be detected by simple pH determination at pH values below 7.2. In order to correct the error in the measurement of total hydrogen ion concentration using the pH glass electrode, Moore and Scarlata (1965) have developed activity coefficients which accurately permit conversion of hydrogen ion activity to hydrogen ion concentration of the gastric contents. Such conversion tables have become common references in gastrointestinal laboratories when rapid and accurate transformations are required of hydrogen ion concentration from pH values.

2.2. The pH Meter–Titration Method

The pH meter–titration procedure measures total acid concentration of the gastric juice. The procedure, which requires precise buffers and a pH meter, involves the use of a known volume of gastric juice for analysis. This sample of gastric contents is titrated to pH 7.0 with dilute sodium hydroxide, 0.1 N NaOH or 0.2 N NaOH. The amount of NaOH (expressed in milliequivalents) needed to attain pH 7.0 divided by the volume of gastric juice in liters is equivalent to the hydrogen ion concentration expressed as milliequivalents of HCL/liter. The volume of gastric secretions multiplied by the hydrogen ion concentration of the gastric juice and divided by the time required to collect the sample is equivalent to the acid output.

To achieve accurate measurements, the pH meter requires daily calibration before use with two standard buffers (e.g., pH 2.0 and pH 7.0). Additional control titrations may be made with a known concentration of hydrochloric acid (e.g., titration of 0.2 ml of 0.1 N HCl).

2.3. Titration with Chemical Indicators

At present, the indicator titration method is not used in psychophysiological research. Indicators used to measure gastric acid change color at a known pH value. There are indicators which change color at or near pH 3.5, such as Topfer's reagent, and indicators which change color at approximately pH 7.0 or pH 8.0, such as neutral red or phenol red. Indicators which change color above (i.e., more alkaline than) pH 7.2 measure titratable acid which is the combination of free and combined acid.

Indicators are considered to have limited usefulness in psychophysiological research since it is difficult to quantify pH changes by this method. The accuracy of this method depends to a degree on the accuracy and precision of the observer.

3. Tests of Gastric Secretory Function

Four types of acid measurement are calculated to assess the range of responsivity of the gastric secretory system: (1) basal acid output, (2) peak acid output, (3) maximal acid output, and (4) calculated maximal acid output. The last three are all ways of estimating the maximum potential of the stomach to secrete acid; they differ only in the procedure used to derive the estimate.

3.1. Basal Acid Output (BAO)

The basal acid output or basal gastric acid secretion refers to the rate of secretion in an unstimulated stomach. It is denoted as the interdigestive or fasting gastric secretion and is determined by collecting the sum of four consecutive 15-min basal acid collections. The result is expressed in milliequivalents per hour.

3.2. Peak Acid Output (PAO), Maximal Acid Output (MAO), and Calculated Maximal Acid Output (CMAO)

PAO refers to the highest rate of acid secretion during the test period following the injection of a stimulant of acid secretion (e.g., histamine acid phosphate, pentagastrin). Generally it is computed as the sum of the two highest 10- or 20-min periods within a 2-hr test session. The results are expressed as milliequivalents per hour. The PAO represents the most reproducible measure of stimulated gastric acid secretion and is a good index of the calculated maximal response of the stomach to secrete acid.

MAO is computed as the sum of the 4 highest 15-min or 6 highest 10-min periods during the 2-hr test period. Baron (1963) considers the MAO to be the total stimulated acid output which occurs during the first postinjection hour.

CMAO assesses the maximal capacity of the gastric acid response following an infinite dose of stimulant. It is computed by measuring the response to multiple doses of a stimulant and extrapolating the maximal response mathmatically (Grossman, 1973).

4. Psychophysiological Measures of Gastric Acid

Clinical methods of gastric acid measurement have been altered to meet the special requirements of psychophysiological research. These requirements are that knowledge of changes in acidity must be available immediately and the measurement procedure should involve as little discomfort as possible so that repeated or prolonged measurement under conditions approximating normal are possible. Currently, there are two classes of measurement methods which have been adopted for human research: intragastric pH measurement and external pH measurement methods. Intragastric measures include intragastric pH telemetry, the intragastric pH electrode, and intragastric titration.

4.1. Intragastric Measures

4.1.1. pH Telemetry

Radio telemetry pH probes are devices for the remote measurement of intragastric pH (Stacher & Stärker, 1975). An encapsulated transmitter broadcasts signals to an FM receiver which is located near the subject's abdomen. The signal is transformed into an electrical equivalent of pH and can be recorded on a strip chart recorder. (See also Chapter 8.)

Norman (1969) published early psychological research with humans using pH telemetry. In his study of the effects of shock avoidance on stomach acid secretion, subjects swallowed a Heidelberg capsule which was tethered to the side of the mouth with tape. The capsule was positioned in the fundus of the stomach by watching pH changes as the capsule passed from the relatively alkaline esophagus and cardia of the stomach (pH 7.0) into the acid-producing regions of the fundus and body of the stomach (pH 2.0). A sharp rise in pH after that would signal the passage of the capsule through the pylorus into the alkaline duodenum, requiring readjustment back into the stomach.

The tethered pH telemetry probe has the distinct advantage of being unobtrusive, independent of shielded cables, and capable of allowing the subject a full range of motion. Furthermore, when swallowed, it creates relatively slight stimulation for the production of acid, especially when compared with intragastric pH electrodes and nasogastric tubes.

The pH transmitter possesses some disadvantages. It is reportedly capable of measuring pH between 1.5 and 9.0. However, there is evidence indicating that the probe is inaccurate below pH 2.0 (e.g., Exenved & Walan, 1975). The Heidelberg capsule (AEG Telefunken) has been found to measure pH accurately to 2.0, although below this level recorded pH values are lower than values obtained by aspiration methods. Precise positioning of the transmitter in the stomach is difficult. Accidental contact with the alkaline mucosa or envelopment in the stomach folds is a major source of artifact with this device.

Alternate uses have been successfully developed for the pH transmitter. It has been useful in measuring the pH from the esophagus and small intestine.

4.1.2. Intragastric pH Electrode

An alternate method of measuring intragastric pH involves the use of the intragastric pH electrode (Beckman Instruments No. 39042). This small glass electrode with an electrically shielded cable is passed orally and positioned in the dependent portion of the stomach. The reference electrode is usually placed in a solution of potassium chloride in which the subject has immersed his hand (Rovelstad, Owen, & Magath, 1952). The new MI 506 combination pH and reference electrode (Londonderry Microelectronics, Londonderry, New Hampshire) is smaller and apparently more reliable than the Beckman pH electrode. Gorman and Kamiya (1972) used this technique in a biofeedback study in which subjects were asked to alter intragastric pH. Changes in pH were monitored by subjects on a pH meter.

The intragastric pH electrode has the advantage of providing immediate and continuous information of gastric pH changes. It has the disadvantage of providing no information about the volume or acid concentration of the gastric contents since it is a measure of only free or dissociated hydrogen ions. It does not measure combined or bound hydrogen ions which have joined to other molecules in the stomach. It has the additional disadvantage of being a logarithmic measure of acid concentration. Therefore, a change from pH 4.0 to pH 3.0 represents a change in acid concentration 10 times less than a change from pH 3.0 to pH 2.0 (Gambescia, Krawiec, Desiderio, & Polish, 1967).

Other disadvantages exist in the use of the intragastric pH electrode. The probe is extremely expensive for the amount of use obtainable from it. It is designed to accurately record pH for 10 intragastric placements. The hostile environment of the stomach quickly erodes the shielding of the probe creating a short life span. Unlike the pH telemeter transmitter, the electrode accurately measures pH below 2.0. Yet it shares a similar problem in that it is difficult to identify the exact placement of the electrode in the stomach. Electrode cables have been known to accidentally curl in the stomach and end in the esophagus. Moreover, changes in pH may result from changes in gastric pH or from the accidental contact with more alkaline portions of the stomach wall. The probe may also become engulfed in the viscous mucus or the folds of the stomach, creating measurement artifact.

Whitehead, Renault, and Goldiamond (1975) attempted to avoid direct contact with the mucosa by constructing a cuff around the pH electrode bulb. Viscous and adherent mucus coming in contact with the pH bulb could be washed away periodically with an injection of a small quantity of water. Both methods are impressive attempts to solve a rather difficult measurement problem and to some extent they serve their purpose. However, they create additional problems. Close shielding of the pH bulb reduces the exposed surface of the probe to the gastric contents and may actually act as a trap for mucus. Infusing water across the face of the bulb may flush off the unwanted materials, but water alters the pH of the gastric contents.

A possible solution to these measurement difficulties may involve the use of a controlled, expandable umbrella cage to protect the probe from direct contact with the mucosa which should be sufficiently large to permit a free flow of materials through it. Air injections could remove unwanted materials from the surface of the electrode.

4.1.3. Intragastric Acid Titration

Titration of acid within the stomach is a method of analyzing changes in acid secretion over short intervals. The method involves the placing of a pH probe into the stomach and then infusing a specific quantity of bicarbonate solution to neutralize the contents to pH 7.0. The amount of bicarbonate needed to achieve neutrality becomes the measure of acid secretion. Norman's procedure (1969) involved locating a pH telemetry capsule in the fundus and then requiring the subject to swallow 30 milliliters of saturated potassium bicarbonate ($KHCO_3$). The result was a shift in the pH toward neutral or slightly alkaline condition. The time required to return to the basal pH level served as the measure of acid secretion rate. The method has been shown to be an accurate measure of acid secretion rate (e.g., Noller, 1962; Stavney, Hamilton, Sircus, & Smith, 1966).

Whitehead, Renault, and Goldiamond (1975) also used intragastric titration to measure acid secretion changes. In their study, in which subjects were reinforced for changes in pH, sodium bicarbonate (1 N) was infused each time pH declined to 2.0. The amount of sodium bicarbonate required to repeatedly neutralize the contents to pH 7.0 became the measure of acid secretion in milliequivalents per minute.

Intragastric acid titration has the advantage of providing immediate information of acid changes and avoids the necessitity of aspirating stomach contents for *in vitro* titrations. However, infusing fluids into the stomach, especially alkaline solutions, stimulates acid secretion. Inflated acid production and loss of the contents through the pylorus can result. In order to reduce the tendency for the contents to pass quickly into the duodenum, potassium bicarbonate may be used instead of sodium bicarbonate for infusion. Potassium bicarbonate ions tend to retard gastric emptying while sodium ions stimulate it (Connell & Waters, 1964; Hunt, 1959).

The intragastric titration measurement procedure suffers from the same source of artifact observed with pH telemetry and intragastric pH electrode measurement.

4.2. External Measurement of Gastric Acid

A method of avoiding the difficulties of measuring pH and acid concentration within the stomach involves collecting the contents for measurement outside of the stomach. Analyzing acid secretions outside of the stomach requires aspirating the contents, which are then monitored with a pH glass electrode. Secretions are removed through a nasogastric tube under low vacuum and either analyzed on line or collected for later testing.

On-line measures require continuous pH monitoring of gastric juice. Welgan (1974) developed a method of continuously measuring acid as it was aspirated from the stomach by mounting a collection vessel near the subject's face. Acid secretions from the nasogastric tube were collected in the vessel briefly as the pH electrode and reference electrode, which were immersed in the continuously flowing fluids, recorded pH on line. Aspirated acid volumes exceeding 3 ml emptied from the measurement vessel into another container for later *in vitro* measurement of acid concentration and volume. The on-line procedure permitted relatively immediate feedback of information to duodenal ulcer patients who were reinforced for pH changes.

Moore and Schenkenberg (1974) have also reported using an external pH measurement procedure in their study of the effect of biofeedback on gastric acid changes. In their study, acid contents were aspirated under low, periodic vacuum and collected for *in vitro* measurement. There was no attempt to continuously measure pH changes. Rather, the acid information was presented at 10-min intervals during training as biofeedback information on preceding gastric acid secretions within that interval.

The external measurement of acid pH avoids the inherent problems of intragastric measurement (e.g., inadvertent electrode contact with the stomach wall and entrapment in the stomach folds). A fluoroscopically controlled placement of the nasogastric tube enables virtually total retrieval of the gastric contents as they collect in the antrum. Further, no fluids are infused into the stomach, thereby eliminating an otherwise potent stimulus to acid secretion and motor activity. The pH apparatus is also considerably less expensive than either pH telemetry or internal electrodes.

There are also disadvantages to external measurement of acid. The tip of the nasogastric tube is subject to occassional blockages. Infusing air through the tube, however, tends to remove the obstructions and vacuum pressure levels which are low (3–5 mm Hg) or periodic suction reduces the risk of such blockages. Higher pressures are likely to draw the mucosa around the tube. In this event, reducing the pressure and manually pulling the tube up slightly will free it and restore normal circulation.

In research requiring a continuous measurement of acid pH, subjects displaying a relatively high rate of basal acid secretion may be favored. This ensures a relatively continuous flow of acid contents from the stomach for analysis. Welgan (1974, 1976, 1977) used duodenal ulcer patients in his studies of learned control of acid secretions since they are known to produce high rates of acid secretion. Subjects were selected if they secreted at least 10 cc of acid per 30-min period.

In research requiring rapid information of acid changes such as biofeedback, aspiration of contents to an on-line electrode assembly can produce a delay which is a function of the viscosity of the fluid. Welgan has estimated the transport time from the stomach to the pH electrode to be between 3 and 30 sec.

As with any intubation procedure, there may be some discomfort during the placement of the nasogastric tube. Subjects who have habituated to the procedure report little or no discomfort. The tube placement can stimulate acid secretions since the tube is a foreign body in the stomach. However, the magnitude of the gastric response tends to be less than to infusion of buffer solutions into the stomach.

Titration of aspirated acid outside of the stomach follows traditional testing procedures in gastroenterology. While Welgan (1974) analyzed the pH of acid secretions on line, the secretions were later titrated for total acid content and volume. Samples from the collections were titrated with 0.1 N NaOH and the results expressed as milliequivalents of HCl per liter.

The disadvantage of this method of analysis lies in its inability to furnish rapid feedback for biofeedback research. The problem could be resolved in future research by implementing two improvements. First, an on-line titration procedure could be constructed similar to that used with intragastric titration. In this case, titrations would be made at the site of the collection vessel and pH electrode. A much simpler method of obtaining acid concentration measures would involve programming a computer to transform on-line pH measurements to acid concentration based on the transformation formulas of Moore and Scarlata (1965).

5. Subject Considerations in Gastric Research

5.1. Subject Selection

Subjects for the study of acid secretions have generally been healthy with no history of gastric disease (Gorman & Kamiya, 1972; Moore & Schenkenberg, 1974; Norman, 1969; Whitehead, Renault, & Goldiamond, 1975). Welgan (1974), on the other hand, used duodenal ulcer patients to obtain maximal acid output per unit of time. The relatively high acid output of duodenal ulcer patients (Baron, 1963) provided the high acid secretory rate necessary to obtain continuous acid measurement.

5.2. Subject Preparation

Food is a potent stimulus of acid secretion. Therefore, the subject should fast from 8 to 12 hr prior to acid measurement. No analysis should be performed with food in the stomach.

All medications affecting gastric secretion should be discontinued at least 24 hr prior to testing. Several medications have been found to affect gastric secretions including cholinergic drugs (Koelle, 1965), anticholinergic drugs (Henn, Isenberg, Maxwell, & Sturdevant, 1975), histamine H-receptor antagonists such as cimetidine (e.g., Henn, Isenberg, Maxwell, & Sturdevant, 1975), bromazepam (Stacher & Stärker, 1975), diazepam (Birnbaum, Karmeli, & Tefera, 1971), trimipramine (Myren & Berstad, 1975), and carbonic anhydrase inhibitors (Linder, Cohen, Berkowitz, & Janowitz, 1964).

Studies of circadian cycles indicate that there are circadian effects on gastric secretions (Moore & Englert, 1970). Therefore, subjects should all be tested at the same time each test period. Repeated measures on the same subject should also be conducted at the same time each day. Generally, the subject should fast overnight and undergo testing the following morning before breakfast.

Saliva, when swallowed, can alter the acid concentration of the stomach contents. Therefore, during the gastric acid analysis, saliva should be removed from the mouth with a sputum ejector under low vacuum. Expectoration of saliva is also common, although this method is not recommended in studies requiring a minimum of body movement.

Proper positioning of the subject is necessary for comfort and accurate measurement of acid secretions. Prolonged discomfort can stimulate acid secretions. Further, a poorly positioned subject may promote unwanted emptying of the gastric contents through the pylorus or promote bile reflux from the duodenum into the stomach raising pH markedly and reducing acid concentration in the stomach. Hector (1968) has shown that placing the subject in a recumbent position on the left side allows optimal collection of gastric contents. Welgan (1974) and Whitehead, Renault, and Goldiamond (1975) used a similar subject position. In other studies, Welgan (1976, 1977) had subjects sit in a semireclining position in a chair and obtained acid secretions from the antrum without difficulty.

5.3. Intubation Procedure

There are several nasogastric and orogastric tubes available for aspiration. The more effective tubes contain a second side tube for an air bleed to improve gastric aspiration. Air entering the stomach through the tube tends to prevent tube blockages from stomach fold enclosures and mucus.

Fluoroscopic placement improves acid collection. The tip of the tube is usually placed in the most dependent portion of the gastric antrum. Frequently, the tip of the tube will coil in the fundus, esophagus, or the tracheobronchial tree (Baron, 1963). Flouroscopic placement can eliminate these hazards. If fluoroscopy is not available, the tube can be placed so the tip is approximately 55–60 cm from the nares. Gastric contents are then aspirated, and 30 to 60 ml of water are infused through the tube. A correctly placed tube will allow 90% of the water to be retrieved. Retrieval of less than this volume indicates that the tube is not in the dependent portion of the antrum (Isenberg, 1978).

Gastric aspiration may be accomplished by manual suction or with a suction pump. Suction pumps generally offer the advantage of producing steady retrieval rates conveniently. Suction pumps are designed to aspirate periodically or continuously. Period suction usually occurs at 2- or 3-min intervals. While these retrieval cycles can be adapted to some types of psychophysiological research, continuous suction is recommended when rapid aspiration of acid is needed. Low suction (3–5 mm Hg) will reduce the likelihood of tube blockages under continuous vacuum. Occasional infusion of air will also help to keep the tube free from blockages.

6. References

Baron, J. Studies of basal and peak acid output with an augmented histamine test. *Gut*, 1963, *4*, 136–144.
Beaumont, W. *Experiments and observations on the gastric juice and the physiology of digestion.* Plattsburg: F. P. Allen, 1833.
Birnbaum, D., Karmeli, F., & Tefera, M. The effects of diazepam on human gastric secretion. *Gut*, 1971, *12*, 616–618.
Connell, A., & Waters, T. Assessment of gastric function by pH telemetering capsule. Lancet, 1964, 2, 227–230.
Cummins, A. Applied anatomy and physiology of the stomach. In H. L. Bockus (Ed.), *Gastroenterology* (Vol. 1). Philadelphia: W. B. Saunders, 1963.
Ekenved, G., & Walan, A. In vitro studies on the neutralizing effect of antacids using the Heidelberg capsule. *Scandinavian Journal of Gastroenterology*, 1975, *10*, 267–272.
Gambescia, J., Krawiec, J., Desiderio, V., & Polish, E. Gastric pH *in situ* with multiple electrodes. In C. M. Thompson, D. Berkowitz, & E. Polish (Eds.), *The stomach*. New York: Grune & Stratton, 1967.
Gordon, O., & Chernya, Y. Physiology of the gastric secretion in man: Studies on patients with gastric fistula and artificial esophagus. *Klinicheskaya Meditsina*, 1940, *18*, 63–71.
Gormon, P., & Kamiya, J. *Biofeedback training of stomach pH*. Paper presented at the Western Psychological Association Meeting, San Francisco, 1972.
Grossman, M. What do you do with basal acid in dose-response studies? A suggested answer. *Gastroenterology*, 1973, *65*, 341.
Grossman, M. Control of gastric secretion. In M. Sleisenger & J. Fordtran (Eds.), *Gastrointestinal disease*. Philadelphia: W. B. Saunders, 1978.
Hector, R. Improved technique of gastric aspiration. *Lancet*, 1968, *1*, 15–16.
Henn, R., Isenberg, J., Maxwell, V., & Sturdevant, R. Inhibition of gastric acid secretion by cimetidine in duodenal ulcer patients. *New England Journal of Medicine*, 1975, *293*, 371–375.
Hunt, J. Gastric emptying and secretion in man. *Physiological Review*, 1959, *39*, 491–553.
Isenberg, J. Gastric secretory testing. In M. Sleisinger & J. Fordtran (Eds.), *Gastrointestinal disease*. Philadelphia: W. B. Saunders, 1978.
Koelle, G. Parasympathomimetic agents. In L. Goodman & A. Gillman (Eds.), *The pharmacological basis of therapeutics*. New York: Macmillan, 1965.

Linder, A., Cohen, N., Berkowits, J., & Janowitz, H. A note on the oral dose of acetazolamide required to inhibit acid secretion. *Gastroenterology*, 1964, *46*, 273-275.

Moore, J., & Englert, E. Circadian rhythm of gastric acid secretion in man. *Nature*, 1970, *226*, 1261-1262.

Moore, J., & Scarlata, R. The determination of gastric acidity by the glass electrode. *Gastroenterology*, 1965, *49*, 178-188.

Moore, J., & Schenkenberg, T. Psychic control of gastric secretion: Response to anticipated feeding and biofeedback training in man. *Gastroenterology*, 1974, *66*, 954-959.

Myren, J., & Berstad, A. The early effect of trimipramine (surmontil) on gastric secretion in man. *Scandinavian Journal of Gastroenterology*, 1975, *10*, 817-189.

Noller, H. Results of examinations of stomach functions with the Endo-Radio capsule—The Heidelberg capsule—A new appliance for assisting stomach diagnosis. *Fortschritte der Medizin*, 1962, *9*, 351-355.

Norman, A. Response contingency and human gastric acidity. *Psychophysiology*, 1969, *5*, 673-681.

Richet, C. Des propriétés chimiques et physiologiques du suc gastrique chez l'homme et les animaux (Appendix A). *Journal of Anatomy and Physiology*, 1878, *14*, 170-333.

Rovelstad, R., Owen, C., & Magath, T. Factors influencing the continuous recording of in situ pH of gastric and duodenal contents. *Gastroenterology*, 1952, *20*, 609-624.

Stacher, G., & Stärker, D. Inhibitory effect of bromazepam on insulin-stimulated gastric acid secretion in man. *American Journal of Digestive Disease*, 1975, *20*, 156-161.

Stavney, L., Hamilton, T., Sircus, W., & Smith, A. Evaluation of the pH sensitive telemetering capsule in the estimation of gastric secretory capacity. *American Journal of Digestive Diseases*, 1966, *11*, 753-760.

Welgan, P. Learned control of gastric acid secretions in ulcer patients. *Psychosomatic Medicine*, 1974, *36*, 411-419.

Welgan, P. Biofeedback control of stomach acid secretions and gastrointestinal reactions. In J. Beatty & H. Legewie (Eds), *Biofeedback and behavior*. New York: Plenum Press, 1976.

Welgan, P. *Short term and long term conditioning of gastric acid secretions*. Paper presented at the 1st International Conference on Biofeedback, Tübingen, W. Germany, November 1977.

Whitehead, W., Renault, P., & Goldiamond, I. Modification of human acid secretion with operant conditioning procedures. *Journal of Applied Behavior Analysis*, 1975, *8*, 147-156.

Wolf, S. *The stomach*. New York: Oxford University Press, 1965.

Wolf, S., & Welsh, J. The gastrointestinal tract as a response system. In N. Greenfield & R. Sternbach (Eds.), *Handbood of psychophysiology*. New York: Holt, Rinehart & Winston, 1972.

Wolf, S., & Wolff, H. *Human gastric function*. New York: Oxford University Press, 1943.

8

TELEMETRIC AND ISOTOPE METHODS OF MEASURING GASTRIC ACID SECRETION, MOTILITY, AND EMPTYING

GEORG STACHER

1. Measurement of Gastric Acid Secretion by Intragastric Titration and a Telemetering pH Sensor

The classical methods of measuring gastric acid secretion by means of a nasogastric tube and extra- or intracorporal titration are of limited value in psychophysiological investigations. The stimuli arising from the tube impose considerable stress on the subjects and often induce retching and nausea. The stimuli, thereby, can alter the physiological state of the whole organism including the function of the organ under study.

A procedure which causes much less discomfort and strain to the subjects employs intragastric titration and a telemetering capsule as an intragastric pH sensor. Out of various pH-sensitive telemetric devices described so far (Ardenne & Sprung, 1958b; Collins, Martel, Well, & Hamilton, 1972; Jacobsen & Mackay, 1957; Kitigawa, Nishigor, Murata, Nishimoto, & Takada, 1966; Meldrum, Watson, Riddle, Bown, & Sladen, 1972) only one (Nöller, 1960) is commercially available at present (AEG-Telefunken). This device, known as the Heidelberg Capsule, consists of a high-frequency transmitter, a pH sensor, and a power supply, which are encased in an acrylic capsule measuring 20 × 6 mm. The transmitter operates on a Hartley circuit with a carrier frequency of about 1.9 megahertz. It is powered by a miniature battery assembly activated before use by

---

GEORG STACHER • Psychophysiology Unit at the Psychiatric and at the First Surgical Clinic, University of Vienna, A-1090 Vienna, Austria.

an electrolyte, that is, isotonic saline. The pH sensor consists of an external antimony electrode in direct contact with the surrounding gastric contents, and a silver chloride electrode inside the capsule. The electrodes are separated by a dialysis membrane permeable to ions but not to large molecules. Changes in the pH of the surrounding fluid alter the output voltage of the sensor battery, which in turn modulates the frequency of the transmitter circuit. The frequency shift per pH unit is about 16 kilohertz (kHz), that is, about 80 kHz for the range from pH 2 to pH 7. If the capsule is calibrated prior to use in buffer solutions of pH 2, 5, and 7 at body temperature, it is possible to determine the pH of an unknown solution from the frequency of the transmitter circuit.

The signal of the capsule is received by an antenna system consisting of three aerials polarized at right angles to each other. The antenna is associated with an amplifying receiver and a pen recorder. As the commercially available receiver is very unsatisfactory, a new receiver was developed (Klaus & Stacher, 1983) which is devised also to measure the strength of the directional electromagnetic field emitted by the capsule. As the direction of the field varies with the movements of the stomach wall, it is possible to record the occurrence of gastric movements. However, this magnetometric method, although very sensitive, does not allow inferences on the extent of movements, which are detected even when no pressure elevations are present. The life span of the capsule is limited by battery and varies between 8 and 18 hr. The frequency drift can be as great as 20–28 kHz per 4 hr which, however, can be compensated for. As the capsule is radiopaque, its position within the body can be determined fluoroscopically. To avoid high-frequency interference, it is recommended to perform the measurements in a screened room.

The calibrated capsule with a thin silk thread attached to it is swallowed, and its arrival in the stomach is indicated by the recording of an acidic pH. The thread then is fixed to the cheek or nose of the subject to prevent the capsule from being transported further downstream. The subject is placed in a bed or comfortable chair in a semirecumbent or recumbent position and slightly turned to the left.

The intragastric titration begins with the neutralization of the gastric contents with 2 ml of molar potassium bicarbonate ($KHCO_3$) administered orally with a syringe. When enough gastric acid is produced to bring the gastric pH back to the original acidic level, another 2 ml $KHCO_3$ are administered and the monitoring of gastric acid secretion begins. During the time of investigation, doses of 2 ml $KHCO_3$ are administered whenever the level of pH 5.0 is reached. The times from one neutralization to the next are measured. Each interneutralization time is assumed to be identical with the time during which 2 millimole (mmol) of hydrochloric acid are produced by the stomach. From these interneutralization times, acid output in mmol per unit of time is calculated. The smaller the amount of $KHCO_3$ administered per titration the higher is the temporal resolution of the intragastric titration technique.

KHCO$_3$ is chosen as a titrant as it has been shown that potassium tends to inhibit gastric emptying and thereby to limit the error arising from the loss of gastric contents through the pylorus. Sodium, by contrast, tends to accelerate gastric emptying (Hunt & Pathak, 1960). The titration endpoint of pH 5.0 was chosen because the probability of error caused by the presence within the stomach of carbon dioxide produced by the titration is not great at this pH (Christiansen, 1980).

Although various authors comparing the intragastric titration method with the tube method reported a high correlation between the acid outputs measured with the two techniques (Connell & Waters, 1964; Stack, 1969; Stavney, Hamilton, Sircus, & Smith, 1966; Yarborough, McAlhany, Cooper, & Weidner, 1969), the values obtained by intragastric titration tend to be slightly higher than those obtained by tube suction. This might be caused by the fact that acidic gastric juice reaching the duodenum when the aspiration method is employed inhibits gastric acid output (Spenney, 1979), while the neutralized gastric contents reaching the duodenum during intragastric titration cause no inhibition. Provided the subjects under study are instructed appropriately, the doses of bicarbonate to be administered for titration can be given also during states of deep relaxation, hypnosis, and even sleep without major disruption of the prevailing state of activation (Stacher, Presslich, & Stärker, 1975).

The intragastric titration method with an endoradiosonde as a pH sensor has proved to be a reliable tool not only in physiological (Ekenved & Walan, 1975; Johannesson, Magnusson, Sjöberg, & Skov-Jensen, 1973; Stacher & Dinstl, 1973; Stacher & Stärker, 1974; Stacher & Stärker, 1975; Stacher, Bauer, Brunner, & Grünberger, 1976; Stacher, Bauer, Schulze, Pointner, & Landgraf, 1976) but also in psychophysiological investigations (Berner & Stacher, 1971; Stacher, Berner, & Naske, 1973; Stacher, Berner, Naske, Schuster, Bauer, Stärker, & Schulze, 1975). By recording the electromagnetic field strength of the capsule the method also provides a qualitative measure of the movements of the gastric wall. Unfortunately, the high cost of equipment and the necessity of a screened room have impeded, until now, a broader application of this reliable and rather unintrusive method.

2. Measurement of Intragastric Pressures by Means of a Telemetering Capsule

The direct measurement of gastric contractile activity generally requires the passage of tubes through the nose, mouth, or artificial opening into the stomach. Those used for collecting gastric acid cause discomfort, emotional distress, and even nausea to the subject and can result in changes in the function of the organ being studied. Nausea has been shown to be accompanied by a marked inhibition of gastric motility (Wolf, 1943). The use of ingestible pressure-sensitive telemetering capsules, by contrast, permits the measurement of gastric pressures under relatively "natural" conditions.

A variety of pressure sensitive capsules has been described (Ardenne & Sprung, 1958a; Farrar, Zworykin, & Baum, 1957; Fink & Stacher, 1972; Mackay & Jacobson, 1957; Rowlands & Wolff, 1960; Silverstone, Smith, & Stunkard, 1968; Thompson, Valori, & Wingate, 1982). However, mainly due to the limited potential market, no such device is commercially available at present. Pressure-sensitive radio pills consist basically of a transistorized oscillator powered by a replaceable tiny mercury battery and a pressure sensor.

The capsule in use in our laboratory (Fink & Stacher, 1972) employs a pressure sensor consisting of a gold membrane bonded to a piece of iron, which is moved by the pressure changes within the coil of a tuned circuit. This in turn modulates the frequency of the oscillations generated by the transmitter. The oscillations are detected by an assembly of three unidirectional antennas located over the abdomen of the subject. A frequency-modulation receiver (Klaus & Stacher, 1983) demodulates and amplifies the signals, and the pressure fluctuations are recorded on paper and/or magnetic tape. As the capsule radiates only a small amount of energy and the movements of the device in the stomach result in changes of signal strength at the antenna, the receiver automatically increases amplification as the signal fades and, thereby, indicates correct pressure even at very low signal strengths. When the signal becomes too weak, another antenna providing better detection can be selected manually (a switch) or automatically. The recording of the strength of the signal, which depends on the orientation of the capsule and its distance from the antenna, provides information on the movements of the gastric wall. This technique is sensitive enough to record minute movements even when no pressure elevations are present. No inference, however, can be drawn as to the extent of the movement, and only the number of movements per unit of time can be evaluated.

The capsules in use in our laboratory operate on a carrier frequency of about 1.9 MHz and respond to a pressure change of 10 mm of mercury (mm Hg) with a frequency change of about 1 kHz. The frequency changes linearly in response to pressure changes between -30 and $+600$ mm Hg. The maximum frequency response is above 300 Hz. The capsule measures 35 × 6 mm and has a weight of 8 g. To allow measurements over a long period of time the capsule is powered by two mercury hearing aid batteries (Mallory Type MS-13 H/1.5 V). It is calibrated prior to the beginning and possibly after a study by a manometer at body temperature. Immediately after calibration, the subject swallows the capsule. To ensure a position within the stomach, a surgical silk thread can be attached to the capsule to allow an "anchoring" of the device. The subject lies in a bed or sits on a chair throughout the experiment or can even move freely in the room. To prevent high-frequency interference, it is necessary to perform all measurements in a screened room and to install choke filters in the electricity supply.

Upon completion of the study, the subject is instructed to save all stools until the capsule is recovered. The capsule is cleaned with germicidal agents, and new batteries are installed before reuse. The "life" of the capsules is determined mainly by the life of the diaphragm and can last for 5 to 15 passages. When the capsule is used for the measurement of gastric pressures only and is withdrawn from the stomach by the thread, the durability of the membrane is much longer.

3. Measurement of Gastric Motility and Emptying by a Radioisotope Technique

The measurement of gastric emptying under approximately physiological conditions poses more problems than that of gastric contractile activity. Recently, a noninvasive technique has been introduced which allows recording of gastric emptying together with antral contractile activity (Akkermans, Jacobs, Hong-Yoe, Roelofs, & Wittebol, 1980; Jacobs, Akkermans, Hong-Joe, Hoekstra, & Wittebol, 1982). The subjects are given a semisolid test meal thoroughly mixed with a low dose of a nonabsorbable radioactive tracer. Gastric emptying is recorded by a gamma camera and a digital computer system by counting the decrease in radioactivity over the stomach. Contractile activity is recorded by measuring the phasic changes of radioactivity in two or more small regions over the antrum. Thereby, modulation depth, which corresponds to the amplitude of contractions, frequency, and propagation velocity of antral contractions can be determined. However, as this method requires the ingestion of a radioisotope, ethical problems could arise when its employment in healthy subjects is considered.

4. References

Akkermans, L. M. A., Jacobs, F., Hong-Yoe, O., Roelofs, J. M. M., & Wittebol, P. A noninvasive method to quantify antral contractile activity in man and dog. In J. Christensen (Ed.), *Gastrointestinal motility*. New York: Raven Press, 1980.

Ardenne, M. v., & Sprung, H. B. Über Versuche mit einem verschluckbaren Intestinalsender. *Naturwissenschaften*, 1958, *45*, 154–155. (a)

Ardenne, M. v., & Sprung, H. B. Über den verschluckbaren Intestinalsender mit pH-Wert-Signalisierung. *Naturwissenschaften*, 1958, *45*, 654–565. (b)

Berner, P., & Stacher, G. Zur Reproduzierbarkeit von Angstzuständen und deren Auswirkung auf die Magensäureproduktion. *Zeitschrift für Psychosomatik und Medizinische Psychoanalyse*, 1971, *17*, 356–362.

Christiansen, J. *In vivo* intragastric titration. *Gastroenterology*, 1980, *78*, 423–424.

Collins, W. J., Martel, A. J., Well, R. F., & Hamilton, G. B. Use of the Corning pH capsule to evaluate the duration of effectiveness of various doses of an aluminum–magnesium hydroxide preparation. *Gastroenterology*, 1972, *62*, 736.

Connell, A. M., & Waters, T. E. Assessment of gastric function by pH telemetering capsule. *Lancet*, 1964, *2*, 227–230.

Ekenved, G., & Walan, A. *In vivo* studies on the neutralizing effect of antacids using the Heidelberg capsule. *Scandinavian Journal of Gastroenterology*, 1975, *10*, 267-272.

Farrar, J. T., Zworykin, V. K., & Baum, J. Pressure-sensitive telemetering capsule for study of gastrointestinal motility. *Science*, 1957, *126*, 975-976.

Fink, G., & Stacher, G. Eine neue Endoradiosonde zur Messung intraluminaler Drucke im Magendarmtrakt. *Acta Chirurgica Austriaca*, 1972, *4*, 1-6.

Hunt, J. N., & Pathak, J. D. The osmotic effects of some simple molecules and ions on gastric emptying. *Journal of Physiology*, 1960, *154*, 254-269.

Jacobson, B., & Mackay, R. S. A pH-endoradiosonde. *Lancet*, 1957, *1*, 1224.

Jacobs, F., Akkermans, L. M. A., Oei Hong Yoe, Hoekstra, A., & Wittebol, P. A radioisotope method to quantify the function of fundus, antrum, and their contractile activity in gastric emptying of semi-solid and solid meal. In M. Wienbeck (Ed.), *Motility of the digestive tract*. New York: Raven Press, 1982.

Johannesson, E., Magnusson, P. O., Sjöberg, N. O., & Skov-Jensen, A. Intragastric pH evaluation with radiotelemetry. *Scandinavian Journal of Gastroenterology*, 1973, *8*, 65-69.

Klaus, R., & Stacher, G. A new amplifying receiver for use with telemetering capsules recording pH and pressure in the gastrointestinal tract. Manuscript in preparation, 1983.

Kitagawa, K., Nishigor, A., Murata, N., Nishimoto, K., & Takada, H. Radiotelemetry of the pH of the gastrointestinal tract by glass electrode. *Gastroenterology*, 1966, *51*, 368-372.

Mackay, R. S., & Jacobson, B. Endoradiosonde. *Nature*, 1957, *179*, 1239-1240.

Meldrum, S. J., Watson, B. W., Riddle, H. C., Brown, R. L., & Sladen, G. E. pH profile of gut as measured by radiotelemetry capsule. *British Medical Journal*, 1972, *2*, 104-106.

Nöller, H. G. Die Endoradiosonde zur elektrischen pH-Messung im Magen und ihre klinische Bedeutung. *Deutsche Medizinische Wochenschrift*, 1960, *39*, 1707-1713.

Rowlands, E. N., & Wolff, H. S. The radio pill: Telemetering from the digestive tract. *British Communications and Electronics*, 1960, *7*, 598-601.

Silverstone, J. T., Smith, G. P., & Stunkard, A. J. Gastric pressures recorded by a telemetering capsule. *American Journal of Digestive Diseases*, 1968, *13*, 615-618.

Spenney, J. G. Physical chemical and technical limitations to intragastric titration. *Gastroenterology*, 1979, *76*, 1025-1034.

Stacher, G., Berner, P., & Naske, R. Der Einfluß von Ruhesuggestion in Hypnose auf die Magensaftproduktion. *Wiener Medizinische Wochenschrift*, 1973, *123*, 160-164.

Stacher, G., & Dinstl, K. Die Säureproduktion des resezierten Magens. *Acta Chirurgica Austriaca*, 1973, *5*, 54-58.

Stacher, G., & Stärker, D. Inhibitory effect of bromazepam on basal and betazole-stimulated gastric acid secretion in man. *Gut*, 1974, *15*, 116-120.

Stacher, G., Berner, P., Naske, R., Schuster, P., Bauer, P., Stärker, D., & Schulze, D. Effect of hypnotic suggestion of relaxation on basal and betazole-stimulated gastric acid secretion. *Gastroenterology*, 1975, *68*, 656-661.

Stacher, G., Presslich, B., & Stärker, H. Gastric acid secretion and sleep-stages during natural night sleep. *Gastroenterology*, 1975, *68*, 1449-1455.

Stacher, G., & Stärker, D. Inhibitory effect of bromazepam on insulin-stimulated gastric acid secretion in man. *American Journal of Digestive Diseases*, 1975, *20*, 156-161.

Stacher, G., Bauer, P., Brunner, H., & Grünberger, J. Gastric acid secretion, serum-gastrin, and psychomotor function under the influence of placebo, insulin-hypoglycemia, and/or bromazepam. *International Journal of Clinical Pharmacology*, 1976, *13*, 1-10.

Stacher, G., Bauer, P., Schulze, D., Pointner, H., & Landgraf, M. Effect of alterations of blood glucose levels on gastric acid secretion, plasma gastrin, and plasma osmolality in man. *American Journal of Digestive Diseases*, 1976, *21*, 563-568.

Stack, B. H. R. Use of the Heidelberg pH capsule in the routine assessment of gastric acid secretion. *Gut,* 1969, *10,* 245–246.

Stavney, L. S., Hamilton, T., Sircus, W., & Smith, A. N. Evaluation of the pH-sensitive telemetering capsule in the estimation of gastric secretory capacity. *American Journal of Digestive Diseases,* 1966, *11,* 753–760.

Thompson, D. G., Valori, R. M., & Wingate, D. L. Radiotelemetry of human jejunal pressure activity; Retrospect and prospect. In M. Wienbeck (Ed.), *Motility of the digestive tract.* New York: Raven Press, 1982.

Wolf, S. The relation of gastric function to nausea in man. *Journal of Clinical Investigation,* 1943, *22,* 877–882.

Yarborough, D. R., III., McAlhany, J. C., Cooper, N., & Weidner, M. G., Jr. Evaluation of the Heidelberg pH capsule: Method of tubeless gastric analysis. *American Journal of Surgery,* 1969, *117,* 185–192.

9

RESPONSIVENESS OF THE STOMACH TO ENVIRONMENTAL EVENTS
ROBERT M. STERN

1. Introduction

I first became interested in the motility of the stomach while working in R. C. Davis's laboratory in 1960. It is my feeling that 20 years later we still know very little about the responsiveness of the stomach to environmental events. I will begin with a discussion of the various reasons for the paucity of knowledge in this area and then describe some of the environment–stomach relationships that have been reported.

2. Causes for Inadequate Information about Stomach Responsiveness

There are at least four factors that have contributed to our lack of understanding of the effects of environmental events on stomach activity. They are as follows:

1. Unreliability of subjective reports
2. Difficulties with all known recording techniques
3. Confounding by digestive functions
4. Confounding by "spontaneous" activity

ROBERT M. STERN • Department of Psychology, The Pennsylvania State University, University Park, Pennsylvania 16802.

2.1. Unreliability of Subjective Reports

The first and most obvious way to obtain data on the responsiveness of the stomach to environmental events from humans is to ask them. In a study published in 1969 (Stern & Higgins, 1969), we reported the results of a questionnaire, the Somatic Perception Questionnaire (SPQ; see Figure 1 for a revised form) which was administered to over 600 college students, their siblings, and

---

Below you will find a list of 10 reactions to stress which was obtained from a previous Psychology 2 class. On the scale opposite each response indicate by circling the appropriate number the degree to which you are aware of that response in situations such as (a) before an important interview, (b) before making a speech or presentation in front of strangers, (c) before going to or while waiting in a medical doctor's or dentist's office, or (d) any other situation you find stressful.

	Always				Never
Face feels hot or flushed	1	2	3	4	5
Nervous stomach	1	2	3	4	5
Sweating palms	1	2	3	4	5
Lump in throat or dryness in mouth	1	2	3	4	5
Cold hands and/or feet	1	2	3	4	5
General restlessness	1	2	3	4	5
General body sweating	1	2	3	4	5
Increased heart rate	1	2	3	4	5
Frequent urination or urge to urinate	1	2	3	4	5
Awareness of heart beat	1	2	3	4	5

Figure 1. Somatic Perception Questionnaire.

parents. The purpose of the study was to examine the effects of sex, age, and familial occurrence on an individual's perceived somatic reactions to stress. In brief, the results demonstrated that sex and age were important determiners of perceived bodily responses to stress. Reports of a particular bodily reaction by the parents but not by the same-sexed sibling, greatly increased the probability of a student reporting the occurrence of that same reaction.

Two aspects of that study are germane to this discussion. Table 1 displays a summary of the basic questionnaire data. As can be seen, for college students and their siblings, but not as great a degree for their parents, the most common bodily reaction reported to stressful situations was "nervous stomach." Some time after collecting these data, I interviewed a sample of the subjects who had reported "nervous stomach" as their predominant response to stress in an attempt to learn more about their gastrointestinal reactions. The great majority of these college students described for me vague aches and pains which occur in their stomachs while pointing to the area of their abdomen over their intestines. I have discussed these results with a gastroenterologist who said that more than half of his patients complain of vague aches and pains in their stomach but that his subsequent examination usually indicates that the difficulty is in the intestine. I think that it is interesting how the stomach has become so predominant in reported gastrointestinal symptomatology in the United States.

In 1975, working together with three colleagues at Penn State (Guthrie, Verstraete, Deines, & Stern, 1975), we gave an expanded version of the SPQ to

Table 1
Percentage Subjects Reporting Each Stress Reaction as a Function of Sex and Age[a]

Stress reaction	Sex		Age	
	Males	Females	Students and siblings	Parents
1. Face feels hot or flushed	19	32	27	24
2. Nervous stomach	55	66	68	45
3. Sweating (palms)	48	41	54	27
4. Lump in throat or dryness in mouth	23	21	20	26
5. Cold hands and/or feet	14	32	28	13
6. General restlessness	60	58	60	57
7. General body sweating	26	25	27	24
8. Increase heart rate	51	50	53	46
9. Frequent urination or urge to urinate	16	24	17	27
10. Awareness of heartbeat	43	53	51	42

[a]From Stern and Higgins (1969).

French, American, Filipino, and Haitian college students. These samples enabled us to examine differences by sex, language (French in Haiti, and English in the Philippines), and level of industrialization, with the United States and France as highly industrialized societies. Table 2 shows the expanded questionnaire and

Table 2
Analysis of Variance: F Ratios for Main Effects and Interactions of Sex (S), Industrialization (I), and Language (L) for 33 Items of Questionnaire ($N = 823$)[a]

Item (abbreviated)	F Ratio					
	S	I	L	S × I	S × L	I × L
1. Flushed face	3.22	1.84	9.10[b]	6.65	.00	9.75[b]
2. Excess gas	6.35	30.66[b]	11.17[b]	2.80	.43	19.90[b]
3. Cold hands	11.65[b]	39.03[b]	37.56[b]	2.27	1.50	.77
4. Oppressed	5.36	2.88	24.37[b]	.01	8.87[b]	2.77
5. Lump in throat	.90	5.80	1.09	2.01	1.00	.21
6. Memory stops	4.37	1.22	.47	2.03	3.96	.23
7. Stutters	1.42	47.78[b]	8.97[b]	.02	1.49	1.77
8. Aware of heartbeat	19.58[b]	.22	.54	.66	.00	.28
9. Breath short	.02	23.73[b]	.03	.33	.03	2.57
10. Diarrhea	6.78[b]	2.97	5.40	.03	2.36	13.74[b]
11. Thoughts confused	3.41	15.35[b]	3.83	1.43	.42	.76
12. Sweaty palms	.34	8.50	2.62	.05	5.92	.16
13. Heartbeat quick	10.37[b]	.59	.16	.03	.95	2.35
14. Feels guilty	.00	19.59[b]	13.72[b]	.44	1.11	12.34[b]
15. Urge to urinate	0.41	23.37[b]	.03	3.20	2.66	6.56
16. Nightmares	20.30[b]	13.90[b]	22.29[b]	.69	.49	5.60
17. Rashes and pimples	.89	21.30[b]	2.33	4.41	.43	33.15[b]
18. Knot in stomach	30.63[b]	29.72[b]	1.46	.28	.08	8.64[b]
19. Feels weak	15.29[b]	45.08[b]	.10	.82	.30	8.66[b]
20. Can't concentrate	16.01[b]	6.81[b]	4.08	.37	.29	8.29[b]
21. Body sweat	.93	.20	18.15[b]	1.29	5.61	2.62
22. Hands shake	17.32[b]	1.29	5.48	.80	.61	5.97
23. Worries	42.84[b]	.79	11.85[b]	1.15	1.94	.02
24. Sighs	12.58[b]	50.64[b]	.87	6.80[b]	.21	3.89
25. Feels restless	20.19[b]	24.20[b]	.23	.22	2.56	22.95[b]
26. Acid stomach	0.48	6.45	6.16	.20	1.18	8.15[b]
27. Bites nails	.11	.80	10.41[b]	.45	1.41	28.27[b]
28. Mouth dry	4.67	.92	1.02	.11	.00	14.14[b]
29. Trouble sleeping	15.18[b]	1.87	.03	1.81	.43	5.00
30. Muscle twitches	1.99	53.90[b]	36.99[b]	.65	.91	11.69[b]
31. Headaches	10.94[b]	29.19[b]	27.13[b]	.09	.36	49.47[b]
32. Feels no good	18.63[b]	1.03	7.97[b]	1.67	2.57	.97
33. Feels dizzy	2.15	89.33[b]	41.94[b]	6.94[b]	3.02	42.67[b]

[a] From Guthrie et al. (1975).
[b] $p < .01$.

a summary of results. The aspect of this study relevant to this discussion is that a gastrointestinal factor which was clearly defined in the data from English-speaking subjects was not found in the reports of the French and Haitian students. I have more recently asked French-speaking students if they ever experience abdominal aches or pains during stress. They indicated that indeed they did, pointed to the same general area of their intestines as did my students, and told me the difficulty was with their liver.

Let us look more directly at the issue of the frequent lack of correspondence between an individual's report of visceral activity and actual body changes. In Figure 2, I have attempted to summarize some of the factors which may intercede between an actual bodily change and a person's perception of such activity. It is suggested here that a person who perceives himself as a stomach responder may show greater actual stomach reactivity and/or greater sensitivity to the feedback of his stomach activity. This sensitivity is thought to have two separable components: feedback threshold and cognitive factors (such as the degree to which an individual pays attention to his stomach).

Feedback threshold is used here to refer to the ability of a person to discriminate changes in his stomach activity (or sweating, intestinal activity, etc.). Two studies have been reported by Stunkard and his associates (Griggs & Stunkard, 1964; Stunkard & Koch, 1964) comparing obese and normal subjects first on the relationship of their reports of hunger to gastric motility and secondly on their ability to detect their own motility. The basic procedure used by Stunkard was based on the theory of signal detectability (Swets, Tanner, & Birdsall, 1961). The main advantage of using this procedure is that one can separate out the effects on detection of (1) physiological sensitivity and (2) psychological bias in terms of the criterion of responding. (Cf. Chapter 6 in this volume.) For example, Griggs and Stunkard reported that their obese subject could perceive his

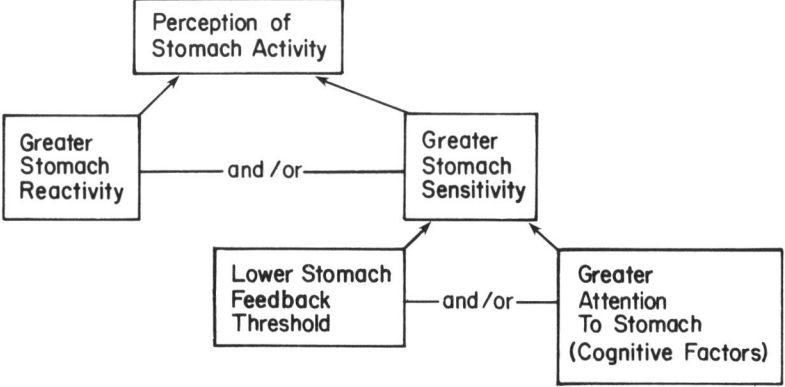

Figure 2. Factors which may contribute to the perception of stomach activity.

stomach motility as well as their normal subject, but the obese subject had a strong response bias; he usually denied the presence of contractions. This study is important because of its introduction into psychophysiology of the methodology of the theory of signal detection. Whitehead and Drescher (1980) conducted studies using a procedure similar to that used by Stunkard and his associated to measure the ability of subjects to perceive contractions of their stomachs, and they examined the relationship of this ability to the control of gastric motility.

Referring again to Figure 2, *cognitive factors* that might cause an individual to pay greater than normal attention to his stomach activity include past as well as more recent events. It seems obvious that a person who shows a very high level of stomach reactivity and/or low threshold for stomach feedback will pay attention to his stomach. But, in addition, it is suggested here that some individuals may show little stomach reactivity and a relatively high stomach feedback threshold but still pay a great deal of attention to their stomachs (consider themselves stomach responders) because of operant conditioning, probably at an early age (Miller, 1969), imitative behavior, or because of a recent experience such as the death of a friend or relative from stomach cancer.

This discussion of some of the factors which may intercede between actual bodily changes and the individual's report of them is presented for two purposes. The first is as a warning to researchers trying to relate environmental events to stomach activity who would use subjective reports as their measure of stomach activity. The second purpose is to alert clinicians to the many factors that may lie between their patients' reports of stomach distress and their actual bodily changes.

2.2. Difficulties with All Known Recording Techniques

By way of presenting my second excuse for not knowing more about the responsiveness of the stomach to environmental events, I want to describe very briefly some of the difficulties inherent in the various methods of recording stomach activity. (For an extensive listing of articles which describe the recording of gastric motility see Stern & Davis, 1982; and Chapter 5 of this volume.)

Most methods involve putting something inside the gastrointestinal tract which stimulates local activity (i.e., balloons, catheters, collection tubes, magnets, endoradiosondes, and endoscopes). X-ray methods cannot be used over an extended period of time and, futhermore, the subject must swallow barium. An additional problem with magnets and endoradiosondes is that it is difficult to identify the precise location from which to record. The solution to this problem commonly used—anchoring the device with a premeasured piece of thread which is tied to the subject's tooth—frequently brings about the gag reflex, which can be a stronger stimulus than the environmental event under study. The EGG, or surface electrogastrogram, has its own problems of interpretation. At this time, I think it is safe to say that the frequency of the EGG is a valid indicator of the frequency of the basic electrical rhythm or electrical control activity. The relationship of the amplitude of the EGG to actual motor activity of the stomach is, however, still not well understood.

Perhaps the best way to study the effects of environmental events on gastric activity is to examine individuals with a complete constriction of the esophagus and, therefore, an abdominal fistula into the stomach. The difficulty with using this method is that, thanks to modern medicine, such persons are now usually provided with an artificial esophagus. Examples of this approach are Beaumont's (1833) account of Alexis St. Martin, Carlson's (1912) description of his research with Fred Vlcek, or Wolf and Wolff's (1947) well-known and often quoted account of Tom. I personally feel that there is a great deal to learn from these accounts even though they lack experimental rigor and may not be highly generalizable.

2.3. Confounding by Digestive Functions

Numerous investigators have refuted the claims of Cannon and Washburn (1912) and Carlson (1912) that large contractions of the empty stomach give rise to the sensation of hunger. (See, for example, Bloom, Filion, Stunkard, Fox, & Stellar, 1970.) However, nobody would question the statement that eating has profound effects on the motility and secretory activity of the stomach. Therefore, if we desire to learn more about the effects of environmental events on the stomach, we must control or at least take into account the effects of eating. To do otherwise would be as ridiculous as trying to study the effects on the cardiovascular system of attentional factors of subjects some of whom are standing while others are down on all fours in the starting position assumed by sprinters just prior to a race.

The effects of thinking about eating, discussing eating, or seeing stimuli associated with eating are much the same as the effects of eating—an increase in gastric secretions and motility. Pavlov (1927) described in some detail the "psychic secretions" of his dogs, and each of us is capable of conjuring up an image which will produce the same results. Wolf and Wolff (1947) reported that when they discussed food with their famous subject, Tom, they could observe an increase in the redness of the mucosa, an increase in acid secretion, and an increase in motility.

The effects on the stomach of eating cannot be studied with most methods of recording gastric activity since most methods involve putting something, for example, a balloon, catheter, endoscope, or radiosonde, into the stomach that would not stay in one place and/or would cause the subject to regurgitate the food which he/she just consumed. Davis, Garafolo, and Kveim (1959) used the surface EGG method of recording to study the effects of eating. They found an increase in the occurrence of 3 cpm waves and a large increase in the amplitude of the waves. They reported no change in frequency. It should be kept in mind that Davis and his associates believed that their surface-recorded records were measures of stomach contractions.

Nelsen and Kohatsu (1968) have more recently studied the effects of eating in both man and dogs. These investigators also recorded EGGs from the surface of the skin but interpreted them differently. They argued that the EGG is a measure of the frequency of the basic electrical rhythm or electrical control activity but not of contractions. The results of their study showed that the frequency increased in both species following eating. Nelsen and Kohatsu did not examine amplitude changes.

In my laboratory at Penn State University and that of my colleague, C. M. Davis, at Simon Fraser University, we have consistently found a large increase in the amplitude of the EGG after eating. Figure 3 shows a typical record from my laboratory. The subject was a healthy 25-year-old male. The active EGG electrode was placed approximately 1 cm above the navel and 1 cm to the left; the reference electrode was attached to the subject's left leg. Relatively low amplitude 3 cpm activity can be seen prior to eating, but note the large increase in amplitude after eating commenced.

A factor related to eating that might influence stomach motility is the time of day one normally eats. I hypothesized that long-term temporal conditioning might take place such that at the time one normally eats, there might be an increase in motility, secretion, and the like. I collected EGG data from 100 healthy male subjects at the time of their awakening in the morning. Of the

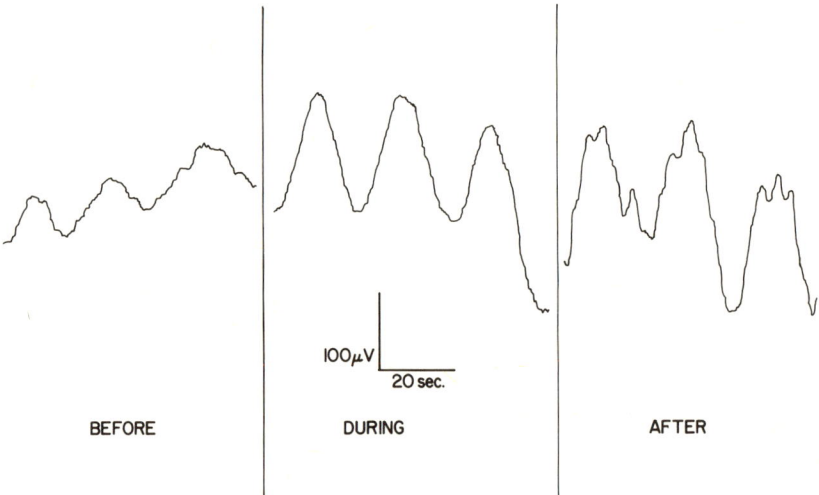

Figure 3. Typical EGG recorded from healthy human subject before, during, and after eating.

subjects, 50 ate breakfast every morning, and 50 never ate breakfast. My results were disappointing. The group mean amplitudes were not significantly different; they were all uniformly low. Time since eating appeared to be an overpowering variable.

I started this section by discussing the confounding of digestive functions with the response of the stomach to environmental events. Most investigators deal with this problem by having their subjects be 4–6 hr hungry. However, I would like to raise the issue that this may be an inappropriate solution since there may exist in the real world very meaningful interactions between hours since eating and the response to certain stimuli or external stressors. What I am suggesting is that by doing laboratory tests only on fasting subjects, we might be obtaining very limited data on the effects of environmental stimuli on the stomach.

2.4. Confounding by Spontaneous Activity

In this last category of confounding variables, I have placed nondigestive factors that affect the activity of the stomach and are not directly related to environmental events.

Anyone who has observed the stomach of a resting subject, either directly through an endoscope or indirectly via one of the recording methods described previously, has observed that contractions and secretions occur occasionally in the absence of any known stimulus. Sometimes this activity is aperiodic and very difficult to account for. Central nervous system explanations may be suggested such as the possibility that the subject was just thinking about eating a delicious meal. Peripheral explanations may also be given such as the possibility that some momentarily trapped food particles worked loose in the upper gastrointestinal tract and thereby stimulated stomach activity. The explanation for so-called spontaneous activity is not of importance to most researchers, but the existence of spontaneous activity in the stomach is of procedural importance to all who are interested in the responsiveness of the stomach to environmental events. Obviously, care must be taken not to confound spontaneous activity with the response to an external stimulus.

I have placed the effects on stomach activity of sleep in this section for lack of a better place to put it. Baust and Rohrwasser (1969) recorded gastric pH from eight healthy subjects during night sleep. The subjects swallowed an endoradiosonde at the beginning of the session. Basically, the experiments found that with respect to wakefulness, gastric acidity increased with depth of sleep. Kales and Tan (1969) recorded sleeping gastric acidity levels from normals and ulcer patients. They found acid secretion to be greater during rapid eye movement (REM) sleep than during other stages of sleep in the ulcer patients but not in the normals.

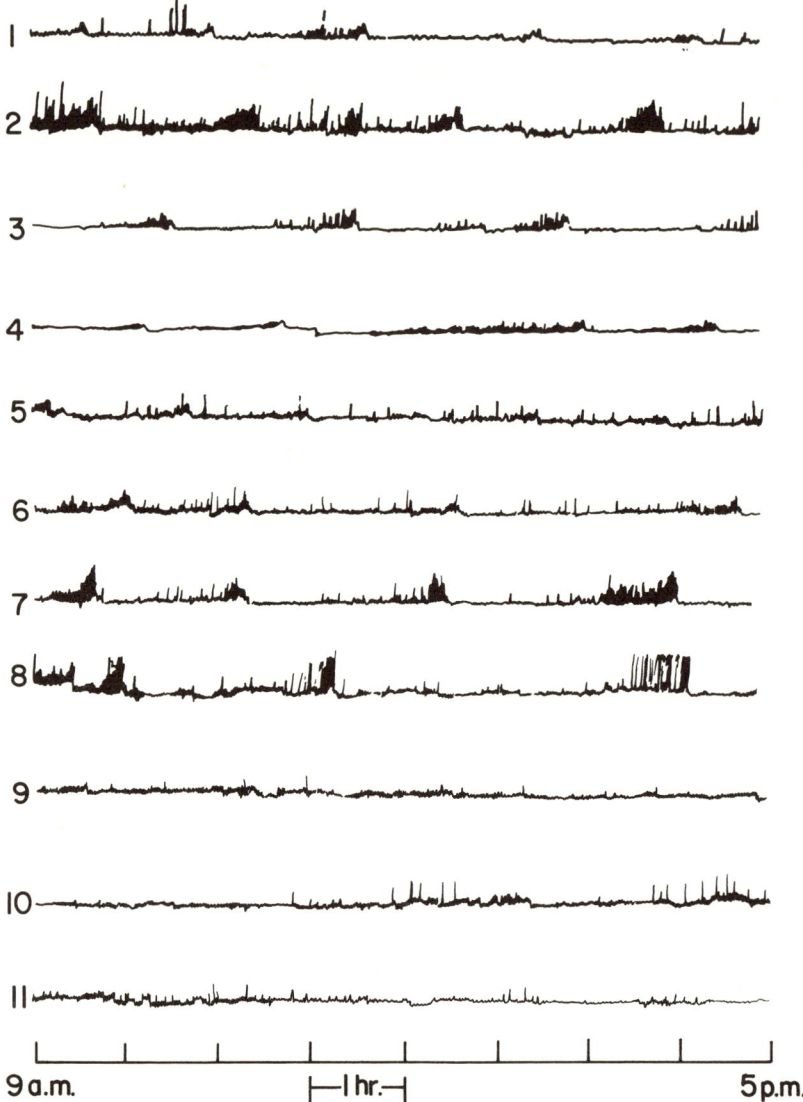

Figure 4. Direct gastric pressure records. Each line is the 8-hr stomach recording from one subject, condensed to show contraction periods. (Reproduced by permission from Hiatt & Kripke, 1975.)

Baust and Rohrwasser (1969), in the same study mentioned previously, also recorded gastric motility from their sleeping subjects with an endoradiosonde. They reported that gastric motility decreased with depth of sleep but increased during REM sleep. The authors expressed some surprise at finding the opposite effect of depth of sleep on gastric pH and motility.

To confuse matters further, Yaryura-Tobias, Hutcheson, and White (1970) also used an endoradiosonde to measure gastric motility from normal sleeping subjects and obtained quite different results. They reported the greatest motility during the lightest and deepest stages of sleep and did not report finding an increase during REM sleep. Considering the state of our knowledge in this area, I think that the best advice to researchers interested in the responsiveness of the stomach to environmental events is to make sure that subjects are awake before presenting stimuli.

The function of REM sleep, a sleep stage that occurs every 90–120 min, has been of interest to sleep researchers for approximately 20 years. Kleitman (1963) has suggested that this ultradian rhythm is identifiable in waking as well as sleep. Activity cycles of 90–120 min have since been demonstrated for a wide variety of physiological functions during sleep and less distinctly in brain functions during wakefulness.

Hiatt and Kripke (1975) conducted a study of ultradian rhythms in waking gastric activity. Stomach motility was recorded by the balloon method from 11 normal, fasted subjects for 8 hr. Figure 4 shows the intraluminal gastric pressure records obtained from the subjects. Note the tendency for periods of intense gastric contraction to recur at regular intervals in most records. The typical subject had 4–5 cycles of gastric activity in 8 hr. Contraction periods lasted from 5–40 min, with a mean of approximately 18 min. The stomach contraction periods shown in Figure 4 are striking in the clarity of their rhythm and in their resemblance to the time plots of REM sleep periods. They are also something else to be aware of when studying responsiveness of the stomach to environmental events. The electrical correlate of this cyclic recurrence of periods of contractions alternating with periods of complete quiet has been the subject of much recent research (e.g., Code & Marlett, 1975; Smout, van der Schee, & Grashuis, 1980) and has been designated as the migrating myoelectric complex or the interdigestive myoelectric complex.

Now that I have completed my introduction, I would like to describe some of the effects of environmental events on the stomach that have been reported in the literature. I have divided this material into two sections—passive responding to external situations and active responding to external stimuli.

3. Passive Responding to External Situations

In this section on passive responding I have included the effects of temperature, tones and lights, fear and anger, and other emotional states.

3.1. Temperature

If asked to generalize about the effects of environmental temperature on eating behavior, most of us would indicate that in the cold we eat more whereas during very hot weather we decrease our food intake. One of the first laboratory studies which examined the relationship between environmental temperature and emptying time of the stomach was conducted by Sleeth and Van Liere (1937). Four dogs exposed to temperature averaging $-10°C$ showed an average decrease of 17% in the emptying time of the stomach. When the same animals were exposed to temperatures averaging 32°C they showed an average increase of 10% in the emptying time of the stomach. Sleeth and Van Liere concluded: "This work gives experimental evidence for the basis of the recognized fact that an individual often feels more hungry during cold weather and less hungry in extremely warm weather" (p. 275). Obviously these workers assumed a causal relationship between stomach emptying time and eating behavior.

Henschel, Taylor, and Keys (1944), using 17 normal human subjects, also examined the relationship between environmental temperature and gastric emptying time. The 17 men were placed in rooms with temperatures of 25°C and 49°C on different days. X-rays were used to trace the time course of gastric emptying. Contrary to the findings with dogs by Sleeth and Van Liere, in all but one of the human subjects, gastric emptying time was faster at the high temperatures. Henschel *et al.* (1944) concluded that decreased appetite during hot weather cannot be explained on the basis of decreased gastric motor function but may be related to decreased general activity. However, it should be noted that we now know that increased gastric emptying time might accompany *increased* gastric motor function in cases where there is closure of the pylorus. Henschel *et al.* point out that whenever possible, we tend to be less active when the environmental temperature is high. Henschel *et al.* reported that they had observed approximately 100 men working in their laboratory at temperatures of 49°C and that they showed very good appetites, except for those who suffered from heat exhaustion.

Wolf and Wolff (1947) presented evidence from their fistulated subject, Tom, in support of the findings of Henschel *et al.* of increased gastric activity under higher temperatures. Wolf and Wolff opened the windows in their laboratory in order to lower the temperature and observed that Tom's gastric mucosa paled. When they closed the window and allowed the room to warm again, they observed that Tom's mucosa became redder, acid production accelerated, and vigorous contractions commenced. Wolf and Wolff suggested that these physiological changes might explain why we tend to eat when we come in out of the cold in the winter. An alternative explanation is that we eat when we come indoors in winter because (1) that is where the food is and (2) we were very active when we were outside. It should be kept in mind that in all the studies discussed above the effects of environmental temperature and not body temperature were examined.

Hölzl, Schroder, and Kiefer (1979) investigated the effects of having the subject immerse his hand in ice water at 0–3°C for brief periods. Both EGG and magnetogastrogram recordings showed significant increases in the amplitude of 3 cpm activity in response to this stimulus.

Next, I will discuss the effects of swallowed hot and cold substances on gastric activity. Gershon-Cohen, Shay, and Fels (1940), who used fluoroscopy to study gastric emptying, reported that cold meals leave the stomach almost immediately and that hot meals leave more slowly. They also reported that this difference in rate of emptying disappears rapidly as the temperature of the ingested food is normalized in the stomach. Bisgard and Nye (1940) recorded gastric motility with intragastric balloons before and after ingestion of hot and cold water. In contrast to the results reported by Gershon-Cohen *et al.*, Bisgard and Nye reported an increase in stomach motility when hot water was swallowed and a decrease when cold water was swallowed. In a more recent study, Williams and Walike (1975) infused water and liquid diet formula at varying temperatures into feeding tubes implanted in the stomachs of rhesus monkeys. With the monkeys awake and restrained, gastric motility was recorded using a strain gauge sutured to the stomach wall. The temperature of the liquid did not significantly alter gastric motility or gastric emptying time.

A final study to be discussed in this section describes the effects of changes in environmental and body temperature on gastric motility. Diefenbach (1975) studied gastric motility as a function of temperature in crocodiles. Gastric motility was recorded using a balloon inserted through a cannula into the stomach. Six animals were tested after a 3-week fast, during feeding of mice, and for an additional 5–10 days. Records were obtained while the crocodiles were in tanks of water maintained at 20°, 25°, and 30°C. Prior to eating, the fasting crocodiles showed almost no contractions. Following eating, all crocodiles showed contractions but those maintained in water of 30°C showed much greater amplitude and frequency than those who were kept in 20°C water. In summary, for crocodiles, gastric contractions increase in frequency and amplitude with temperature or upon feeding.

3.2. Tones and Lights

Jungmann and Venning (1952) conducted one of the first systematic studies of the effects of sensory stimuli on the stomach. Radiological observations of the stomach of 55 human subjects were made before and after the presentation of an unexpected gunshot. Momentary changes in the rate and amplitude of contractions were seen in approximately 50% of the subjects. In most cases in which rate changed following the stimulus, the change consisted of suppression of the next wave or waves (usually 2 or 3). Jungmann and Venning did not record respiration, but it is my feeling that the momentary suppression in gastric contractions was probably mediated by sympathetic activity stimulated by the deep breath that most subjects take following a sudden loud noise (Stern & Anschel, 1968).

Davis, Garafolo, and Kveim (1959) used surface EGG recording from the upper left abdominal quadrant to examine the effects of a bright light on the stomach activity of 18 college students. The subjects lay on a cot in a darkened room for 25 min; then the experimenter turned on a 200-W lamp in a reflector about 1.3 m above the subject's face. Some of the subjects had recently eaten and the others had fasted for about 12 hr. The EGGs during the 25-min rest period showed significantly greater amplitude from the subjects who had recently eaten than from the fasting subjects. More to the point, all subjects showed a significant increase in amplitude during the 5 min of visual stimulation. Again, no respiration data were reported, and we do not know how noxious the stimulus was for the subjects.

In the early 1960s, I conducted a study (Stern, 1964) the purpose of which was to investigate the effects of three different stimulus conditions on stomach activity. Under the first condition, subjects were exposed to absolute sensory reduction, that is, no visual or auditory stimulation; under the second condition, vision was not restricted and a low auditory input was constantly present; under the third condition, the same auditory input was present but diffusion lenses restricted visual input to unpatterned stimulation. Surface recording of EGG served as the dependent variable. The hypothesis tested was that gastric activity would decrease in all groups during a 40-min experimental period, but that the group receiving diffuse visual stimulation would show the slowest rate of change. This hypothesis was based upon previous work in my laboratory and upon the results of sensory deprivation studies conducted in other laboratories. Previous experimenters who used diffuse stimulation observed disturbances in both physiological and behavioral variables; no such changes were reported when the absolute levels of visual and auditory inputs were reduced to a minimum. All 16 subjects were male undergraduate students from the introductory psychology class at Indiana University. Time since eating varied from subject to subject, but was the same for the two sessions of any one subject. All subjects participated in the diffuse stimulation condition and one of the other two conditions.

As predicted, the results showed that gastric activity recorded under conditions of diffuse stimulation was consistently greater than that recorded from the same subjects in either of the other conditions. Statistical tests indicated that the differences between the groups were significant for Minutes 20, 30, 40, but not for Minute 10. The failure to obtain a significant difference at the first sample is thought to be due to the fact that subjects were not, at this point, under different stimulus conditions for a sufficient length of time to produce differential effects.

In the study just described, evidence was presented indicating that variations in visual and auditory stimulation have a significant effect on the EGG, as measured with surface electrodes. This first study dealt with the effects of three constant levels of stimulation. In the next study conducted (Stern, 1965), my interest was in determining the effects of contrast in stimulation, or in other words, the effects of the immediately preceding level of stimulation on the gastric response to a moderate level of stimulation. It was hypothesized that a change to a moderate level of stimulation would result in a decrease in activity below baseline level for a group which was responding at a high level to high stimulation and an increase in level of responding for a group which was responding at a previously low level to low stimulation.

Forty male university students were assigned, according to a randomized groups design, 20 subjects to a high-stimulation group and 20 subjects to a low-stimulation group. Subjects were instructed to lie quietly on a cot and to pay careful attention to any changes in visual and auditory stimulation. Subjects wore diffusion lenses which permitted only unpatterned visual stimulation to reach their eyes; auditory stimulation was presented over earphones. The EGG was recorded with surface electrodes attached to the skin of the abdomen, and a reference electrode was attached to the calf of the left leg. The stimulation schedules for the two groups were: moderate-high-moderate and moderate-low-moderate. The total recording session lasted 40 min; 10 min were allowed at the beginning for the subjects to adapt to the experimental situation, and each stimulation period lasted 10 min. The auditory stimulation was a 500-Hz tone presented at 70 db during high stimulation and 40 db during moderate stimulation. No tone or light was presented during low-stimulation periods. The approximate illumination actually reaching the subject's eyes, as measured with a Macbeth illuminometer, was 64 mL for high stimulation and 12 mL for moderate stimulation.

The records of gastric activity were read for the maximum amplitude within each consecutive 1-min period, this being the measure which had been found to be most sensitive to changes in external stimulation. Figure 5 shows three-point sliding means for the high stimulation and low stimulation groups for Period 2 and Period 3 expressed as a percentage of each subject's mean activity for Period

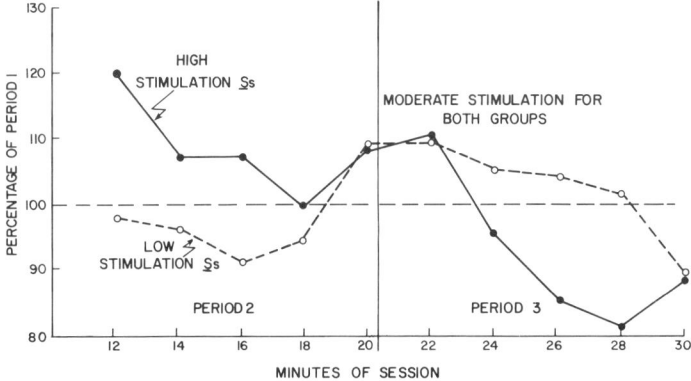

Figure 5. Sliding means for amplitude of gastrointestinal activity during Periods 2 and 3 expressed as a percentage of Period 1. (Reproduced by permission from Stern, 1965.)

1. As can be seen, the relative activity of the two groups reversed. That is, for Period 2, subjects receiving high stimulation responded at a higher level than subjects receiving low stimulation, but for Period 3 the relative amplitude of activity of the two groups reversed. It appears that the stomach activity of the two groups did differentiate in the predicted manner except at the end of Period 2 and the beginning of Period 3. At Minute 19, both groups showed an increase in activity, which can probably best be explained in terms of expectation of a change in stimulation. These elevated levels of activity persisted until the third minute of Period 3, Minute 23, for both groups. This finding was somewhat of a surprise, since it was expected that the change in stimulation at Minute 20 would cause a rapid reversal in relative levels of activity of the two groups. It appears that at least for the stomach, any change in stimulation is activating for 2 to 3 min regardless of the direction of the change. It is not until this initial effect of the abrupt change dissipates that the contrast effect can be seen.

3.3. Fear, Anger, and Other Emotional States

Ever since William James published his theory of emotion in 1884, psychologists and others have been searching for specific bodily changes that give rise to our feelings of fear, anger, joy, and other emotions. Even though numerous studies have been conducted in which every imaginable bodily change has been recorded, little support for James's theory has accumulated. Probably the strongest support has come from studies that have looked at the relationship of fear, anger, and related emotional states to stomach activity.

Over a hundred years ago Beaumont (1833) reported that the stomach of Alexis St. Martin, his fistulated subject, emptied more slowly when he was fearful. Cannon (1909), in one of his early papers pointed out that fear, worry, or anxiety inhibits the secretion and motility of the stomach. To quote from Cannon:

> The foregoing exposition of the influence of emotions on the activities of the stomach and intestines has shown how profoundly the mental state may affect favorably or unfavorably the secretions of the stomach, so important for the continuation of the digestive process, and how quickly and directly the mental state may entirely check the onward movement of food. (p. 486)

The major interests of Wolf and Wolff (1947) in their studies of their fistulated subject, Tom, were in the effects of emotional stimuli on gastric activity. Figure 6 shows the effects on Tom's mucosa and secretion of a fearful or anxiety producing situation. Note the decrease in acid secreted and the decrease in reddening of the gastric mucosa. This, of course, agrees with the earlier reports of Cannon, Beaumont, and others. Perhaps the more interesting finding was that when Tom was made angry, he showed an increase in secretion,

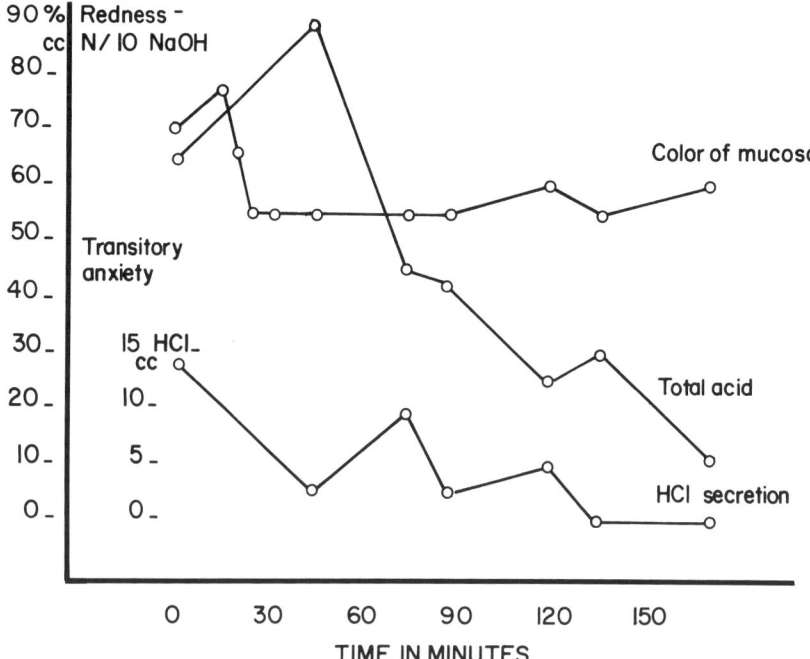

Figure 6. Decreases in reddening of gastric mucosa and in gastric acidity accompanying transitory anxiety. (Reproduced by permission from Wolf & Wolff, 1943.)

motility, and reddening of the gastric mucosa (Figure 7). To repeat, when he was fearful, motility decreased, but when he was angry, his motility increased.

Soon after Wolf and Wolff's classic work appeared, several lines of research suggested that epinephrine and norepinephrine are selectively released in different emotional states. Funkenstein (1956) and others reported that epinephrine was the predominant response in fearful or anxious or "anger inward" situations. Norepinephrine was thought to be the primary secretion in "anger outward" situations. These findings tend to fit in very nicely with the results obtained by Wolf and Wolff. When Tom felt fearful, we might assume that his primary secretion was epinephrine. Epinephrine is known to inhibit gastric secretion and the motility of smooth muscle. Unfortunately, more recent studies on human subjects do not support the assumption that epinephrine and norepinephrine are selectively released in different emotional states. Frankenhaeuser (1975) has reported that epinephrine is secreted in a variety of emotional states, including anger and fear. Similarly, a rise in norepinephrine may occur in a variety of emotional states, but the threshhold for norepinephrine release in emotional situations is generally much higher than for epinephrine secretion.

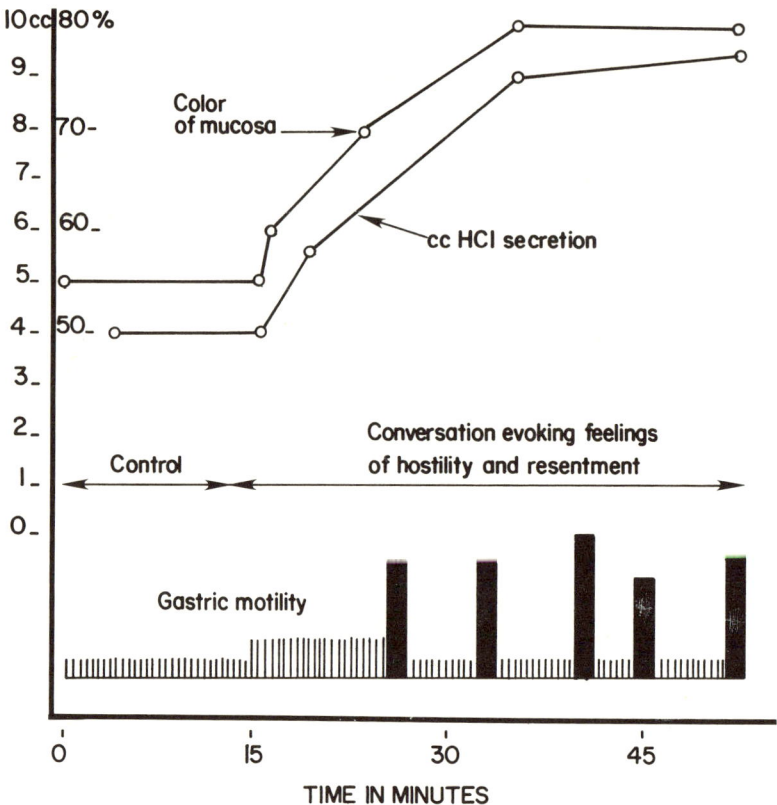

Figure 7. Increases in gastric motility, reddening of gastric mucosa, and gastric acidity, accompanying feelings of hostility and resentment. (Reproduced by permission from Wolf & Wolff, 1943.)

Weiner (1977) summarizes more recent reports of the effects of various emotions on human stomach activity; he indirectly supports the claims of Frankenhaeuser and fails to support the findings of Wolf and Wolff or the theory of James. According to Weiner, anxiety, anger, guilt, and feelings of humiliation are all accompanied by an increase in gastric secretion and a nonsystematic increase or decrease in motility. On the other hand, Hall, Herb, and Brady (1967) and Kehoe and Ironside (1964) have produced differential effects on gastric secretory output in human subjects using hypnosis to create different emotional states. Anger was associated with the highest mean secretory rate, anxiety and contentment were associated with moderate rates, and feelings of depression, helplessness, and hopelessness with the lowest rates of gastric secretion.

The major difficulty in assessing studies in this area and comparing results, even more difficult than measuring the changes in stomach activity, is in understanding what the various authors meant by fear, anger, anxiety, and other constructs. The manner in which their subjects interpreted the different situations, that is, the quality and intensity of their emotions, is even a greater problem and probably the greatest cause of the confusion which exists in this area.

4. Active Responding to External Stimuli

Included in this section is a discussion of the effects on gastric activity of exercise and mental arithmetic. Also to be discussed is stress and ulcer development.

4.1. Exercise

Hellebrandt and Tepper (1934) used a fluoroscopic procedure to study the influence of exercise on gastric motility. Their initial finding was that mild exercise tends to hasten gastric emptying time, especially if it follows immediately the ingestion of the meal. Their second finding was that violent exercise inhibits stomach motility, but this may be followed by a period of augmented activity so that final emptying time is not much altered. The authors conclude as follows: "In the end, exercise closely associated with meal-time does not seem detrimental as far as digestion is concerned. It delays it, (violent exercise) but the transitory inhibition appears to do no harm" (p. 362).

In a related study, Hellebrandt and Dimmitt (1934) examined the effects of exercise on the relations between secretory and motor functions of the stomach. The single subject used in the study swallowed a double tube, one side of which was used to measure motility with a gastric balloon and the other side to obtain samples of gastric contents. The authors reported that mild exercise facilitated not only gastric motility but also acid secretion, and violent exercise inhibited gastric motility and also acid secretion.

A third report from Hellebrandt's laboratory (Hellebrandt, Brogdon, & Hoopes, 1935) asked the question: What happens to gastric inhibition with repetition of violent exercise? In the six subjects studied, they found a very rapid disappearance of the inhibition of gastric secretion which normally accompanies violent exercise. The authors concluded that this disappearance was not a training effect in the usual sense of that word. They indicated that it happened too early, and once the gastric inhibition was overcome, it was not possible again to induce it even with much more extreme grades of the same exercise. The authors credit Professor Ragsdale of the Psychology Department of the University of Wisconsin with suggesting that the phenomenon might be explained in terms of "visceral learning." What Professor Ragsdale meant by this was that at first the subjects made a quite diffuse visceral response, but after only a few trials they made adjustments so that their reactions were more appropriate to the situation. I was surprised and interested to come across this use of the term "visceral learning" in the 1930s in light of its use today by investigators such as Neal Miller working in the area of biofeedback.

4.2. Mental Arithmetic

Davis, Berry, and Paden (1960) investigated the effects of mental arithmetic on gastrointestinal activity. The subjects were 19 college students; gastrointestinal activity was recorded with surface EGG. Simultaneous recordings were attained from the following three locations: upper left quadrant (stomach), upper right quadrant (duodenum), and centrally just below the navel (transverse colon). After a 15-min rest period, the subjects did mental arithmetic problems for 10 min, giving the answer to each problem as they worked and receiving immediate feedback as to whether it was right or wrong. A 10-min final rest period followed the mental arithmetic period. The mean amplitude of the EGG from all three recording sites increased during the mental arithmetic task, and for two of the three locations EGG amplitude decreased during the final rest period.

In an effort to separate the effects of doing mental arithmetic from the effects of being evaluated for one's accuracy of doing mental arithmetic, Davis *et al.* repeated their experiment using 17 new subjects and did not have the subjects reveal their answers. Unlike the first group of subjects, this group showed no increase in amplitude during the task period.

More recently Hölzl and his associates (Hölzl *et al.*, 1979) looked at the effects of mental arithmetic on gastric motility using conjoint spectral gastrography. Their six subjects had to add and subtract six one-digit numbers at a pace of one every 1.2 sec followed by a brief pause to write down the answer. Errors cost the subjects part of their earnings. Hölzl *et al.* reported that mental arithmetic increased gastric activity when compared with a rest period and was more effective than electric shock but less effective than the cold pressor test.

4.3. Stress and Ulceration

Weiner (1977) noted that in recent years, studies of gastrointestinal pathology have focused on the mechanisms by which psychological states are translated into gastrointestinal responses. A classic investigation in this tradition was the so-called "executive monkey" study reported by Brady, Porter, Conrad, and Mason (1958). This study will be the focal point for the remainder of this chapter, that is, I will trace lines of research which had their origins in some aspect of the executive monkey study.

Brady *et al.* (1958) described a study in which four pairs of rhesus monkeys were kept in restraining chairs for periods of up to seven weeks. During these weeks, the four pairs of animals were exposed to a Sidman avoidance schedule;

that is, to a procedure in which electric shocks were presented, without warning, at regular intervals, but these could be postponed by a lever press response from an experimental animal. Through each 24 hr the monkeys experienced alternate 6-hr periods of "avoidance" and rest. The animals had been trained by exposure to an electric shock repeated at 20-sec intervals: A lever could be pressed by either monkey of the pair, and when this was appropriately manipulated both animals avoided the next shock. The more efficient of the two, that is, the first animal to learn the avoidance response, was selected as the experimental or "executive" monkey, the less efficient being the "control" animal who subsequently had no opportunity to manipulate a lever effective for avoidance, but was exposed to any shocks which, because of the "executive's" inefficiency, were delivered to both animals. When these yoked pairs were in one of the 6-hr "avoidance" periods, this was signaled by a red light. Within a few hours, the "executives" developed stable avoidance response rates of 15–20 lever presses per min, and received not more than two shocks per hr. During rest periods, avoidance response rates dropped. Brady et al. (1958) reported the deaths of three of their "executives" after 9, 23, and 25 days, the fourth being sacrificed in a moribund state after seven weeks. All "executives" had extensive gastric lesions and ulcers, while the "controls" remained unaffected.

Subsequent publications reported that examination of gastric secretion, monitored by means of a fistula preparation, revealed reductions of activity during avoidance activity, but increases during the rest periods: there were, however, individual differences in this aspect of the response to testing. The six hours on/off schedule seemed particularly relevant for the production of gastric pathology, and it was suggested that poststressor rebound interacted with rhythmic variation in function to explain the pathology of "executive" monkeys.

After the report of Brady et al. (1958), attention turned to the possibility that the human EGG might be used to examine gastrointestinal motility during Sidman avoidance sessions. Davis and Berry (1963) examined the EGGs of 12 pairs of male and 12 pairs of female students before, during, and after a 10-min session of noise avoidance. "Executive" and "control" subjects were randomly assigned to their respective roles, and the latter group was reported to be unaware of the task being undertaken by the former. Amplitude of the EGG waves was measured, and the executive subjects showed a larger response than the controls in the avoidance and post-avoidance rest sessions. This result was somewhat surprising in view of Cannon's (1909) description of reduced gastrointestinal activity in fear and the evidence from monkeys of suppressed secretory activity during test sessions. Brady (1963), however, suggested that, contrary to assumptions of covariation between secretion and motility, there may be questions raised about selective effects on secretion and motility. As Brady also observed, there were critical differences between the monkey and the human studies: the most obvious was the marked reduction in testing time from days to minutes of involvement. The theme of secretory/motility variation in executive-type tasks was pursued through a number of subsequent publications from the early 1960s.

White (1964) used a procedure similar to that used by Davis and Berry (1963) and reported a reduction of amplitude in avoidance sessions, and the possibility of decreased secretory activity as evidenced by a shifting baseline record. Evidence of reduced secretory function, recorded with the aid of an endoradiosonde, was reported by Norman (1969) from a study of avoidance responding.

Meanwhile, research continued to be conducted in the Indiana University laboratory on the effects on gastrointestinal activity recorded with the EGG during the noise-avoidance procedure devised by Davis and his colleagues. Fedor and Russell (1965) found greater amplitude of 3 cpm waveforms when human subjects had been unsuccessful in avoidance of the aversive noise. I (Stern, 1966) introduced into the design the situation of each subject being his own control, being successively "executive" and "control" when exposed to alternating periods of noise-avoidance (or "response-contingent stimulation") and to similar amounts of auditory stress randomly presented. Amplitude was examined in periods of response-contingent and random scheduling and during the successful or unsuccessful avoidance of noise. As can be seen in Figure 8,

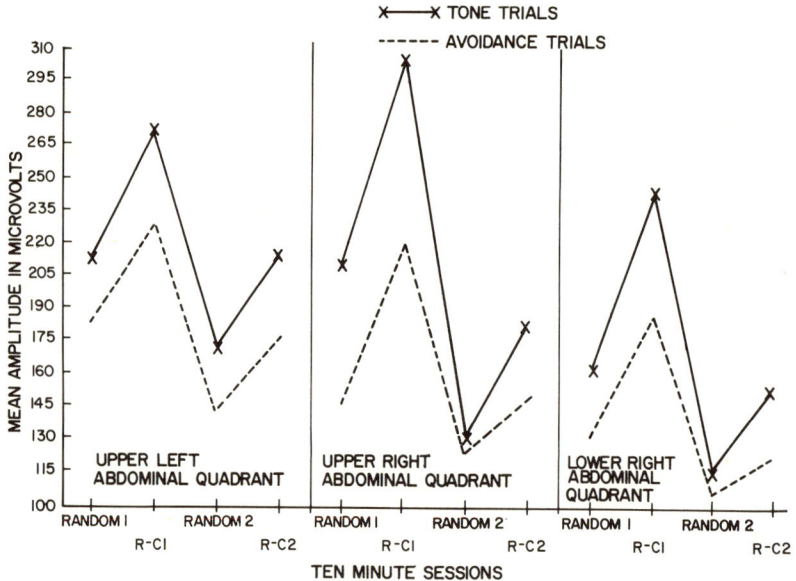

Figure 8. Mean amplitude of gastrointestinal motility for tone and avoidance trials, for four consecutive treatment sessions, and for three abdominal positions. (Reproduced by permission from R. M. Stern, 1966.)

there was greater amplitude of EGG waveforms during unsuccessful responses, and there was greater amplitude during the response-contingent than during the random stimulation. In summary, the second half of the 1960s saw no resolution of the apparent discrepancy between motility data and executive-type tasks.

Recently, there have been some changes in the method originally suggested by Davis, and described by Russell and Stern (1967) for recording the EGG. In my laboratory, we now place a single electrode at the intersection of the midline and epigastric line (line connecting the lower ribs of the left and right sides). This point, in most supine subjects, is over the antrum of the stomach. Details of the revised technique are available in Stern, Ray, and Davis (1980), which also discusses quantification of EGG records and limitations in relating them to actual contractions in light of the work of Nelsen and Kohatsu (1968), Daniel and Irwin (1968), and others.

Using the newer techniques of EGG recording and analysis a pilot study of gastric activity during response-contingent stress was undertaken in my laboratory. Power spectral analysis showed that 3 cpm activity tended to increase during a half-hour's rest following a standard meal, while such activity was reduced when a noise-avoidance task was undertaken in the postprandial period. A study in which yoked controls receive noise stimuli but do not undertake avoidance activity is now needed before we can adequately answer the question, originally posed by the Davis studies, of the direction of change in gastrointestinal activity which accompanies "executive" function in a Sidman avoidance situation.

The control subject in the Sidman avoidance situation is helpless; he/she is exposed to an unavoidable stimulus. Work by Seligman and his colleagues has highlighted the consequences of such exposure to unavoidable trauma, "learned helplessness" (Miller, Rosellini, & Seligman, 1977).

Weiss has conducted a series of elegant studies which, while relevant to Seligman's experimental findings, also contribute to the "executive monkey" saga. Weiss argues that a psychological factor of importance in determining the somatic consequences of such traumatic stimulation is the amount of control experienced. In 1968, Weiss demonstrated that "executive" rats having some control over the presentation of shock stimulation exhibited significantly less gastric erosion than yoked animals exposed to shock stimulation identical to that of the "executives." Restrained rats were tested in matched groups of three. The third of the triplet was merely restrained and not exposed to shock, and it exhibited minimal gastric erosion. Thus "control" rather than shock was regarded as the factor relevant for protection of the "executive." This is, of course, in marked contrast to the "executive" monkey finding. In 1971 Weiss more closely followed the original paradigm of Brady and his colleagues by using an unsignaled Sidman avoidance schedule. In a range of studies Weiss has repeatedly demonstrated that "executive" rats show less gastric erosion, and so has necessitated a reappraisal of the original monkey findings.

Weiss (1977), for example, suggested that selection for the "executive" role of those monkeys who more rapidly learned to avoid shock stimuli resulted in more emotional animals being "executives," and thus animals more susceptible to the development of gastrointestinal pathology. Weiss argues that gastric lesion development can be precisely predicted from assessment of two factors: (1) the number of responses made in the testing situation and (2) the amount of relevant feedback received after a coping attempt. Thus, lesions increase with increased responding and decreased information feedback. In a Sidman avoidance situation there is little such feedback. There are no external signals which are terminated by a correct response. Thus, Weiss argues, the "executive" monkeys of Brady *et al.* (1958) were selected because they had high response rates and were in a Sidman avoidance situation, both factors being ulcerogenic. When Weiss selected rats who had high response rates and exposed them to the low-feedback condition of Sidman avoidance, they too developed the "executive" ulcers. So, Weiss argues, the "executive" role is not necessarily associated with increased risk of gastrointestinal pathology, only in the somewhat exceptional situation of combining high rate of responding with low information about efficacy. And the general message for us from Weiss's rat studies is, perhaps, that the experience of control has prophylactic value, that the executive is not the prime candidate for psychosomatic disorders if he feels that he is the master of his fate!

As a postscript to this section, I would like to summarize some of Natelson's (1977) comments from a paper entitled, "The Executive Monkey Revisited." Natelson points out that even though the results of the original Brady *et al.* study were never replicated, it was a classic in the sense that it was the first demonstration of an animal model for chronic peptic ulcer disease in which only afferent inputs to the brain had been manipulated. In his own research using aversive behavioral paradigms with monkeys, Natelson has shown that aversive schedules do produce self-limiting lesions (not chronic peptic ulcers) whose frequency is related to the psychological demands imposed on the subject.

5. Summary and Conclusions

In the first part of this chapter, I discussed why we do not know more about this topic. Four explanations given for the paucity of knowledge in this area are as follows: (1) the unreliability of subjective reports of stomach activity, (2) the difficulty with gastric recording techniques, (3) confounding of digestive and environmental factors, and (4) confounding of other ongoing activity with the response to environmental events. Studies reviewed which dealt with the responsiveness of the stomach to environmental events were divided into two sections—passive responding and active responding. In the first category, I included studies which examined the effects on stomach activity of temperature, tones, and lights, and fear, anger, and other emotions. In the second section I reviewed reports which dealt with exercise, mental arithmetic, and stress and ulcers. In conclusion, I feel that we know very little about the responsiveness of the stomach to environmental events because of our difficulty in obtaining unobtrusive, continuous measures of gastric activity. Either we need more "Toms" or we need more investigators like Hölzl, who will devote their energies to the development of better recording techniques.

6. References

Baust, W., & Rohrwasser, S. Gastric motility and pH during natural human sleep. *Pflueger's Archives*, 1969, *305*, 229–240.

Beaumont, W. *Experiments and observations on the gastric juice and the physiology of digestion.* Plattsburgh, New York: F. P. Allen, 1833.

Bisgard, J. D., & Nye, D. The influence of hot and cold application upon gastric and intestinal motor activity. *Surgical Gynecology and Obstetrics*, 1940, *71*, 172.

Bloom, P. B., Filion, R. D., Stunkard, A. J., Fox, S., & Stellar, E. Gastric and duodenal motility, food intake and hunger measured in man during a 24-hour period. *American Journal of Digestive Diseases*, 1970, *15*, 719–725.

Brady, J. V. Further comments on the gastrointestinal system and avoidance behavior. *Psychological Reports*, 1963, *12*, 742.

Brady, J. V., Porter, R. W., Conrad, D. G., & Mason, J. W. Avoidance behavior and the development of gastroduodenal ulcers. *Journal of the Experimental Analysis of Behavior*, 1958, *1*, 69–73.

Cannon, W. B. The influence of emotional states on the functions of the alimentary canal. *American Journal of Medical Science*, 1909, *137*, 480–487.

Cannon, W. B., & Washburn, A. L. An explanation of hunger. *American Journal of Physiology*, 1912, *29*, 441–454.

Carlson, A. J. Contributions to the physiology of the stomach. 1. The character of the movements of the empty stomach in man. *American Journal of Physiology*, 1912, *31*, 151–168.

Code, C. F., & Marlett, J. A. The interdigestive myo-electric complex of the stomach and small bowel of dogs. *Journal of Physiology*, 1975, *246*, 289–309.

Daniel, E. E., & Irwin, J. Electric activity of gastric musculature. In C. F. Code (Ed.), *Handbook of physiology, alimentary canal* (Vol. IV). *Motility*. Washington, D.C.: American Physiological Society, 1968.

Davis, R. C., & Berry, F. Gastrointestinal reactions during a noise avoidance task. *Psychological Reports*, 1963, *12*, 135–137.

Davis, R. C., Garafolo, L., & Kveim, K. Conditions associated with gastrointestinal activity. *Journal of Comparative and Physiological Psychology*, 1959, *52*, 466–475.

Davis, R. C., Berry, F., & Paden, A. *The effect of certain tasks and conditions on gastro-intestinal activity.* Bloomington, Indiana: Indiana University, 1969. (Technical Report)

Diefenbach, C. O. Gastric function in Caiman crocodilus (Crocodylia: Reptilia). I. Rate of gastric digestion and gastric motility as a function of temperature. *Comparative Biochemistry and Physiology*, 1975, *51*, 259–265.

Fedor, J. H., & Russell, R. W. Gastrointestinal reactions to response-contingent stimulation. *Psychological Reports*, 1965, *16*, 95–113.

Frakenhaeuser, M. Experimental approaches to the study of catecholamines and emotion. In L. Levi (Ed.), *Emotions: Their parameters and measurement*. New York: Raven Press, 1975.

Funkenstein, D. H. Nor-epinephrine-like and epinephrine-like substances in relation to human behavior. *Journal of Mental Disorders,* 1956, *1244,* 58–68.
Gershon-Cohen, J., Shay, J. H., & Fels, S. S. The relation of meal temperature to gastric motility and secretion. *American Journal of Roentgenology, Radium Therapy and Nuclear Medicine,* 1940, *43,* 237–242.
Griggs, C., & Stunkard, A. The interpretation of gastric motility. II. Sensitivity and bias in the perception of gastric motility. *Archives of General Psychiatry,* 1964, *11,* 82–89.
Guthrie, G. M., Verstraete, A., Deines, M., & Stern, R. M. Symptoms of stress in four societies. *Journal of Social Psychology,* 1975, *95,* 165–172.
Hall, W. H., Herb, R. W., & Brady, J. P. Gastric function during hypnosis and hypnotically induced gastrointestinal symptoms. *Journal of Psychosomatic Research,* 1967, *11,* 263.
Hellebrandt, F. A., & Dimmitt, L. Studies on the influence of exercise on the digestive work of the stomach. III. Its effect on the relation between secretory and motor function. *American Journal of Physiology,* 1934, *107,* 364–369.
Hellebrandt, F. A., & Tepper, R. H. Studies on the influence of exercise on the digestive work of the stomach. II. Its effect on emptying time. *American Journal of Physiology,* 1934, *107,* 355–363.
Hellebrandt, F. A., Brogdon, E., & Hoopes, S. L. The disappearance of digestive inhibition with the repetition of exercise. *American Journal of Physiology,* 1935, *112,* 442–450.
Henschel, A., Taylor, H. L., & Keys, A. Gastric emptying time of man at high and normal environmental temperatures. *American Journal of Physiology,* 1944, *141,* 205–208.
Hiatt, J. F., & Kripke, D. F. Ultradian rhythms in waking gastric activity. *Psychosomatic Medicine,* 1975, *37,* 320–325.
Hölzl, R., Schroder, G., & Kiefer, H. Indirect gastrointestinal motility measurement for use in experimental psychosomatics: A new method and some data. *Behavior Analysis and Modification,* 1979, *3,* 77–97.
James, W. What is emotion? *Mind,* 1884, *9,* 188–204.
Jungmann, H., & Venning, P. Radiological investigation of stomach changes following a loud auditory stimulus. *British Journal of Radiology,* 1952, *25,* 202–208.
Kales, A., & Tan, T. L. Sleep alterations associated with medical illness. In A. Kales (Ed.), *Sleep: Physiology and pathology.* Philadelphia: Lippincott, 1969.
Kehoe, M., & Ironside, W. Studies on the experimental evocation of depressive response using hypnosis. III. The secretory rate of total gastric acid with respect to various spontaneous experiences such as nausea, disgust, crying, and dyspnea. *Psychosomatic Medicine,* 1964, *26,* 224–249.
Kleitman, N. *Sleep and wakefulness* (2nd ed.). Chicago: University of Chicago Press, 1963.
Miller, N. E. Learning of visceral and glandular responses. *Science,* 1969, *163,* 424–445.
Miller, W. R., Rosellini, T. A., & Seligman, M. E. P. Learned helplessness and depression. In J. D. Maser & M. E. P. Seligman (Eds.), *Psychopathology: Experimental models.* San Francisco: W. H. Freeman, 1977.
Natelson, B. H. The executive monkey revisited. In F. P. Brooks & P. W. Evers (Eds.), *Nerves and the gut.* Thorofare, New Jersey: Black, 1977.
Nelsen, T. S., & Kohatsu, S. Clinical electrogastrography and its relationship to gastric surgery. *American Journal of Surgery,* 1968, *116,* 215–222.
Norman, A. Response contingency and human gastric acidity. *Psychophysiology,* 1969, *5,* 673–682.
Pavlov, I. P. *Conditioned reflexes. An investigation of the physiological activity of the cerebral cortex* (G. V. Anrep, Trans.). London: Oxford University Press, 1927.
Russell, R. W., & Stern, R. M. Gastric motility: The electrogastrogram. In P. H. Venables & I. Martin (Eds.), *A manual of psychophysiological methods.* Amsterdam: North Holland, 1967.
Sleeth, C. K., & Van Liere, E. J. The effect of environmental temperature on the emptying time of the stomach. *American Journal of Physiology,* 1937, *118,* 272–275.

Smout, A. J. P. M., van der Schee, E. J., & Grashuis, J. P. Postpranadial and interdigestive gastric electrical activity in the dog recorded by means of cutaneous electrodes. In J. Christensen (Ed.), *Gastrointestinal motility*. Raven Press, 1980.

Stern, R. M. Effects of variation in visual and auditory stimulation on gastrointestinal motility. *Psychological Reports*, 1964, *14*, 799–802.

Stern, R. M. Effects of contrast in stimulation on gastrointestinal motility. *Psychological Reports*, 1965, *16*, 156–158.

Stern, R. M. A reexamination of the effects of responsive-contingent aversive stimulation on gastrointestinal activity. *Psychophysiology*, 1966, *2*, 217–223.

Stern, R. M., & Anschel, C. Deep inspirations as stimuli for responses of the autonomic nervous system. *Psychophysiology*, 1968, *5*, 132–141.

Stern, R. M., & Davis, C. M. *Gastric motility: A selectively annotated bibliography*. Stroudsburg, Pennsylvania: Hutchinson Ross, 1982.

Stern, R. M., & Higgins, J. D. Perceived somatic reactions to stress: Sex, age, and familial occurrence. *Journal of Psychosomatic Research*, 1969, *13*, 77–82.

Stern, R. M., Ray, W. J., & Davis, C. M. *Psychophysiological recording*. New York: Oxford University Press, 1980.

Stunkard, A., & Koch, C. The interpretation of gastric motility. I. Apparent bias in the reports of hunger by obese persons. *Archives of General Psychiatry*, 1964, *11*, 74–82.

Swets, J. A., Tanner, W. P., & Birdsall, T. G. Decision processes in perception. *Psychological Review*, 1961, *68*, 301.

Weiner, H. *Psychobiology and human disease*. New York: Elsevier, 1977.

Weiss, J. M. Effects of coping responses on stress. *Journal of Comparative and Physiological Psychology*, 1968, *65*, 251–260.

Weiss, J. M. Effects of coping behavior with and without a feedback signal on stress pathology in rats. *Journal of Comparative and Physiological Psychology*, 1971, *77*, 22–30.

Weiss, J. M. Ulcers. In J. D. Maser & M. E. P. Seligman (Eds.), *Psychopathology: Experimental models*. San Francisco: W. H. Freeman, 1977.

White, E. H. Additional notes on gastrointestinal activity during avoidance behavior. *Psychological Reports*, 1964, *14*, 343–347.

Whitehead, W. E., & Drescher, V. M. Perception of gastric contractions and self-control of gastric motility. *Psychophysiology*, 1980, *17*, 552–558.

Williams, K. R., & Walike, B. C. Effect of the temperature of tube feeding on gastric motility in monkeys. *Nursing Research*, 1975, *24*, 4–9.

Wolf, S., & Wolff, H. G. *Human gastric function*. New York: Oxford University Press, 1947.

Yaryura-Tobias, J. A., Hutcheson, J. S., & White, L. Relationship between stages of sleep and gastric motility. *Behavioral Neuropsychiatry*, 1970, *2*, 22–24.

10

TREATING STOMACH DISORDERS
Can We Reinstate Regulatory Processes?
BARBARA B. WALKER

1. Introduction

Like the simple cell membrane of the protozoan, the gastrointestinal system is responsible for extracting all of our nutritional needs from the environment. Given the wide variety of substances we ingest, this is a remarkable accomplishment. It is the result of a highly integrated system with regulatory mechanisms distributed at every level of the organism. At times the gastrointestinal system becomes disregulated, leading to various gastrointestinal and behavioral disturbances. These disorders are among the most common of all afflictions; half of our population suffers from acute gastrointestinal illnesses every year. More than 10% have chronic diseases of the digestive tract, and these diseases are a major cause of absenteeism from work (Hill & Kern, 1977).

In order to organize and present information about the gastrointestinal tract, the system is usually divided into discrete segments. Although the focus of this paper is on the stomach, it should be emphasized that the stomach, along with the salivary glands, esophagus, and intestines are best conceptualized as small portions of a highly integrated system rather than as separate entities. For this reason, throughout this paper the focus will be on the stomach as it is integrated with activity in other portions of the gastrointestinal system as well as the nervous system. A brief introduction to the structure, function, and disorders of the stomach follows. After that, conceptualizations of regulation and disregula-

---

BARBARA B. WALKER • Ann Arbor Veterans Administration Medical Center and University of Michigan, Ann Arbor, Michigan 48105.

tion will be discussed, and the major question of this paper will be addressed, that is, can we reinstate regulatory processes?

2. Structure, Function, and Disorders of the Stomach

The functions of the stomach are complex because it is concerned not only with storing and transporting food, but also with modifying the food so that it is in a form capable of being delivered to the small intestine where absorption takes place. The stomach must adjust the pH, temperature, consistency, and osmolarity of food as well as begin protein digestion. To perform these functions, it is equipped with an exquisite network of motor and secretory equipment which is subject to an elaborate set of neural and hormonal controls.

The stomach is basically a reservoir where food is soaked in gastric juice containing enzymes and hydrochloric acid and then released by peristalsis into the duodenum. The esophagus meets the stomach at a point which is known as the cardiac or fundus of the stomach. The stomach then curves downward and to the right, incorporating the body of the stomach. The distal portion which leads to the duodenum has been termed the antrum. Both of the openings to the stomach are guarded by sphincters.

There are several types of cells in the gastric mucosa. The most notable are the chief cells which secrete pepsinogen (the precursor to pepsin) and the parietal cells which secrete hydrochloric acid. Hydrochloric acid appears in such high concentrations that gastric juice has a pH ranging between 1 and 5, and it has been estimated that at least 1500 calories are necessary to produce one liter of juice with this acidity (Langley, 1971). This degree of acidity is critical for digestion since pepsin, the enzyme for protein digestion, is only active in an acid environment. If acidity is less than normal, protein digestion will be impaired. Mucous is secreted in large quantities to buffer the acid and serve as a protective barrier between the contents of the stomach and the stomach wall. The mucosa of the duodenum continually monitors the chemical and physical properties of the material that comes from the stomach and helps to maintain hormonal and neural regulation of gastric activity.

The mechanisms involved in the neural and hormonal regulation of gastric activity are complex and highly interdependent. For this reason, most investigators prefer to discuss these mechanisms as they relate to various phases of gastric secretion. One phase, the "interdigestive" or "basal" period, refers to secretions that occur in the absence of known stimuli. Only a small amount of secretion is apparent, and it appears to be stimulated by both vagal and hormonal mechanisms. The "cephalic" phase refers to the secretory response to stimuli such as the sight of food. These may be either conditioned or unconditioned responses and are completely eliminated by vagotomy, indicating that this phase is entirely neurogenic. In the "gastric" phase, gastric activity is stimulated by both hormonal and neural activity in the stomach. In this phase, mechanical and chemical stimuli elicit the release of gastrin from the antrum which stimulates hydrochloric acid secretion. In contrast to other phases, the "intestinal" phase is thought to be exclusively hormonal. This phase occurs when food is delivered to the intestine and enterogastrones are released which serve to inhibit gastric activity.

The primary neural and hormonal mechanisms for controlling gastric activity are shown in Figures 1 and 2. As shown in Figure 1, the cortex, thalamus, hypothalamus, and brain stem have all been implicated in the regulation of gastric activity. Although autonomic innervation is primarily parasympathetic, sympathetic activity also plays a role in regulation. Whereas vagal stimulation and the release of adrenocorticotropic hormone (ACTH) stimulate gastric activity, sympathetic stimulation inhibits activity. The sensation of pain is related to the sympathetic afferent fibers whereas sensations of hunger and satiety are associated with the vagal afferent fibers.

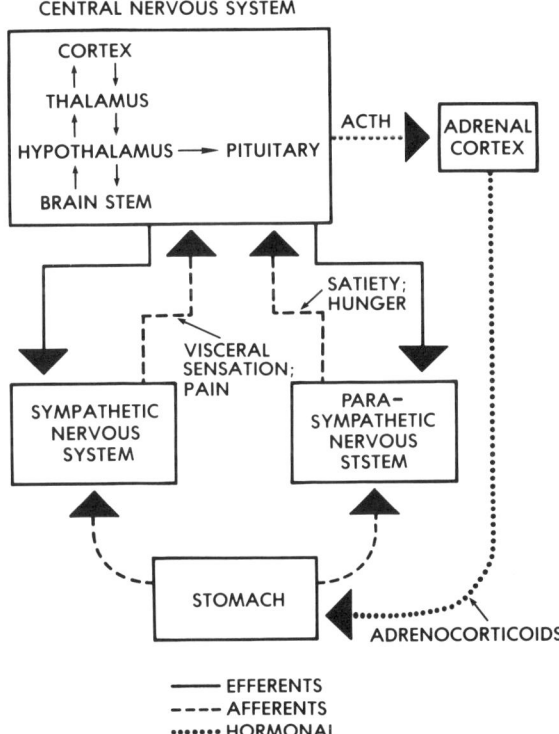

Figure 1. Neural mechanisms for controlling gastric activity.

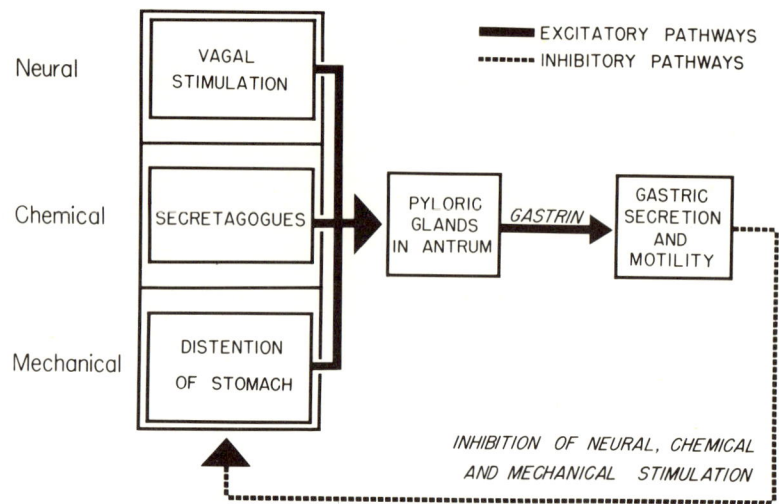

Figure 2. Integration of neural, chemical, and mechanical activity for regulating gastric activity.

Figure 2 illustrates some of the relationships among different systems and stresses the importance of feedback in controlling gastric activity. Neural stimuli (e.g., vagal stimulation), chemical stimuli (e.g., secretagogues) and mechanical stimuli (e.g., distention of the stomach) are each capable of stimulating the pyloric glands in the antrum of the stomach to secrete gastrin. In the normal process of digestion, all of these stimuli are present. Gastrin is a potent elicitor of gastric secretion and motility. As food is digested and moved into the duodenum, enterogastrones are released, the mechanical and neural stimuli are removed, and gastric activity is inhibited.

These figures illustrate only small portions of the highly integrated network of activity involved in digestion. As discussed earlier, at times these regulated processes become disregulated leading to a variety of gastrointestinal and behavioral disorders. Almost every type of lesion in the gastrointestinal system has been termed "peptic ulcer" at one time or another, and it has generally been assumed that "peptic ulcers" are the result of excess secretion of hydrochloric acid (Greenberger & Winship, 1976). It seems clear, however, that ulcers are not all alike; there are fundamental differences among ulcers occurring in different portions of the gastrointestinal system. Our understanding of ulcers has suffered greatly from efforts to attribute a common etiology to all types of ulcers.

Eighty percent of ulcers occur in the duodenum, and sufficient evidence has accumulated to support the hypothesis that duodenal ulcers are related to excess hydrochloric acid secretion. Epigastric pains experienced by the duodenal ulcer patient are rhythmic and usually occur when the stomach is empty. The pains generally subside after ingesting food or an antacid, providing support to the idea that it is the acid content of the stomach that is the inciting factor. Gastric ulcers usually occur in the antral portion of the stomach and, unlike duodenal ulcers, are more related to the integrity of the mucosa than to increases in hydrochloric acid. In fact, the mean secretory rate in patients with chronic gastric ulcers may be *less* than that of healthy subjects (Greenberger & Winship, 1976). It has been suggested that the mucosal membrane in these patients is incapable of secreting a layer of mucous that can serve as adequate protection. The pain associated with gastric ulcers is similar to that associated with duodenal ulcers but it lacks the periodicity observed in duodenal ulcer patients, and food and antacids do not provide as much relief to gastric ulcer patients.

A number of drugs can damage the gastric mucosa and are therefore thought to be ulcerogenic. Corticosteroids, for example, have been used to treat rheumatoid arthritis and frequently lead to gastric ulcers by irritating the mucosal barrier. Salicylates also cause severe damage to the mucosal barrier, leading to inflammation, bleeding, and erosion (Woodbury, 1970). Smoking may also play a role in the pathogenesis of ulcers because nicotine inhibits pancreatic secretion which can result in inadequate neutralization of gastric acid (Bynum, Solomon, Johnson, & Jacobson, 1972).

A disorder for which massive gastric hypersecretion is clearly responsible is the Zollinger–Ellison syndrome. In this syndrome, a gastrin-producing tumor continuously stimulates parietal cells to secrete hydrochloric acid. This marked acid secretion can total 5–6 liters in 12 hr, completely overwhelming all neutralizing mechanisms. Patients with this syndrome often have multiple lesions of the esophagus, stomach, duodenum, and small intestine.

With this brief introduction, we now turn to the major question to which this paper addresses itself: Can we reinstate regulatory processes? To answer this question, it is first important to clarify conceptualizations of regulatory and disregulatory processes.

3. Regulation

Walter B. Cannon's (1939) notion of the "emergency reaction" and Hans Selýe's (1946) formulation of a "general adaptation syndrome" have provided the basis for classical views regarding regulation. Although Cannon focused on autonomic changes that occur in response to stress, and Selýe was concerned primarily with biochemical changes, both scientists held a similar view of the relationship between the environment and the organism. This view emphasized that the brain dictates bodily responses to environmental stimulation. The body responds to orders from the brain.

This view gave rise to a conceptualization of psychosomatic disorders as diseases that result from a disturbance of emotions. Dunbar (1935) suggested that various personality patterns may be associated with different psychosomatic disorders, and later Alexander (1950) suggested that specific emotions might give rise to specific types of pathology. Regardless of the etiology, however, treatment of psychosomatic disorders focused on the emotional responses of the individual. Since the mind was thought to control bodily functions, the mind became the focus of therapeutic attempts. Usually this took the form of psychoanalysis.

In the past 20 years it has become clear that the relation between bodily processes and environmental events is much more complex than Cannon and Selýe initially described. Afferent fibers which complete visceral feedback systems with the central nervous system play an important role in psychological as well as physiological processes. This has given rise to a model of regulation which stresses the importance of information that the brain continuously receives from the body. Afferent impulses contribute to determining a context with which the brain receives and processes information. Personality factors, cognitive activity, heredity, and learning also play a role in determining this context. As a result, perception is an active process which involves physiological as well as psychological processes. This idea dates back to William James (1890), and several lines of evidence have now accumulated to support this model. Evidence for this model can be divided into two categories: the role of efferent activity and the role of afferent activity in regulation.

3.1. The Role of Efferent Activity in Regulation

Cannon (1939) believed that the same physiological responses occur in pain, hunger, fear, and rage, but experimental evidence has not supported this idea. Ax (1953), for example, demonstrated that patterns of responses associated with fear could be differentiated from those associated with anger. Other investigators (Davis, Buchwald, & Frankmann, 1955; Lacey, 1959) have also described a variety of different physiological reactions that occur in response to a variety of stimuli. Further evidence suggests that individuals exhibit different patterns of autonomic responses to stress (Engel, 1960; Engel & Bickford, 1961; Lacey, 1959). Lacey (1959) demonstrated that, regardless of the stressor, individuals respond maximally with changes in the same physiological system. Furthermore, patients with specific disorders respond to stress maximally with changes in the symptomatic system (Malmo & Shagass, 1949; Moos & Engel, 1962; Walker & Sandman, 1977).

The evidence cited above indicates that different stressors elicit different patterns of responses, and different individuals show idiosyncratic patterns of physiological responses. As such, heredity, cognitive activity, learning, and personality factors are important considerations when attempting to understand the interactions among the brain, the viscera, and the environment. Schachter, for example, has proposed that emotional states can be manipulated by changing the cognitive set or the physiological reactions of subjects (Schachter & Singer, 1962). Similarly, Lazarus (1967) has emphasized the importance of appraisal and cognitive factors in emotion. He and his colleagues (Lazarus, Speisman, Mordkoff, & Davison, 1962) have demonstrated that physiological responses and emotional states can be influenced by changing the instructional sets that are given to subjects. Further, it has long been known that certain individuals are genetically predisposed to various disorders (Gardner, 1972), and that autonomic activity is subject to the principles of learning (Miller, 1969; Pavlov, 1927). In fact, much theorizing and research about psychosomatic disorders has recently focused on attitudes (Graham, 1972) and learning (Miller, 1969; Miller & Dworkin, 1977).

3.2. The Role of Afferent Activity in Regulation

Although most investigations have focused on the role of the brain in regulating autonomic activity, a substantial amount of data has accumulated to indicate that visceral afferent activity affects a variety of perceptual and cognitive processes. Most of the research regarding the behavioral significance of visceral activity has focused on the cardiovascular system and is a direct result of inferences stemming from a series of studies carried out by the Laceys and their colleagues. Lacey, Kagan, Lacey, and Moss (1963) found that both heart rate and blood pressure differentiated between tasks requiring attention to input (e.g., detecting flashes) from those in which attention to the environment would be detrimental to performance (e.g., mental arithmetic). These authors suggested that "mental concentration" is accompanied by transient hypertensive states whereas attention to the environment is accompanied by brief hypotensive states. Experiments demonstrating that faster reaction times are associated with slower heart rates (Coquery & Lacey, 1966; Lacey & Lacey, 1970; Obrist, Webb, & Sutterer, 1969) provided initial support for this speculation, and the relation between heart rate and behavior has since been demonstrated in a variety of paradigms such as complex problem solving (Kaiser & Sandman, 1975), visual search (Coles, 1972), auditory threshold (Saxon & Dahle, 1971), and viewing stressful stimuli (Hare, 1973; Sandman, 1975; Walker & Sandman, 1977).

The relationship between heart rate and behavior has also been demonstrated in two studies using operant conditioning paradigms to change heart rate. In one study, subjects perceived tachistoscopic stimuli more accurately during conditioned cardiac deceleration than during cardiac acceleration (McCanne & Sandman, 1974). In another, subjects were able to generate more counterarguments to persuasive messages (indicating facilitated cognitive processing) during cardiac acceleration than during deceleration (Cacioppo, Sandman, & Walker, 1978). Furthermore, other data indicate that spontaneous changes in heart rate are related to perception (Sandman, McCanne, Kaiser, & Diamond, 1977) as well as electrocortical activity (Walker & Sandman, 1979). These data, taken together, indicate that decreases in heart rate are related to increased attention to the environment whereas increases in heart rate are related to a rejection of environmental input and possibly to enhanced cognitive activity.

Although these studies have dealt primarily with cardiovascular changes and attention, there is little reason to doubt that afferent activity is equally important in the regulation of other physiological and behavioral processes. In fact, 90% of the 30,000 fibers in the vagi are afferent (Agostoni, Chinnock, Daly, & Murray, 1957; Evans & Murray, 1954). With respect to the gastrointestinal system, Ádám and his colleagues have reported several intriguing experiments regarding afferent activity. They have demonstrated, for instance, that intestinal stimulation induces electrocortical changes and changes in the wakefulness–sleep balance in cats (see Ádám, 1978). Inflating a balloon in the duodenum of dogs and humans leads to desynchronization of electrocortical activity (Ádám, Heffler, Kovacs, Nagy, & Szigeti, 1965; Preisich & Ádám, 1964), and individuals can be taught to perceive visceral stimulation that they were unable to perceive prior to conditioning (see Ádám, 1978). Thus, it seems clear that visceral afferent impulses from systems other than the cardiovascular system also exert extrahomeostatic influences on the brain and behavior. The role of these afferent impulses in maintaining states of behavioral and physiological regulation has only begun to be explored (cf. Chapters 17 and 18 of this volume).

By now it should be clear that both afferent and efferent activity constantly work together to maintain regulation. Regulatory processes rely heavily upon feedback systems to communicate and, as Schwartz (1977) has pointed out, lack of appropriate feedback or the inability to interpret feedback often leads to disregulation.

4. Disregulation of the Stomach

How does disregulation occur in the gastrointestinal tract? Within the organism itself, there are regulatory feedback mechanisms operating from the cellular level to the cortex that can be disrupted. For example, the stomach is equipped with complex autoregulatory mechanisms that can control secretion even in the absence of external factors (Brooks, 1970). Acetylcholine and antral distension stimulate the release of gastrin, but when pH in the antrum falls below 3, gastrin release is inhibited (Brooks, 1970; Davenport, 1966). Superimposed upon these gastric regulatory mechanisms are central, autonomic, and hormonal regulatory systems. Afferent fibers in the vagi, for example, encode changes in pH, osmotic pressure, and distension, and efferent vagal impulses can stimulate the parietal cells directly. In addition, the small intestine plays a role in control of secretion in that acid entering the duodenum inhibits gastric secretion.

In addition to these feedback systems contained within the gastrointestinal tract itself, there are behavioral and psychosocial feedback networks that interact with the organism and play a role in regulation. Each level of organization contains autoregulatory mechanisms that can be modulated by activity occurring at higher levels. Gastric secretion, for example, is controlled locally by nervous reflexes and hormonal activity. The autonomic nervous system imposes another level of control, and autonomic activity is, of course, subject to rigorous control by central nervous system activity. The relation between central and autonomic activity, however, depends to some extent upon events occurring outside of the organism. As discussed earlier, the brain is constantly taking in and processing environmental events, and these processes coincide with autonomic changes. Thus, it is easy to understand why physiological and psychosocial factors are best conceptualized as "complementary" with respect to the etiology and progression of illness. It is the interaction of physiological and psychosocial feedback systems that ultimately determines the outcome.

There have been relatively few experiments that have attempted to examine these complex interactions. As with studies of regulation, most investigators have focused on efferent activity. Typically, these studies have examined the changes in the gastrointestinal system that occur as a result of stress, and the most well-known experiments demonstrating a relationship between stress and gastrointestinal activity have focused on changes in the stomach.

In 1958, Brady and his colleagues (Brady, 1958; Porter, Brady, Conrad, Manson, Galambos, & Rioch, 1958) demonstrated that they could induce ulcers in monkeys who had to press a lever at least once every 20 sec to prevent shocks to themselves and control monkeys. They called this monkey the "executive monkey," and the phenomenon gained considerable attention in both basic research and applied clinical settings. It appeared that these studies provided experimental evidence that ulcers were related to decision making; the individual responsible for making decisions was the most likely to develop an ulcer.

There are several problems with the interpretation of these findings, however, that need to be pointed out. First, the only schedule that induced ulcers was one involving 6 hr of rest and 6 hr of lever-pressing. Other schedules did not lead to chronic ulcers (cf. Natelson, 1977). Secondly, rather than selecting the animals randomly, monkeys that showed the most initiative in pressing the lever were chosen as "executive monkeys" and more passive monkeys served as controls. Furthermore, the "executive monkeys" did not merely develop ulcers; they died while in the apparatus, and the ulcers were later determined upon autopsy. Subsequent studies that involved the use of fistulas revealed that increases in gastric acid occur during the rest period rather than during performance of an avoidance task (Brady, 1963; Polish, Brady, Mason, Thack, & Niemack, 1962). All of these factors contributed to the fact that several studies failed to replicate the original "executive monkey" phenomenon (Foltz & Millet, 1964; Natelson, 1977).

Weiss (1977) has presented findings that are in direct opposition to those of the "executive monkey" study and has developed a model which seems to reconcile the two sets of results. These data and the model provide interesting evidence to support the idea that information feedback systems play a critical role in disregulation. The model suggests that gastric lesions are a function of the amount of relevant feedback available as well as the number of responses that are made. Gastric lesions decrease as the amount of relevant feedback increases, but increase as the number of responses increases. The model is a pyramid with only two edges as the base. One edge of the base represents the number of responses made and the other edge represents the amount of relevant feedback. The amount of ulceration can be determined by finding the intersection of these two points and measuring the height of the pyramid above that point. If, for example, many responses are made and the amount of feedback is low, the intersection occurs below a high point in the pyramid and severe ulceration can be predicted. On the other hand, if few responses are made with a large amount of feedback, the points intersect below the lowest point in the pyramid and ulceration will be minimal.

One implication of this model is that information feedback elicits organized patterns of behavior which serve as coping responses and lessen the impact of a stressor. Weiss' studies, for example, have demonstrated that animals given the opportunity to avoid shock develop less severe gastric lesions than those denied the opportunity (see Weiss, 1977). Furthermore, fighting can be induced in rats by shocking their tails, and animals allowed to fight show less severe gastric ulceration (Weiss, Pohorecky, Salmon, & Gruenthal, 1976) than animals who are alone and therefore unable to fight. Even rats who are merely allowed to make aggressive responses toward each other without physical contact (because of a plexiglass grid between them) show a significant reduction in gastric lesions (Weiss *et al.*, 1976).

Whereas organized behavior patterns serve as coping responses and diminish physiological responses to stress in lower animals, it appears that cognitive activity can serve a similar function in humans (Lazarus, 1967). In view of this, it is interesting that ulcer patients have been described as "oral-aggressive" by Alexander (1950), and as having an attitude of one who "has been deprived of what he is due and wants revenge" (Grace & Graham, 1952). Like rats who are prevented from fighting and develop gastric lesions, ulcer patients may have developed coping styles which prevent them from adequately expressing aggressive impulses. Lazarus (1966) has found that physiological responses to stress change dramatically when coping responses are manipulated, and perhaps changes in coping style would lead to physiological changes that are therapeutically beneficial for ulcer patients. The situation is complicated, however, because changes in physiological activity can also lead to changes in coping responses.

Regardless of the relation between coping processes and physiological activity, it seems clear that ulcer patients display different physiological responses to stress than other individuals. In one study done in our laboratory, duodenal ulcer patients, rheumatoid arthritics, and healthy subjects were exposed to mildly stressful cognitive and affective stimuli while a variety of autonomic measures were recorded (Walker & Sandman, 1977). The ulcer patients were consistently the least responsive physiologically. With the exception of increased skin conductance responses while solving arithmetic problems, duodenal ulcer patients were responsive only while viewing slides taken during autopsies, when they showed increases in gastric activity as well as skin conductance responses. Furthermore, while the other groups responded to each set of stimuli with changes in heart rate, the heart rates of ulcer patients remained remarkably stable throughout the session. As mentioned earlier, physiological responses to stress are part of a complex feedback system devoted to maintaining both physiological and psychological regulation. The diminished and atypical physiological responses to stress in ulcer patients suggests a disruption of regulatory processes.

By now it should be apparent that no single cause can be identified for a specific gastrointestinal disorder. Disregulation is multifaceted and as a result, developing treatments for stomach disorders is a complicated task. Different approaches focus on different levels of the organism. The medical approach, for example, focuses on activity within the gut, whereas the psychoanalytic approach focuses on intrapsychic conflicts. In the following section, these two approaches will be reviewed, followed by a discussion of a psychobiological approach which attempts to treat disorders from a more holistic viewpoint.

5. Reinstating Regulatory Processes

5.1. The Medical Approach to Treating Stomach Disorders

The medical approach assumes that there is an identifiable physiological cause for a patient's symptoms that must be diagnosed and treated. Therefore, if a patient complains of gastrointestinal disturbances, the physician looks at the gastrointestinal tract for the cause of the symptoms. Once the cause is identified, the physician can attempt to repair the damage. In the case of the stomach, the disorder is usually an ulcer, and treatment generally entails surgery, drugs, or a change in diet.

5.1.1. Surgery

Approximately 20% of all ulcer patients undergo surgery. Vagotomy, one common surgical intervention, involves severing the two large vagal trunks that innervate the stomach. This surgery decreases secretion but also inhibits peristalsis which leads to difficulties with gastric emptying. As a result, the surgeon may then perform a gastrojejunostomy to widen the pylorus which will assist in emptying. This combination of a vagotomy and a drainage procedure is the simplest operation for peptic ulcer. Unfortunately, there is an extremely high recurrence rate. If the surgeon chooses to do so, an antrectomy may also be performed to remove the portion of the stomach that secretes gastrin. This increases the effectiveness of the surgery since the two major stimuli for parietal cell secretion are then removed and parietal cell mass is reduced.

It is important to mention that chronic complications are often associated with gastrointestinal surgery (see Williams & Cox, 1969). Regardless of the type of surgery, patients may begin to lose weight and strength. Unusual patterns of gastric motility may develop leading to pain, diarrhea, or constipation. Vagotomized patients often suffer from either gastric retention or an inability of the stomach to retain its contents. Both of these situations are associated with intense discomfort. These complications, coupled with the relatively high recurrence rate, illustrate that surgery is not a "cure" for gastrointestinal disorders. Unfortunately, there is often no alternative.

5.1.2. Pharmacological Agents

Since duodenal ulcers have typically been associated with increases in acid secretion, it seems reasonable to suspect that antacids might be effective in treating this type of ulcer. Initial uncontrolled studies and clinical experience suggested that this is the case, but more recent evidence has cast serious doubts. In a double-blind, well-controlled study, Sturdevant, Isenberg, Secrist, and Ansfield (1977) found no differences between antacid and placebo in the time to onset, the degree, or the duration of pain relief in duodenal ulcer patients. Other studies have also reported nonsignificant differences between antacids and placebo (Butler & Gersh, 1975; Hollander & Harlan, 1973). Sturdevant *et al.* (1977) have suggested that the expectation of relief may play an important role in modifying a patient's affective response to pain. Since relief of duodenal ulcer pain by antacids is regularly reported by patients and is supported by some early studies (Bonney & Pickering, 1946; Lawrence, 1952; Palmer, 1927), it is premature to conclude that antacids have no effect on ulcer pain. These new data, however, suggest that factors other than neutralization of gastric acid play a role in the pain associated with duodenal ulcers.

Since the major stimuli inducing gastric acid secretion are gastrin and vagal stimulation, anticholinergics have traditionally been used to block stimulation of the parietal cells. These drugs are effective in reducing basal, nocturnal, and stimulated acid secretion (Fordtran, Morawski, & Richardson, 1973), but because of extreme variation among individuals, the dosage is difficult to determine. Unfortunately, the dosage must be increased until side effects are noted and then reduced. Since all anticholinergics produce side effects, it has been impossible to perform double-blind controlled studies of their effectiveness in the treatment of ulcers. In spite of this problem, some studies have attempted to determine whether these drugs are superior to placebo (Hunt & Wales, 1966; Sun & Ryan, 1970; Walan, 1970), and a majority have found that they are not (see MacGregor, 1977).

Several new agents have recently become available and appear to be effective in healing peptic ulcers (Jeejeebhoy, 1978). Carbenoxolone sodium increases gastric mucosal resistance and accelerates healing in both gastric and duodenal ulcer (Brown, Salmon, & Thien-Htut, 1972; Horwich & Galloway, 1965). Unfortunately, the main effects of the drug are related to sodium retention, which also causes edema, weight gain, and congestive heart failure. Cimetidine, another new pharmacological agent, blocks histamine (H_2) receptors and thus inhibits the stimulating effect of histamine on gastric secretion (Burland & Simkins, 1977). It has been found to significantly increase the rate of healing of duodenal ulcers (Gillespie, Gray, & Smith, 1977) and may even be useful to prevent recurrence (Jeejeebhoy, 1978). Metaclopramide is a drug that hastens gastric emptying and reduces the flow of bile onto the duodenum. It also increases the tone of the gastroesophageal sphincter (Heitmann & Moller, 1970) and helps control reflux esophagitis and ulcerations of the esophagus (Johnson, 1971). In addition, it seems to have a positive effect on gastric ulceration and gastritis (Jeejeebhoy, 1978). The side-effects of metaclopramide, however, include depression, lethargy, and Parkinsonism, which may limit its usefulness. Currently, carbenoxolone sodium is the drug of choice for gastric ulcer, whereas cimetidine is the drug of choice for duodenal ulcer.

5.1.3. Diet

A bland diet including milk, cottage cheese, and white meat has traditionally been recommended as part of ulcer therapy, but there is little evidence that this diet has any effect on ulcer pain or healing of ulcers (MacGregor, 1977). For example, Doll, Friedlander, and Pygott (1956) found that gastric ulcers were unaffected by bland diets, and other investigators (Lennard–Jones & Babouris, 1965) have shown that milk and cream not only do not decrease gastric acid secretion, but they may actually increase it. Furthermore, Ippoliti, Maxwell, and Isenberg (1976) have recently shown that the calcium in milk can be a potent stimulator of gastric acid secretion.

5.1.4. Summary

It is important to note that these three major forms of medical intervention (surgery, drugs, and diet) also exert powerful influences on other systems. This can be seen more clearly if viewed in terms of the model of regulation emphasized throughout this chapter. Figure 3 illustrates the model as it pertains to the

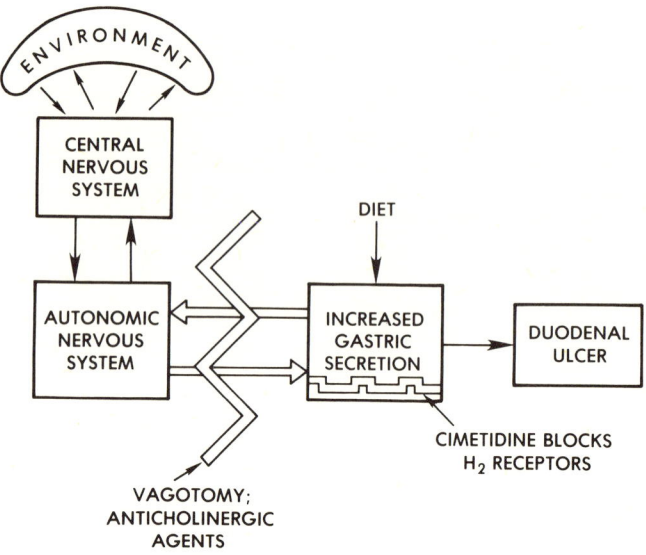

Figure 3. Medical treatment of the gastrointestinal system.

development and medical treatment of duodenal ulcers. The figure illustrates that medical treatments focus on the gastrointestinal system itself: anticholinergic drugs and vagotomies interrupt vagal stimulation, cimetidine inhibits secretion by blocking histamine receptors, and changing the diet directly changes the substances introduced into the stomach and duodenum. The model emphasizes, however, that these treatments can have profound effects on other processes as well. The outcome of vagotomy, for example, may represent more than the loss of parasympathetic stimulation of gastric secretion (see Donahue, Marrie, Krystosek, & Nyhus, 1977). After vagotomy, gastric mucosal cells show changes in the sympathetic nerve terminals. In addition, afferent as well as efferent impulses are severed during vagotomy, and, as discussed above, these impulses are critical for regulating other physiological and behavioral processes. Although cimetidine does inhibit gastric secretion, reports of side effects such as breast changes in males (Hall, 1976) and mental confusion (Delaney & Ravey, 1977; Nelson, 1977) are also beginning to emerge, emphasizing that afferent and efferent systems are both involved, and caution should be taken when prescribing these new substances (Castell, 1978). As seen in Figure 3, these treatments may serve to perpetuate disregulation rather than reinstate regulatory processes.

5.2. The Psychoanalytic Approach to Treating Stomach Disorders

Psychoanalysis, the prevailing psychological approach to the treatment of physical disorders, is a direct outgrowth of the medical approach. Like the medical approach, psychoanalysis focuses on the underlying causes rather than on the symptoms of the disorder. Whereas the physician searches the gastrointestinal tract for the cause, the psychoanalyst focuses on intrapsychic events. One assumption of this approach is that physical symptoms result from disturbances of mental events; when intrapsychic conflicts are resolved, bodily processes will resume normal functioning. In 1965, Alexander and Flagg stated the position clearly: ". . . psychotherapy is the only treatment which can alter the patients' psychic conflict, which constitutes the primary disturbance in the chain of events causing the ulcer" (p. 874). According to Alexander (1950), the critical factor in the development of ulcers is the frustration associated with the wish to receive love. When this wish is rejected, it is converted into a wish to be fed. This then leads to chronic gastric hyperfunction and ultimately, to an ulcer.

There are data from both clinical and psychophysiological studies providing evidence for a relationship between intrapsychic conflicts and stomach disorders. Several clinical investigators, for example, have found evidence of oral-dependent tendencies (Garma, 1958; Streitfeld, 1954; Weisman, 1956) and frustrations associated with demands for love in ulcer patients (Taboroff & Brown, 1954). Fear (Mahl, 1949) and anxiety (Heller, Levine, & Sohler, 1953) have been related to changes in the vascularity of the mucosa of the large intestine in ulcerative colitis (Engel, 1954).

These data suggest that emotions and subconscious processes are related to gastrointestinal disturbances, but evidence regarding the benefits of psychotherapy is sparse. Most of the studies designed to assess the efficacy of psychotherapy have been uncontrolled, and the data are equivocal (see Bräutigan & VonRad, 1977). It seems that traditional forms of psychotherapy contribute to physical and emotional improvements in some individuals but not in others.

It is thus apparent that the medical approach ignores psychological processes whereas the psychoanalytic approach ignores physiological activity. In response to this, a psychobiological approach is beginning to emerge in an attempt to integrate psychological and psychophysiological principles in treating patients with physical ailments.

5.3. The Psychobiological Approach to Treating Stomach Disorders

Figure 4 illustrates the duodenal ulcer patient as conceptualized from a psychobiological perspective. As shown in the figure, central, autonomic, and hormonal mechanisms within the organism regulate gastric activity, but this represents only a portion of the processes involved. There is continuous communication between the environment and the organism which also plays a significant role in regulation. Physiological mechanisms interact with behavioral and psychosocial factors to maintain regulation, and disregulation results from disruption of these systems. Therefore, the goal of a psychobiologically oriented treatment is to reinstate regulatory processes (see Schwartz, 1977). The general

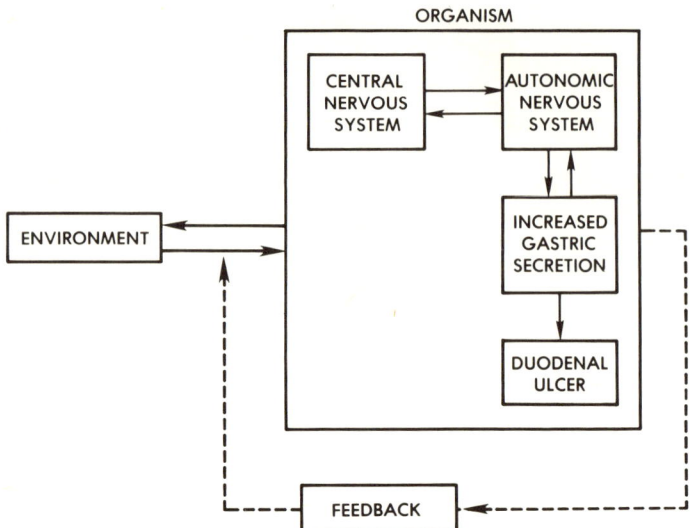

Figure 4. Model of the psychobiological approach to treatment.

strategy of such an approach is first to determine how each portion of the system has been disrupted, and then to design treatment plans accordingly. Unlike other approaches, diagnostic and treatment procedures are carried out at multiple levels, treatment is highly individualized and directly related to assessment, and the patient plays an active role in treatment.

In order to illustrate this type of approach, consider the hypothetical case of a duodenal ulcer patient referred to our Behavioral Medicine Consultation Service at the Ann Arbor Veterans Administration Medical Center. Suppose that despite numerous types of treatments, the patient continues to experience considerable pain, and both physician and patient are confused as to why various treatments have failed. It would be explained to both physician and patient that a more complete analysis must be undertaken not only of gastrointestinal activity, but also of psychological, behavioral, and psychophysiological factors. The following types of assessment would then be carried out:

1. *Medical.* Based upon results of medical diagnostic tests and discussions with the referring physician, the nature of the gastrointestinal disturbance would be clarified. The extent of physical damage, possible mechanisms of action, and responses to different medical treatment would be obtained from the medical record and discussed with both physician and patient.

2. *Psychological.* The patient would be asked to undergo a brief psychological evaluation to obtain some general information regarding his/her personality and level of cognitive functioning. Typically, patients are given the Minnesota

Multiphasic Personality Inventory and a sentence completion test to take home and return on the next visit. This yields information about motivation as well as personality. Tests of cognitive functioning are usually carried out within the hospital.

Since "medical patients" are rarely given a psychological evaluation, results of the psychological assessment are sometimes surprising to the referring physician. An ulcer patient, for example, may show "poor compliance" because he or she is cognitively impaired and unable to understand the physician's instructions. On the other hand, psychological assessment may indicate that poor compliance is an expression of hostility, paranoia, or depression. In each case, treatment will differ.

3. *Behavioral*. Similar to behavioral approaches used for other types of disturbances, an interview is carried out with the patient to specify a "target" which will serve as the focus of the behavioral analyses and treatment (see Melamed & Siegel, 1980). In a duodenal ulcer patient, the target is most likely to be gastric pain. A "functional analysis" is then carried out during which the clinician attempts to gain a clear understanding of the pain as well as the events that precede and follow painful episodes. The patient plays an active role in this process by keeping a log in which each painful episode is recorded. Typically, patients are asked to record what they were "doing, thinking, and feeling before, during, and after each episode."

The importance of this log cannot be overemphasized. First, self-monitoring alone can lead to improvement (see Pomerleau & Brady, 1979). Second, the log often reveals significant factors that cannot be obtained from the patient directly because the patient is unaware of them. For example, pain may be experienced more when the patient is at home than away from home, and the pain may have a significant effect upon family interactions. In this case, the clinician must consider some form of family intervention. Third, the log helps establish a base line from which changes can be measured. In the hands of a skilled clinician and a cooperative patient, the log can provide extremely useful information for evaluating the degree of disruption in different feedback systems as well as the effects of different types of treatment on these systems.

4. *Psychophysiological*. Based upon results of the medical, psychological, and behavioral assessments, a protocol for psychophysiological evaluation is determined for each patient individually. During this evaluation, a variety of autonomic responses are measured while the patient engages in various types of activities. Although the protocol differs for each patient, cognitive stressors (e.g., arithemetic problems), affective stressors (e.g. slides taken during autopsies), an interview, and some imagery exercises are usually included in the battery.

This type of evaluation serves several purposes. From a psychophysiological perspective, it allows the clinician to observe the patient's responses to different real and imaginary situations. In the initial interview, for example, patients frequently link "anxiety and tension" with gastric disturbance, but are unable to explain the nature of their feelings from either a psychological or somatic point of view. In a psychophysiological evaluation, the clinician can observe which types of stressors lead to changes in different autonomic systems. This is important for designing some form of intervention using biofeedback. From a more psychological point of view, the evaluation serves as a format for introducing the patient to psychophysiological concepts and techniques, for answering questions, and for reducing anxiety that is frequently induced by psychophysiological procedures.

An individualized treatment plan is then designed based upon these types of assessments. A plan for an ulcer patient might include a psychological treatment such as behavior therapy, a medical treatment such as pharmacotherapy, and a psychophysiological treatment such as biofeedback. Attempts are made to integrate the various types of treatment in an effort to teach the patient self-regulation. The hope is that as this goal is approached, the need for medication will diminish and surgical intervention will be avoided.

5.4. Biofeedback and Gastric Activity

Because disregulation occurs when feedback systems are disrupted, reinstating regulation involves manipulating different types of feedback. Figure 4 illustrates how one type of feedback can be provided to give a patient information about bodily changes. This type of feedback has been termed biofeedback, and in conjunction with operant conditioning techniques, is being explored as a treatment for gastrointestinal disorders.

A study recently completed in our laboratory illustrates how the biofeedback paradigm can be used to teach individuals to control electrogastric activity (Walker, Lawton, & Sandman, 1978). The purpose of the study was to examine the possibility that individuals can modify electrogastric activity specifically as it is reflected by the tonic component of the electrogastrogram (EGG). This was of interest because in a previous study (Walker & Sandman, 1977) it was the tonic component that differentiated healthy subjects from those with duodenal ulcers. It is possible that specific control of tonic EGG activity could be therapeutic for certain duodenal ulcer patients.

Eight fasting male subjects participated in two sessions on two consecutive mornings. Transducers were attached to enable monitoring of EGG, respiration, heart rate, digital blood flow, and abdominal EMG. Each subject was instructed that when a light was illuminated they were to try to move the needle on a meter in front of them to the right (indicating a negative deflection of the EGG) without changing respiration or tensing any muscles. They were also told that the electrical activity of their stomachs would control the meter during each trial. During the second session, they were asked to try to move the needle on the meter to the left (indicating a positive deflection of the EGG). This order was reversed for half the subjects. The experimental procedure is illustrated in Figure 5.

The results of the study indicated that individuals can modify tonic EGG activity. Changes in the negative direction were more easily obtained than changes in the positive direction. Consistent with other investigations of the gastrointestinal system (Whitehead, Renault, & Goldiamond, 1975) some subjects evidenced discriminative control while others did not. Those who showed the least amount of abdominal EMG activity and reported being the most relaxed and "indifferent" were the ones who evidenced discriminative control.

Weiss (1977) has speculated that increases in skeletal muscle activity may be related to the vulnerability of an individual to gastric ulceration, and its seems possible that muscle activity plays an important role in the feedback system related to the regulation of gastrointestinal activity. There are some data to suggest that EMG biofeedback and relaxation training may be effective in treating duodenal ulcers (Aleo & Nicassio, 1978; Beaty, 1976) and functional colitis (Weinstock, 1976).

Several experiments have demonstrated that the biofeedback paradigm can be used to teach healthy individuals to modify other gastrointestinal activity. Moore and Schenkenberg (1974), for example, found that a subject could increase and decrease gastric acid secretion when provided with feedback but could not continue when the feedback was removed. These authors used a nasogastric tube to collect gastric contents and provided the subjects with feedback of their

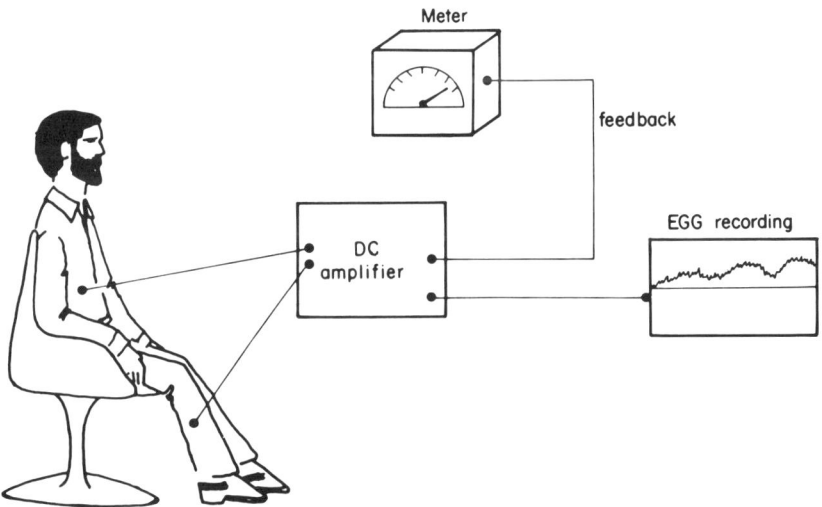

Figure 5. Experimental procedure for biofeedback.

success approximately every 10 min. Other investigators (Gorman & Kamiya, 1972; Whitehead et al., 1975) found that healthy subjects can learn to control gastric acid secretion when gastric pH is recorded using a pH electrode located within the stomach.

These data, in conjunction with data from studies with animals, have led to attempts to apply biofeedback techniques to the treatment of ulcers. As mentioned earlier, it seems clear that excess hydrochloric acid plays a primary role in duodenal ulcers whereas diminished mucosal resistance plays a primary role in gastric ulcers. Since it is difficult to measure mucosal activity in intact humans, feedback studies have focused on the control of gastric secretion in duodenal ulcer patients.

Welgan (1974) asked duodenal ulcer patients to decrease gastric acid secretion while receiving feedback provided by continuous aspiration of gastric contents. Although the concentration of acid decreased from the base-line period, no differences were observed between subsequent periods of feedback and no-feedback. Later studies (Welgan, 1977) suggested that pH feedback results in changes in the volume of secretions rather than in acid concentration. Welgan (1977) has pointed out the many technical difficulties with these measurements, and it seems that resolution must await technical advances (cf. Chapter 7, this volume).

6. Summary

In this chapter evidence has been presented to indicate that the gastrointestinal system does more than respond passively to commands from the brain. There are complex feedback systems between the central and autonomic nervous system which serve to regulate both physiological and behavioral processes. Both afferent and efferent activity work together to maintain regulation, and when communication is disrupted, disregulation occurs.

Since disregulation is multifaceted and no single cause can be identified for any specific gastrointestinal disorder, developing treatments is a complicated task. Medical, psychological, and psychobiological approaches to treatment have been examined. The medical approach looks to the gastrointestinal tract for the cause of disregulation and attempts to remedy the disorder by surgery, drugs, or change in diet. Although this approach has the advantage of providing some immediate relief, the treatments often lead to other forms of disregulation (see Figure 3). The psychoanalytic approach also searches for underlying causes but assumes them to be intrapsychic events. Unfortunately, there is little evidence to support the contention that resolving mental conflicts is therapeutic for patients with gastrointestinal disorders. The psychobiological approach represents an attempt to incorporate physiological and psychological perspectives in assessing and treating stomach disorders. This approach relies heavily upon behavioral and psychophysiological techniques. While it is still too early to assess, the evidence to date suggests that psychobiological approaches to treating stomach disorders will lead to significant theoretical and clinical advances.

7. References

Ádám, G. Visceroception, awareness, and behavior. In G. E. Schwartz & D. Shapiro (Eds.) *Consciousness and self-regulation* (Vol. 2). New York: Plenum Press, 1978.

Ádám, G., Heffler, J., Kovacs, A., Nagy, A., & Szigeti, A. Electrographic test for the discrimination of intestinal stimuli. *Acta Physiologica Academiae Scientiarum Hungaricae*, 1965, *27*, 145–147.

Agostoni, E., Chinnock, J., Daly, M., & Murray, J. Functional and histological studies of the vagus nerve, its branches to the heart, lungs, abdominal viscera in the cat. *Journal of Physiology*, 1957, *135*, 182.

Aleo, S., & Nicassio, P. *Auto-regulation of duodenal ulcer disease: A preliminary report of four cases.* Paper presented at the Ninth Annual Meeting of the Biofeedback Society of America, Albuquerque, March 1978.

Alexander, F. *Psychosomatic medicine: Its principles and applications.* New York: Norton, 1950.

Alexander, F., & Flagg, G. W. The psychosomatic approach. In B. B. Wolman (Ed.), *Handbook of clinical psychology.* New York: McGraw-Hill, 1965.

Ax, A. F. The physiological differentiation between fear and anger in humans. *Psychosomatic Medicine*, 1953, *14*, 433–442.

Beaty, E. T. Feedback assisted relaxation training as a treatment for peptic ulcers. *Biofeedback and Self-Regulation*, 1976, *1*, 323–324. (Abstract)

Bonney, G. L. W., & Pickering, G. W. Observations on the mechanism of pain in ulcers of the stomach and duodenum. *Clinical Science*, 1946, *6*, 63–89.

Brady, J. V. Ulcers in "executive monkeys." *Scientific American*, 1958, *199*, 95–100.

Brady, J. V. Further comments on the gastrointestinal system and avoidance behavior. *Psychological Reports*, 1963, *12*, 742.

Bräutigan, W., & VonRad, M. Toward a theory of psychosomatic disorders. *Psychotherapy and Psychosomatics*, 1977, *28*, 285–343.

Brooks, F. *Control of gastrointestinal function.* London: Macmillan Co., 1970.

Brown, P., Salmon, P., & Thien-Htut, A. E. Double-blind trial of carbenoxolone sodium capsules in duodenal ulcer therapy based on endoscopic diagnosis and follow-up. *British Medical Journal*, 1972, *3*, 661–664.

Burland, W. L., & Simkins, M. A. (Eds.). Cimetidine (Proceedings of the Second International Symposium on Histamine Receptor Antagonists). *Excerpta Medica*, Oxford, 1977.

Butler, M. L., & Gersh, H. Antacid vs. placebo in hospitalized gastric ulcer patients; a controlled therapeutic study. *American Journal of Digestive Disorders*, 1975, *20*, 803–807.

Bynum, T. E., Solomon, T. E., Johnson, L. R., & Jacobson, E. D. Inhibition of pancreatic secretion in man by cigarette smoking. *Gut*, 1972, *13*, 361–365.

Cacioppo, J. T., Sandman, C. A., & Walker, B. B. The effects of operant heart rate conditioning on cognitive elaboration and attitude change. *Psychophysiology*, 1978, *15*, 330–338.

Cannon, W. B. *The wisdom of the body.* New York: Norton, 1939.

Castell, D. Sense with cimetidine. *Journal of the American Medical Association*, 1978, *240*, 564.

Coles, M. G. Cardiac and respiratory activity during visual search. *Journal of Experimental Psychology*, 1972, *96*, 371–379.

Coquery, J., & Lacey, J. I. *The effect of foreperiod duration on the components of the cardiac response during the foreperiod of a reaction time experiment*. Paper presented at the Annual meeting of the Society for Psychophysiological Research, Denver, October 1966.

Davenport, H. W. *Physiology of the digestive tract*. Chicago: Year Book Medical Publishing, Inc., 1966.

Davis, R. C., Buchwald, A. M., & Frankmann, R. W. Autonomic and muscular responses and their relation to simple stimuli. *Psychological Monographs*, 1955, *69* (No. 20), 1–71.

Delaney, J. C., & Ravey, M. Cimetidine and mental confusion. *Lancet*, 1977, *2*, 512.

Doll, R., Friedlander, P., & Pygott, F. Dietetic treatment of peptic ulcer. *Lancet*, 1956, *1*, 5–9.

Donahue, P. E., Marrie, A. J., Krystosek, R., & Nyhus, L. M. Role of vagotomy in duodenal ulcers. *Postgraduate Medicine*, 1977, *62*, 156–167.

Dunbar, H. *Emotions and bodily changes*. New York: Columbia University Press, 1935.

Engel, B. T. Stimulus–response and individual-response specificity. *Archives of General Psychiatry*, 1960, *2*, 305–313.

Engel, B. T., & Bickford, A. F. Response specificity: Stimulus response and individual response specificity in essential hypertensives. *Archives of General Psychiatry*, 1961, *5*, 478–489.

Engel, G. L. Studies of ulcerative colitis. II. The nature of the somatic processes and the adequacy of the psychosomatic hypotheses. *American Journal of Medicine*, 1954, *16*, 416–433.

Evans, D. H., & Murray, J. Regeneration of nonmedullated nerve fibers. *Journal of Anatomy*, 1954, *88*, 465.

Foltz, E. L., & Millett, F. E. Experimental psychosomatic disease states in monkeys. I. Peptic ulcer—"executive monkeys." *Journal of Surgical Research*, 1964, *4*, 445–453.

Fordtran, J. C., Morawski, S. G., & Richardson, C. J. *In vivo* and *in vitro* evaluation of liquid antacids. *New England Journal of Medicine*, 1973, *288*, 923–928.

Gardner, E. J. *Principles of genetics*. New York: John Wiley & Sons, 1972.

Garma, A. *Peptic ulcer and psychoanalysis*. Baltimore: Williams & Wilkins, 1958.

Gillespie, G., Gray, G., & Smith, I. Short-term and maintenance cimetidine treatment in severe duodenal ulceration. In W. L. Burland & M. A. Simkins (Eds.), Cimetidine. *Excerpts Medica*, 1977.

Gorman, P., & Kamiya, J. *Biofeedback training of stomach pH*. Paper presented to the Western Psychological Association, San Francisco, May 1972.

Grace, W. J., & Graham, D. T. Relationship of specific attitudes and emotions to certain bodily diseases. *Psychosomatic Medicine*, 1952, *14*, 243–251.

Graham, D. T. Psychosomatic medicine. In N. Greenfield & R. Sternbach (Eds.), *Handbook of psychophysiology*. New York: Holt, Rinehart & Winston, 1972.

Greenberger, N. J., & Winship, D. H. *Gastrointestinal disorders: A pathophysiological approach*. Chicago: Year Book Medical Publisher, 1976.

Hall, W. H. Breast changes in males on cimetidine. *New England Journal of Medicine*, 1976, *295*, 841.

Hare, R. D. Orienting and defensive responses to visual stimuli. *Psychophysiology*, 1973, *10*, 453–464.

Heitmann, P., & Moller, N. The effect of metoclopramide on the gastroesophageal junctional zone and the distal esophagus in man. *Scandinavian Journal of Gastroenterology*, 1970, *5*, 620–626.

Heller, M. H., Levine, J., & Sohler, T. P. Gastric acidity and normally produced anxiety. *Psychosomatic Medicine*, 1953, *15*, 509–512.

Hill, R. B., & Kern, F. *The gastrointestinal tract*. Baltimore: Williams & Wilkins, 1977.

Hollander, D., & Harlan, J. Antacids vs. placebo in peptic ulcer therapy: A controlled double-blind investigation. *Journal of the American Medical Association*, 1973, *226*, 1181–1185.

Horwich, L., & Galloway, R. Treatment of gastric ulceration with carbenoxolone sodium: Clinical and radiological evaluation. *British Medical Journal*, 1965, *2*, 1274–1277.

Hunt, J. N., & Wales, R. C. Progress in patients with peptic ulceration treated for more than five years with polidine including a double-blind trial. *British Medical Journal*, 1966, *3*, 13–16.
Ippoliti, A. F., Maxwell, V., & Isenberg, J. I. The effect of various forms of milk on gastric acid secretion. *Annals of Internal Medicine*, 1976, *84*, 286–289.
James, W. *The principles of psychology*. New York: Holt, Rinehart & Winston, 1890.
Jeejeebhoy, K. N. Symposium on peptic ulcer disease: Medical treatment of peptic ulcer. *Canadian Journal of Surgery*, 1978, *21*, 17–18.
Johnson, A. G. Controlled trial of metaclopramide in the treatment of flatulant dyspepsia. *British Medical Journal*, 1971, *2*, 25–26.
Kaiser, D. N., & Sandman, C. A. Physiological patterns accompanying complex problem solving during warning and non-warning conditions. *Journal of Comparative and Physiological Psychology*, 1975, *89*, 357–363.
Lacey, J. I. Psychophysiological approaches to the evaluation of psychotherapeutic process and outcome. In E. A. Rubinstein & M. B. Parloff (Eds.), *Research in psychotherapy*. Washington: American Psychological Association, 1959.
Lacey, J. I., & Lacey, B. C. Some autonomic-central nervous system interrelationships. In P. Black (Ed.), *Physiological correlates of emotion*. New York: Academic Press, 1970.
Lacey, J. I., Kagan, J., Lacey, B. C., & Moss, H. The visceral level: Situational determinants and behavioral correlates of autonomic response patterns. In P. H. Knapp (Ed.), *Expression of the emotions in man*. New York: International Universities Press, 1963.
Langley, L. L. *Physiology of man*. New York: Van Nostrand Reinhold, 1971.
Lawrence, J. S. Dietetic and other methods in the treatment of peptic ulcer. *Lancet*, 1952, *1*, 482–485.
Lazarus, R. S. *Psychological stress and the coping process*. New York: McGraw-Hill, 1966.
Lazarus, R. S. Cognitive and personality factors underlying threat and coping. In M. H. Appley & R. Trumbull (Eds.), *Psychological stress: Issues in research*. New York: Appleton-Century-Crofts, 1967.
Lazarus, R. S., Speisman, J. C., Mordkoff, A. M., & Davison, L. A. A laboratory study of psychological stress produced by a motion picture film. *Psychological Monographs*, 1962, *76* (Whole No. 553).
Lennard–Jones, J. B., & Babouris, N. Effect of different foods on the acidity of the gastric contents in patients with duodenal ulcer. *Gut*, 1965, *6*, 113–117.
MacGregor, I. L. The treatment of peptic ulcer. *New Zealand Journal of Medicine*, 1977, *86*, 86–88.
Mahl, G. F. Effect of chronic fear on the gastric secretion of HCl in dogs. *Psychosomatic Medicine*, 1949, *11*, 30–44.
Malmo, R. B., & Shagass, C. Physiologic study of symptom mechanisms on psychiatric patients under stress. *Psychosomatic Medicine*, 1949, *11*, 25–29.
McCanne, T. R., & Sandman, C. A. Instrumental heart rate responses and visual perceptions: A preliminary study. *Psychophysiology*, 1974, *11*, 283–287.
Melamed, B., & Siegel, L. *Behavioral medicine*. New York: Springer, 1980.
Miller, N. E. Learning of visceral and glandular responses. *Science*, 1969, *163*, 434–435.
Miller, N. E., & Dworkin, B. R. Effects of learning on visceral functions: Biofeedback. *New England Journal of Medicine*, 1977, *296*, 1274–1278.
Moore, J. G., & Schenkenberg, T. Psychic control of gastric acid: Response to anticipated feeding and biofeedback training in man. *Gastroenterology*, 1974, *66*, 954–959.
Moos, R. H., & Engel, B. T. Psychophysiological reactions in hypertensive and arthritic patients. *Journal of Psychosomatic Research*, 1962, *6*, 227–241.
Natelson, B. The "executive monkey" revisited. In F. P. Brooks & P. W. Evans (Eds.), *Nerves and the gut*. Philadelphia: C. B. Slack, 1977.

Nelson, P. G. Cimetidine and mental confusion. *Lancet*, 1977, *2*, 928.
Obrist, P. A., Webb, R. A., & Sutterer, J. R. Heart rate and somatic changes during aversive conditioning and a simple reaction time task. *Psychophysiology*, 1969, *5*, 696–723.
Palmer, W. L. The "acid test" in gastric and duodenal ulcer. *Journal of the American Medical Association*, 1927, *88*, 1778–1780.
Pavlov, I. P. *Conditioned reflexes* (G. V. Anrep, Ed. and trans.). London: Oxford University Press, 1927.
Polish, E., Brady, J. V., Mason, J. W., Thack, J. S., & Niemeck, W. Gastric contents and the occurrence of duodenal lesions in the rhesus monkey during avoidance behavior. *Gastroenterology*, 1962, *43*, 193–201.
Pomerleau, O., & Brady, J. *Behavioral medicine*. Baltimore: Williams & Wilkins, 1979.
Porter, R. W., Brady, J. V., Conrad, D., Mason, J. W., Galambos, R., & Rioch, D. Some experimental observations on gastrointestinal lesions in behaviorally conditioned monkeys. *Psychosomatic Medicine*, 1958, *20*, 379–394.
Preisich, P., & Ádám, G. La discrimination nonconsciente des stimuli duodenaux: Le tes de defferentiation d'habituation electroencephalographique. *Acta Gastro-Enterologica Belgica*, 1964, *27*, 625–629.
Sandman, C. A. Physiological responses during escape and non-escape from stress in field independent and field dependent subjects. *Biological Psychology*, 1975, *2*, 205–216.
Sandman, C. A., McCanne, T. R., Kaiser, D. N., & Diamond, B. Heart rate and cardiac phase influences on visual perception. *Journal of Comparative and Physiological Psychology*, 1977, *91*, 189–202.
Saxon, S., & Dahle, A. Auditory threshold variations during periods of induced high and low heart rates. *Psychophysiology*, 1971, *8*, 23–29.
Schachter, S., & Singer, J. E. Cognitive, social and psychological determinants of emotional state. *Psychological Review*, 1962, *69*, 379–399.
Schwartz, G. E. Psychosomatic disorders and biofeedback: A psychobiological model of disregulation. In J. D. Maser & M. P. Seligman (Eds.), *Psychopathology: Experimental models*. San Francisco: W. H. Freeman, 1977.
Selye, H. The general adaptation syndrome and the diseases of adaptation. *Journal of Clinical Endocrinology*, 1946, *6*, 117–128.
Streitfeld, H. S. The specificity of peptic ulcer to intense oral conflict. *Psychosomatic Medicine*, 1954, *16*, 315–326.
Sturdevant, R., Isenberg, J., Secrist, D., & Ansfield, J. Antacid and placebo produced similar pain relief in duodenal ulcer patients. *Gastroenterology*, 1977, *72*, 1–5.
Sun, D. C., & Ryan, M. L. A controlled study on the use of propantheline and amylopectin sulphate (SM-263) for recurrences of duodenal ulcer. *Gastroenterology*, 1970, *58*, 756–761.
Taboroff, L. H., & Brown, W. H. Study of the personality patterns of children and adolescents with a peptic ulcer syndrome. *American Journal of Orthopsychiatry*, 1954, *24*, 602–610.
Walan, A. Studies on peptic ulcer disease with special reference to the effects of l-hyoscyamine. *Acta Medica Scandinavica Suppl*, 1970, *516*, 1–57.
Walker, B. B., & Sandman, C. A. Physiological response patterns in ulcer patients: Phasic and tonic components of the electrogastrogram. *Psychophysiology*, 1977, *14*, 393–400.
Walker, B. B., & Sandman, C. A. Human visual evoked responses are related to heart rate. *Journal of Comparative and Physiological Psychology*, 1979, *93*, 717–729.
Walker, B. B., Lawton, C. A., & Sandman, C. A. Voluntary control of electrogastric activity. *Psychosomatic Medicine*, 1978, 40, 610–619.
Weinstock, S. A. The reestablishment of intestinal control in functional colitis. *Biofeedback and Self-Regulation*, 1976, *1*, 324–325.

Weisman, A. D. A study of psychodynamics of duodenal ulcer exacerbations with special reference to treatment and the problem of specificity. *Psychosomatic Medicine,* 1956, *28,* 2–42.

Weiss, J. M. Ulcers. In J. Maser & M. Seligman (Eds.), *Psychopathology: Experimental models.* San Francisco: W. H. Freeman, 1977.

Weiss, J. M., Pohorecky, L. A., Salmon, S., & Gruenthal, M. Attenuation of gastric lesions by psychological aspects of aggression in rats. *Journal of Comparative and Physiological Psychology,* 1976, *90,* 252–259.

Welgan, P. R. Learned control of gastric acid secretion in ulcer patients. *Psychosomatic Medicine,* 1974, *36,* 411–419.

Welgan, P. R. Biofeedback control of stomach acid secretions and gastrointestinal reactions. In J. Beatty & J. Legewie (Eds.), *Biofeedback and behavior.* New York: Plenum Press, 1977.

Whitehead, W. E., Renault, P. F., & Goldiamond, I. Modification of human gastric acid secretion with operant conditioning procedures. *Journal of Applied Behavior Analysis,* 1975, *8,* 147–156.

Williams, J. A., & Cox, A. (Eds.). *After vagotomy.* London: Buttersworth, 1969.

Woodbury, D. M. Analgesic-antipyretics, anti-inflammatory agents and inhibitors of uric acid synthesis. In L. Goodman & A. Gilman (Eds.), *The pharmacological basis of therapeutics.* London: Macmillan, 1970.

PART III

COLON
WILLIAM E. WHITEHEAD

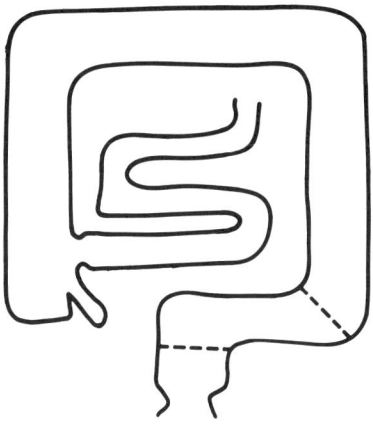

The colon offers psychophysiologists their greatest opportunity to make significant scientific and clinical contributions to gastroenterology: The colon is relatively easy to access for psychophysiological measurement, yet its physiology is poorly understood. As an example, the basic patterns of motility and electromyographic activity which mediate defecation and its disordered states—constipation and diarrhea—are still controversial. Moreover, irritable bowel syndrome and other functional disorders of the colon are prevalent in the population and constitute important clinical syndromes for which treatment is so far inadequate.

Irritable bowel syndrome is usually defined by the presence of abdominal pain and altered bowel habits in the absence of any physical findings adequate to explain the symptoms (cf. Chapter 14). It is an extremely common disorder; 8%–14% of adults report the presence of these symptoms within any given year (Whitehead, Winget, Fedoravicius, Wooley, & Blackwell, 1982; Thompson & Heaton, 1980), and it is estimated that 50%–75% will be affected at some point in their lifetime (Texter & Butler, 1975). The irritable bowel syndrome accounts for 40%–70% of consultations to gastroenterologists (Drossman, Powell, & Sessions, 1977) and for an estimated 115,000 hospital admissions per year (Mendeloff, 1979).

The childhood version of the irritable bowel syndrome, which is called recurrent abdominal pain (Stone & Barbero, 1970), occurs in approximately 14.4% of children aged 6–19 (Oster, 1972). Another colonic disorder believed to be mediated by abnormal colonic motility is diverticular disease, which is characterized by herniations of the intestinal lumen into the muscle layer of the colon creating pockets which may become infected. Diverticular disease is rare in early adult life but increases with age and reaches a prevalence of about 40% in those aged 70 and older (Connell, 1974).

There is a well-documented association of irritable bowel syndrome with psychologial disorders. Of these patients 75% to 90% have psychological scores in the abnormal range, consisting primarily of depression, anxiety, and neurotism (Hislop, 1971; Liss, Alpers, & Woodruff, 1973; Young, Alpers, Norland, & Woodruff, 1976). Moreover, approximately half of irritable bowel patients report a relationship between subjective stress and exacerbations of their symptoms, and about half recall an acute episode of stress immediately preceding the onset of their symptoms (Chaudhary & Truelove, 1962; Hislop, 1971; Waller & Misiewicz, 1969; Wangel & Deller, 1965). Recently we (Whitehead et al., 1982) have called attention to the tendency of these patients to exhibit a pattern of chronic illness behavior characterized by multiple somatic complaints and a history of social rewards for illness.

The psychopathology associated with the irritable bowel syndrome is better understood than its pathophysiology. As Latimer shows in Chapter 13, there is a growing controversy over whether there is any unique physiological response which mediates these symptoms. Latimer argues that the pattern of colonic motility which has been reported in these patients is common to all neurotic patients including those without bowel symptoms. He suggests that many irritable bowel patients have colonic physiology and bowel habits which are within the normal range, and that they are simply neurotics who are preoccupied with normal bowel habits and normal bodily sensations which they exaggerate. Latimer suggests that such patients may constitute one of many types of patients who are currently lumped together as irritable bowel syndrome, and he suggests that there may be a different subgroup of patients with abnormal colonic physiology.

The strongest contender for a biological marker of the irritable bowel syndrome is an abnormal incidence of 3 cpm electromyographic activity in the colon. As Duthie points out in Chapter 12, two groups of investigators have reported that irritable bowel patients show a greater ratio of these electrophysiological events to faster 6 cpm electrical waves compared to normal subjects, and these electrophysiological differences do not disappear when the patient is asymptomatic. If true, this would suggest a biological basis for susceptibility to the symptoms of irritable bowel syndrome (IBS) for which a pharmacological solution might be found. However, other investigators have failed to find any differences in electromyographic activity between IBS patients and normals. Latimer reviews the evidence for and against this abnormal EMG hypothesis in Chapter 13.

A particularly exciting development for psychophysiologists is the skin surface measure of colonic electromyographic activity mentioned in Duthie's chapter. This measure is comparable to the electrogastrogram discussed in an earlier section which has stimulated so much psychophysiological investigation of the stomach. The electrocolonogram requires additional validation, including studies using the signal analysis techniques described by Hölzl and Brüchle in Chapter 5, but it has great potential both in scientific investigation and in biofeedback treatment applications.

Schuster reviews methods of recording colonic motility and compliance in Chapter 11 and describes the use of these procedures in the diagnosis of a variety of medical disorders. In Chapter 14, Schuster describes the application of psychophysiological measures to the biofeedback treatment of the irritable bowel syndrome. Other psychological methods of treatment found to be useful for patients with irritable bowel syndrome are discussed by Latimer in Chapter 13. These psychological treatments include systematic desensitization, cognitive behavior therapy, and behavior modification procedures to change the social consequences of symptomatic complaints. A more detailed discussion of these treatment procedures and the research data supporting their efficacy is given in Whitehead and Schuster (1981).

References

Chaudhary, N. A., & Truelove, S. C. The irritable colon syndrome: A study of the clinical features, predisposing causes, and prognosis in 130 cases. *Quarterly Journal of Medicine,* 1962, *31,* 307–322.
Connell, A. M. Clinical aspects of motility. *Medical Clinics of North America,* 1974, *58,* 1201–1216.
Drossman, D. A., Powell, D. W., & Sessions, J. T., Jr. The irritable bowel syndrome. *Gastroenterology,* 1977, *73,* 811–822.
Hislop, I. G. Psychological significance of the irritable colon syndrome. *Gut,* 1971, *12,* 452–457.
Liss, J. L., Alpers, D., & Woodruff, R. A., Jr. The irritable colon syndrome and psychiatric illness. *Diseases of the Nervous System,* 1973, *34,* 151–157.
Mendeloff, A. I. Epidemiology of the irritable bowel syndrome. *Practical Gastroenterology,* 1979, *3*(3), 12–18.
Oster, J. Recurrent abdominal pain, headache, and limb pains in children and adolescents. *Pediatrics,* 1972, *50,* 429–435.
Stone, R. T., & Barbero, G. J. Recurrent abdominal pain in childhood. *Pediatrics,* 1970, *45,* 732–738.
Texter, E. C., Jr., & Butler, R. C. The irritable bowel syndrome. *American Family Physician,* 1975, *11,* 169–173.
Thompson, W. G., & Heaton, K. W. Functional bowel disorders in apparently healthy people. *Gastroenterology,* 1980, *79,* 283–288.
Waller, S. L., & Misiewicz, J. J. Prognosis in the irritable-bowel syndrome. *Lancet,* 1969, *2,* 753–756.
Wangel, A. G., & Deller, D. J. Intestinal motility in man. III. Mechanisms of constipation and diarrhea with particular reference to the irritable colon syndrome. *Gastroenterology,* 1965, *48,* 69–84.
Whitehead, W. E., & Schuster, M. M. Behavioral approaches to the treatment of gastrointestinal motility disorders. *Medical Clinics of North America,* 1981, *65,* 1397–1411.
Whitehead, W. E., Winget, C., Fedoravicius, A. S., Wooley, S., & Blackwell, B. Learned illness

behavior in patients with irritable bowel syndrome and peptic ulcer. *Digestive Diseases and Sciences,* 1982, *27,* 202–208.

Young, S. J., Alpers, D. H., Norland, C. C., & Woodruff, R. A. Psychiatric illness and the irritable bowel syndrome: Practical implications for the primary physician. *Gastroenterology,* 1976, *70,* 162–166.

11

THE MEASUREMENT OF COLON MOTILITY
MARVIN M. SCHUSTER

1. Introduction

The motor activity of an organ is designed to subserve all of the other functions of the organ. In order to facilitate transit, the esophagus has developed a pattern of motor behavior which we recognize as peristalsis; as soon as a bolus comes into the esophagus, peristalsis very efficiently sweeps it through and moves it out. It would be socially disastrous if that occurred in the colon. The colon can be said to have three functions: dehydration, storage of contents until evacuation becomes socially convenient, and finally evacuation. Each of these three functions is subserved by a special type of physiological motor activity. Segmentation is the major means of effecting storage; and evacuation is achieved, not in a peristaltic manner (because peristalsis rarely occurs in the colon under normal circumstances), but by mass propulsion.

2. Measurement of the Segmenting Contractions of the Distal Colon

2.1. Concept of Paradoxical Motility

Connell (1962) has propounded the concept of the paradoxical motility of constipation and diarrhea and has made the point that segmenting contractions which create the haustral marking one sees on barium X rays are primarily an impeding type of activity. This is the principal type of motility that one encounters in the colon. This physiological activity can be exaggerated either in a

---

MARVIN M. SCHUSTER • The Johns Hopkins School of Medicine and the Division of Digestive Diseases, Baltimore City Hospital, Baltimore, Maryland 21224.

manner of increase or a manner of decrease, and when the segmenting activity is increased, one sees accentuation of these haustral contractions. The barium enema X ray of a patient with constipation shows excessive haustral contractions, which explains the complaint of excessively dehydrated, scybalous stools. This is in sharp contrast to a patient with ulcerative colitis who has the so-called lead-pipe colon in which there is effacement of segmenting, impeding contractions. This situation leads to diarrhea because there is no impeding motility present. Pressures from the colon of a normal subject show much more segmenting activity than in the patient with ulcerative colitis. This also explains the action of the opiates in the treatment of diarrhea. The opiates act to increase the amount of segmenting, impeding contractions.

The two examples of clinical disorders associated with exaggerated segmentation are the irritable bowel syndrome and diverticular disease. One of the disorders associated with diminished activity is ulcerative colitis.

2.2. Recording Techniques

The most common and practical methods of measuring the contractile activity of the distal colon involve pressure measurements. Either an open-tipped, perfused tube or a tube with an attached balloon can be inserted by rectum and the pressure recorded by this means. Open-tipped tubes provide the simplest devices, and they are capable of recording absolute pressures. However, this requires a constant pressure, constant flow pump, and care must be taken to keep the recording tip at the same height as the pressure transducer. Another disadvantage of perfused tubes is that they may become clogged by stool. Balloons have the advantages that they can be used to stimulate colon motility as well as record, no pump is required, and when the balloons are filled with air there is no need to keep them at the same height as the pressure transducers. This disadvantage of balloons is that absolute pressure measurement are not feasible since the elastic properties of the balloon contribute to the recorded pressure. It is possible to use solid-state pressure transducers on the walls of a tube to record intracolonic pressure, but these are liable to be clogged by stool and are not recommended.

A criticism which is often made of pressure measurements is that they are not a direct function of contractions; in order to produce a pressure increase a contraction must occur in a segment of colon which is closed at both ends. It is possible for a contraction in one area to be accompanied by a relaxation in an adjacent area with no net change in pressure.

To deal with this confounding influence Latimer (Latimer, Sarna, Campbell, Latimer, & Daniel, 1981) developed a strain guage which was bonded to the surface of a tube in such a way that it responded to lumen-occluding contractions but not to pressure changes. Small contractions which do not obliterate the lumen, however, may be missed by this technique.

Investigators have also used visual inspection to assess colonic motility. For example, Almy's classic studies of the effects of emotion on the colon were done by observing the colon through a proctoscope during an interview. This is an uncomfortable procedure for the subject, and its reliability of measurement is poor because it depends on subjective judgement under variable conditions of observation. It is more common to infer the presence of colonic spasm from the appearance of barium enema X-rays. This, too, is an unreliable subjective technique and is not practical for psychophysiological investigations.

A serious limitation of all these measurement techniques (except X-ray) is that only the distal 25 cm of the bowel is accessible to observation, even with a proctoscope, and it requires a rigid proctoscope and significant discomfort to reliably advance a tube higher than 15 cm. This is particularly unfortunate since some evidence suggests that the motility of the distal colon differs from that of the rest of the colon (Hardcastle & Mann, 1968). One remedy is to study patients with colostomies.

2.3. Stimulation Techniques

Segmenting contractions of the colon are rare unless some type of provocative stimulus is used (Whitehead, Engel, & Schuster, 1980). We have recorded for as long as 6 hr without seeing any pressure waves. As a result, most investigators have studied the response to pharmacological, psychological, or mechanical stimulation.

There are a number of known gastrointestinal hormones and a number of putative hormones that affect gastrointestinal motility (Table 1). These hormones can either stimulate or inhibit, and their activity may differ in different parts of the gastrointestinal tract. Sphincter muscles behave differently from nonsphincteric muscles (Harvey, 1979). Some of these hormones are released by meals and may play a physiologic role in colonic motility, including the gastrocolic reflex. (This refers to the tendency of meals to elicity colic and/or a bowel movement.)

Snape's group has attempted to standardize evaluation of the response to meals by recording contractile and myoelectric activity for 30 min before and 90 min after a standard meal in a fasted subject. Initially they used a 1,000 calorie meal consisting of a roast beef sandwich and milkshake (Snape, Matarazzo, & Cohen, 1978). Their findings are that the meal elicits an increase in colon motility and myoelectric activity which peaks at about 10 min in normal subjects but only after 60–90 min in patients with irritable bowel syndrome.

Stimulation by psychological events in the form of stressful interviews have been studied by several investigators (e.g., Almy, Hinkle, Berle, & Kern, 1949; Latimer et al., 1981). The basic paradigm is to engage the subject in an interview which moves from neutral topics to topics likely to produce fear or anger and

Table 1
Effects of Gastrointestinal Hormones on Intestinal Motility[a]

Hormones	Effects on gastrointestinal tract		Released by meals
	Stimulate	Inhibit	
Gastrin	yes	—	yes
Secretin	—	yes	yes
Cholecystokinin	yes	—	yes
Glucagon	—	yes	yes
Motilin	yes	—	unsure
Gastric inhibitory polypeptide (GIP)	—	yes	yes
Vasoactive intestinal peptide (VIP)	—	yes	unsure
Pancreatic polypeptide	—	yes	yes

[a] Adapted from Harvey (1979).

back to neutral or pleasant topics while measuring colonic activity. A variation on this technique introduced by Almy and Tulin (1947) was to produce physical pain by tightening a band around the subject's head or immersing his hand in ice water while measuring motor activity. Most investigators report that mobilization of strong affect in this way increases colonic contractile activity, although Latimer et al. (1981) reported no net change for their group because some subjects showed increases while others showed decreases. There is disagreement about the nature of the affect most likely to result in colonic spasm, and there are no consistant differences between patients with irritable bowel syndrome and normal subjects. The major limitation of this technique is the impossibility of standardizing the psychological stimulus.

Our laboratory has developed a mechanical method of stimulating colonic contractile activity which has advantages over pharmacological and psychological stimulation procedures. Using the device shown in Figure 1, we distend a balloon in the rectosigmoid area approximately 15 cm from the anal verge (Whitehead et al., 1980). The distending balloon, which is 5 cm in length, is inflated in a stepwise fashion by adding 20 ml of air every two minutes until a total of 200 ml has been accumulated. The normal response to this distenstion is an immediate active contraction as shown above in Figure 2. However, in patients with irritable bowel syndrome multiple delayed active contractions such as those seen in Figure 3 also occur. These delayed active contractions can be elicited even during asymptomatic periods. Occasional delayed active contractions also occur in two-thirds of normal subjects, but the quantity of such con-

THE MEASUREMENT OF COLON MOTILITY

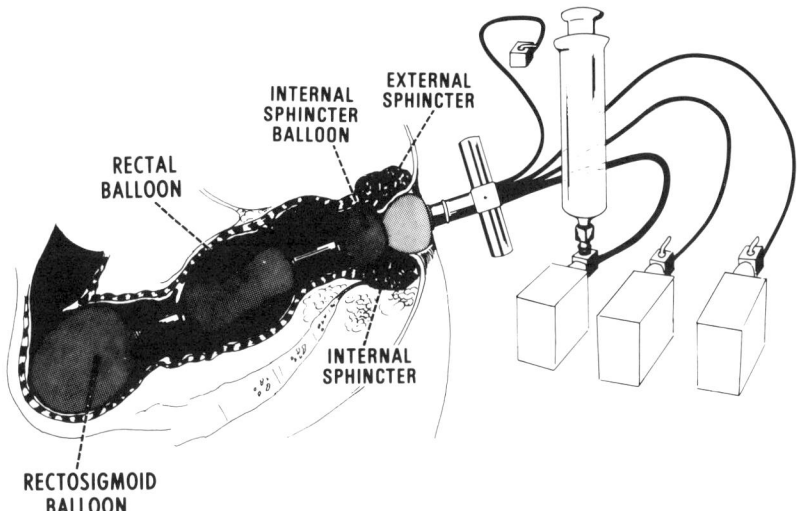

Figure 1. Device for recording colon motility. The most cephalad three balloons are connected to pressure transducers and record contractions of the rectosigmoid junction 15 cm into the bowel, the rectum, and the internal anal sphincter.

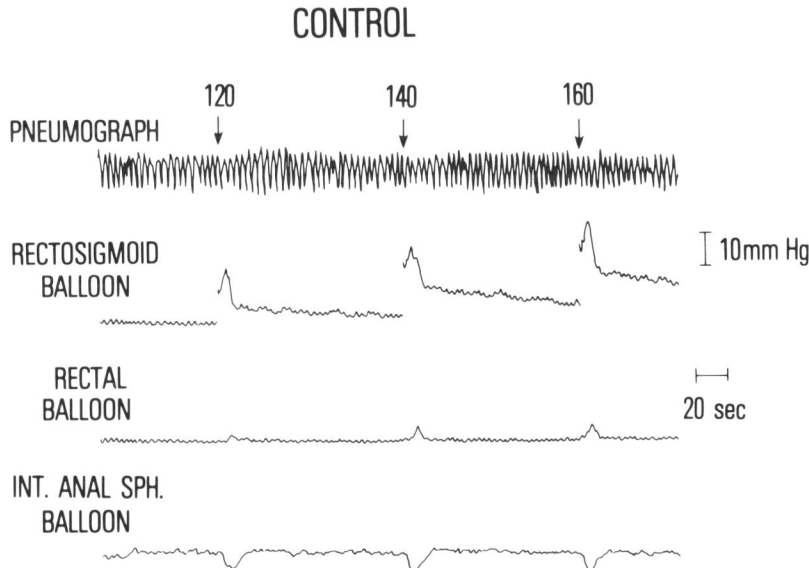

Figure 2. Effects of distending a balloon in the rectosigmoid colon in a normal subject using the device shown in Figure 1. Each increment of air causes an immediate active contraction but no delayed or secondary contractions.

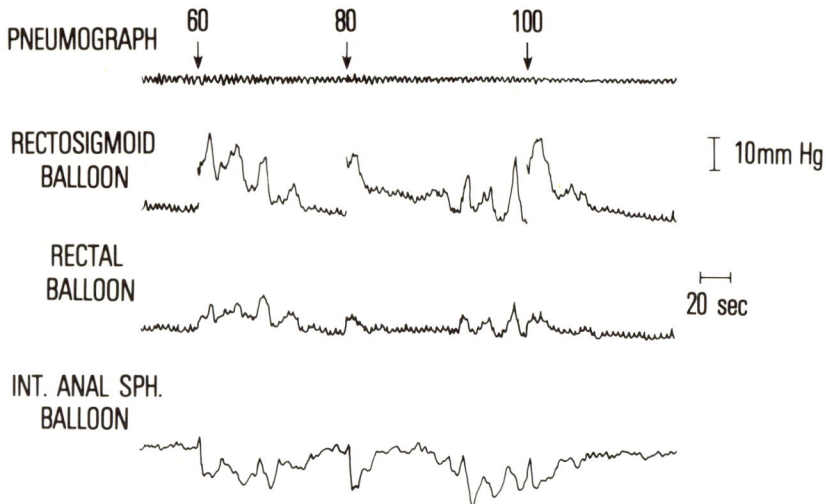

Figure 3. Effects of distending a balloon in the rectosigmoid colon in a patient with irritable bowel syndrome using the device shown in Figure 1. Each increment of air causes both an immediate active contraction and multiple delayed active contractions.

tractions is less and the threshold volume of rectosigmoid distension required to elicit them is higher for normal subjects than for patients with irritable bowel syndrome.

The advantages of this method of eliciting colonic segmenting activity are (1) it is rapidly reversible and repeatable, which is not true for pharmacologic stimuli; and (2) it is more easily standardized than either psychological or pharmacological stimuli. We have obtained excellent agreement between tests run 6 weeks apart as well as between tests repeated in the same session. The stimulus is also physiologic since it mimics the presence of stool or gas in the distal colon.

2.4. Quantification Techniques

The simplest and most frequently used method of quantifying colon motility records is to compute a motility index. This is done by multiplying the amplitude times the duration of each contraction in an interval, adding the products, and dividing this sum by the duration of the measurement interval. This provides an index of the overall amount of activity but provides no information about the types of activity which are occurring. Thus it assumes that pressure waves of all durations (frequencies) are functionally equivalent. This assumption has been challenged (Whitehead et al., 1980).

An alternative approach to quantification is to count the number of pressure waves in different frequency bands which meet some amplitude criterion (e.g., at least 1 mm Hg). Several investigators (Snape, Carlson, Matarazzo, & Cohen, 1977; Taylor, Duthie, Hammond, & Basu, 1978) have suggested that myoelectric slow waves in the frequency band of 0–4 cpm may constitute a greater proportion of total myoelectric activity in the colon of patients with irritable bowel syndrome as compared to normals. Whitehead *et al.* (1980) found that the number of pressure waves in the 0–4 cpm range was also greater in these patients. It, therefore, seems warranted to score separately the number of slow pressure waves in this frequency range.

Motility records are usually scored by hand, and this is a tedious and time-consuming process. It is possible to record pressure measurements on magnetic tape and to score them automatically. Computer programs can be written to provide the conventional indices described above or to generate spectral analysis. However, such computer programs are not currently available.

3. Assessment of Compliance of the Bowel Wall

The second major function of the colon is that of storage. This is subserved by compliance. Figure 4 shows a colon-metrogram performed much in the manner of a cystometrogram by the slow, continuous infusion of a liquid into the

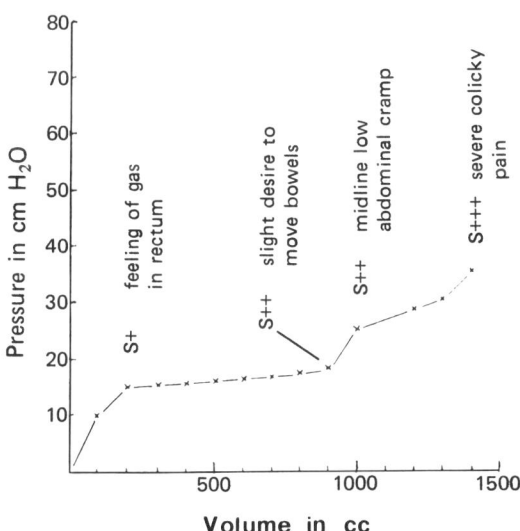

Figure 4. Colonmetrogram performed by steady, gradual instillation of water into the colon. (From White, Verlot, & Ehrentheil, 1940.)

colon (White, Verlot, & Ehrentheil, 1940). On the vertical axis in this illustration are pressures, and on the horizontal axis, the amount that has been instilled. At first there is a gradual increase in pressure until some point at which there appears a slight feeling of distension. Then there is a further increase in pressure with continued filling, and a sense of urgency appears. Continued filling of the colon with water eventually produces a feeling of severe pain. This pressure filling curve shows the compliance of the colon to filling.

One can perform a similar kind of test in a slightly different manner as shown in Figure 5 (Lium, 1939). These are bolus injections of fluid into the colon of a normal subject. A small bolus induces a dramatic but small increase in pressure, and then a plastic adaptation to a new baseline level. At each point on the graph marked with an "I," an additional 10 ml is instilled, and there comes a point, a threshold, at which in addition to this passive change, there occurs an active contraction. That active contraction is associated with marked discomfort and urgency.

Instilling water directly onto the colon provides only a crude measure of compliance because the volume of the container into which it is being instilled varies greatly. The presence of stool or occurrence of spasm can influence the functional capacity of the colon. A somewhat better measure of compliance can be obtained by inflating a balloon in the colon, although one must be careful to allow for the elastic properties of the balloon. Whitehead *et al.* (1980) inflated a balloon in the rectosigmoid area and inferred compliance from the change in pressure which resulted from the addition of a fixed volume of air to the balloon.

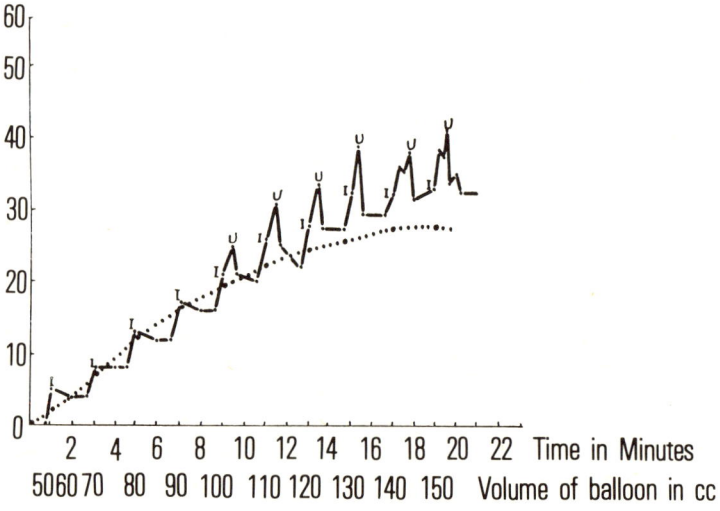

Figure 5. Rectometrogram performed by bolus injections of 10 ml of water every 2 min into a rectal balloon. (From Lium, 1939.)

After subtracting the contribution of the elastic properties of the balloon, normal values were found to be 11.8 mm Hg for 100 ml of air added to the rectosigmoid balloon.

Compliance is an important determinant of the symptoms which result from gastrointestinal disease. In ulcerative colitis, for example, the pressures resulting from rectal distension are much higher because there is decreased compliance (Figure 6). At a lower threshold, high pressures occur which produce a sense of urgency. This is what leads to the symptom of tenesmus, which is the feeling that one has to move the bowels but with the production of only very small amounts, frequently of only muco-sanguinous material or a very small amount of stool. Paralyzing the lower body with either spinal anesthesia or general anesthesia eliminates these active contractions and also eliminates the sensation of urgency.

Exaggerated compliant adaptation is associated with pseudo-Hirschsprung's disease, which is also called idiopathic megacolon, functional megacolon, or psychogenic megacolon. Thus, the primary function subserved by compliance can be either exaggerated or diminished. In ulcerative colitis, compliance is diminished while in megacolon compliance is increased.

4. Assessment of Evacuation

Evacuation is probably achieved by mass propulsion rather than by peristaltic activity (Templeton & Lawson, 1931). Figure 7 is an illustration of that.

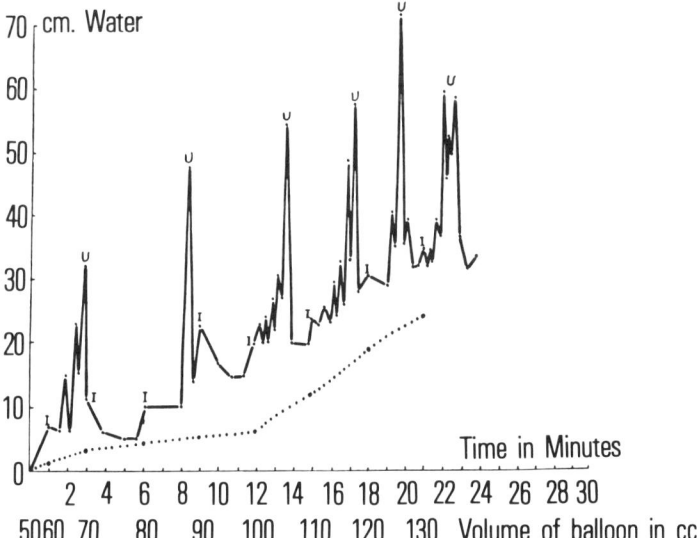

Figure 6. Rectometrogram in patient with ulcerative colitis. (From Lium, 1939.)

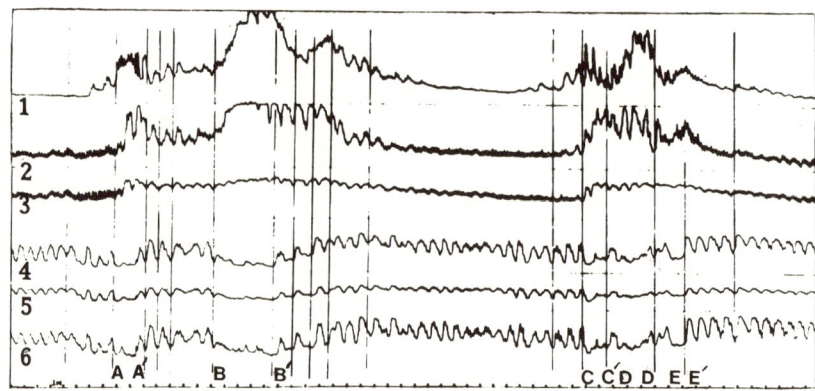

Figure 7. Massive movement in the colon manifested by contraction in the right colon with receptive relaxation in the left. (From Templeton & Lawson, 1931.)

There are three recording tips in the right colon and three in the left. As a massive wave takes place in the right colon, there is a receptive relaxation in the left colon. This results in a mass movement from the zone of high pressure in the right colon to the zone of low pressure in the left colon. This propulsive activity is exaggerated in diarrhea and diminished in constipation.

The physiology of mass movements in the colon has rarely been studied for two reasons: (1) Mass movements occur only once or twice a day and may be easily missed; (2) mass movements do not extend down to the distal 20 cm of bowel and are not accessible to observation. They cease at about 20 cm and are replaced by a preponderance of segmenting activity in the sigmoid colon (Hardcastle & Mann, 1968).

Several indirect measures have been developed for the study of evacuation. The most useful is the radio-opaque marker study described by Martelli, Devroede, Arhan, Duguay, Dornic, and Faverdin (1978). The subject swallows 20 small, radio-opaque rings made by sectioning a nasogastric tube into 1-mm-thick rings, and flat X rays of the abdomen are made at 24-hr intervals. The number and the location of these circles on successive days provides a good estimate of the type and severity of bowel transit disorders, and it can localize obstructions to evacuation. Normally, half the markers are excreted in 24 hr and 80% are excreted by 48 hr. Martelli *et al.* provide normal values for each section of the large bowel. This test is used routinely to evaluate constipated patients, but it has little value as a psychophysiological measure because the radiation hazard makes it impractical to obtain frequent films.

A reasonably good estimate of evacuation parameters can also be obtained by asking the patient to self-monitor and record the frequency and consistency of bowel movements. Although many psychological variables influence the fre-

Table 2
Correlation of Function and Motility

Function	Physiological motor activity	Pathological motor activity	Clinical disorders
Dehydration	Segmentation	Exaggerated or diminished	IBS and divertic ulcerative colitis
Storage	Compliance	Exaggerated or diminished	Megacolon and ulcerative colitis
Evacuation	Mass propulsion	Exaggerated	Diarrhea, ulcerative colitis, and constipation

quency and the self-described consistency of bowel movements (Latimer, 1981), changes in bowel habits can be monitored in this way.

Table 2 summarizes the fact that the three major functions of the colon are subserved by these three types of physiological activity. Each can either be exaggerated or diminished, and can be associated with various types of psychophysiologic disorders (Schuster, 1979).

5. References

Almy, T. P., Hinkle, L. E., Berle, B., & Kern, F. Alterations in colonic function under stress. III. Experimental production of sigmoid spasm in patients with spastic constipation. *Gastroenterology,* 1949, *12,* 437–449.

Almy, T. P., & Tulin, M. Alterations in colonic function in man under stress: Experimental production of changes simulating the "irritable colon." *Gastroenterology,* 1947, *8,* 616–626.

Connell, A. M. The motility of the pelvic colon. Part II. Paradoxical motility in diarrhea and constipation. *Gut,* 1962, *3,* 342–348.

Hardcastle, J. D., & Mann, C. V. Study of large bowel peristalsis. *Gut,* 1968, *9,* 512–520.

Harvey, R. H. Effects of hormones in normal subjects and patients with the irritable bowel syndrome. *Practical Gastroenterology,* 1979, *3*(4), 10–15.

Latimer, P. R. Irritable bowel syndrome: A behavioral model. *Behavior Research and Therapy,* 1981, *19,* 475–483.

Latimer, P. R., Sarna, S., Campbell, D., Latimer, M., & Daniel, E. E. Colonic motor and myoelectrical activity: A comparative study of normal subjects, psychoneurotic patients, and patients with irritable bowel syndrome. *Gastroenterology,* 1981, *80,* 893–901.

Lium, R. Observations on the etiology of ulcerative colitis. IV. The rectometrogram and the rectal reactions of 8 normal subjects and one patient with ulcerative colitis before and after spinal anesthesia. *Journal of the American Medical Society,* 1939, *197,* 841–847.

Martelli, H., Devroede, G., Arhan, P., Duguay, C., Dornic, C., & Faverdin, C. Some parameters of large bowel motility in normal man. *Gastroenterology,* 1978, *75,* 612–618.

Schuster, M. M. Disorders of motility. In P. B. Beeson, W. McDermott, & J. B. Wyngaarden (Eds.), *Cecil textbook of medicine.* Philadelphia: W. B. Saunders, 1979.

Snape, W. J., Jr., Carlson, G. M., Matarazzo, S. A., & Cohen, S. Evidence that abnormal myoelectrical activity produces colonic motor dysfunction in the irritable bowel syndrome. *Gastroenterology,* 1977, *72,* 383–387.

Snape, W. J., Jr., Matarazzo, S. A., & Cohen, S. Effect of eating and gastrointestinal hormones on human colonic myoelectrical and motor activity. *Gastroenterology,* 1978, *75,* 373–378.

Taylor, I., Duthie, C., Hammond, P., & Basu, P. Is there a myoelectric abnormality in the irritable colon syndrome? *Gut,* 1978, *19,* 391–395.

Templeton, R. D., & Lawson, H. Studies in the motor activity of the large intestine. I. Normal motility in the dog recorded by the tandem balloon method. *American Journal of Physiology,* 1931, *96,* 667–676.

White, J. C., Verlot, M. G., & Ehrenthal, O. Neurogenic disturbances of the colon and their investigation by the colon metrogram. *Annals of Surgery,* 1940, *112,* 1042–1058.

Whitehead, W. E., Engel, B. T., & Schuster, M. M. Irritable bowel syndrome: Physiological and psychological differences between diarrhea-predominant and constipation-predominant patients. *Digestive Diseases and Sciences,* 1980, *25,* 404–413.

12

MEASUREMENT OF ELECTRICAL ACTIVITY OF THE COLON IN MAN
HERBERT LIVINGSTON DUTHIE

1. Introduction

The basic changes in smooth muscle fibers connected with contraction have been studied in great detail in animal preparations involving both *in vivo* and *in vitro* techniques (Duthie, 1979). In recent years more attention has been paid to acquiring data from man which will form the basis of this chapter.

2. Methods

2.1. In Vivo

Electrodes placed on the mucosa of the colon have been most frequently used in man. They are mounted on a tube passed into the bowel by means of a sigmodoscope and can be attached to the mucosa by suction (Figure 1; Duthie, 1975) or by means of a spring clip (Snape, Carlson, & Cohen, 1976). Another alternative is to leave the tube free in the lumen and to rely on having groups of three electrodes together to ensure a sufficient contact to obtain a good recording (Bueno, Fioramonti, Ruckebusch, Frexinos, & Coulom, 1980). Pressure recordings can be made simultaneously either by perfusing channels in the rectal tube or by strain gauges attached to the tube. Another type of electrode which has been used in man is fine wire implanted under the serosa of the colon during a surgical operation and left in position for a few days before being removed along with the surgical drain (Sarna, Baradakjian, Waterfall, Lind, & Daniel, 1980).

HERBERT LIVINGSTON DUTHIE • Welsh National School of Medicine, Cardiff, Wales.

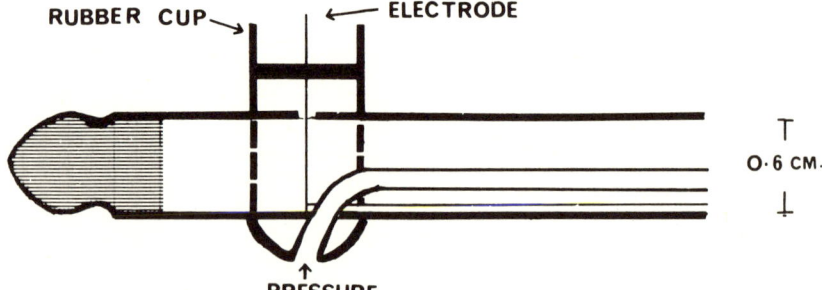

Figure 1. Diagram of the end of the intracolonic probe showing the cup surrounding the needle electrode which is attached to the mucosa by suction. Diametrically opposite to the electrode is a fine catheter filled with saline which is used to detect changes in pressure.

Noninvasive recording has been possible using electrocardiographic electrodes placed on the skin over the sigmoid colon and the right colon. The records obtained show waves of the same frequency as those obtained from the intraluminal electrodes (Taylor, Duthie, Smallwood, & Linkens, 1975). This method cannot be used over the transverse colon because stomach or small gut signals cause confusion.

The electrical signals from the colonic smooth muscle are less regular than those from the rest of the gut and also are of relatively low amplitude. Many workers have used some type of electronic filter to separate the wave forms from the background noise. These filters may be set at different levels to pick out different features of the signals. It has been found useful to record on magnetic tape and use some form of spectral analysis. The most usual is fast Fourier transformation but other techniques such as autoregressive modeling have been used successfully (Linkens, 1978). (For a detailed discussion of signal analysis problems involved here see Chapters 5 and 6.) In general, there have been many more problems with obtaining reproducible records from the colon in humans than from the small bowel or from the stomach, and some of the lack of uniformity of findings between different groups of workers may be due to the different electrodes and the pattern of filters used.

2.2. In Vitro

Standard methods of studying muscle strips from human colon consist of maintaining the strip in a chamber in a physiological solution which has been perfused with a mixture of oxygen and 5% carbon dioxide. Strain gauges are used to measure contraction and either extracellular or intracellular electrodes are used to record changes in electrical potential (Van Merwyk & Duthie, 1980).

3. Normal Electrical Patterns *in Vivo*

Two main types of electrical activity have been observed in the smooth muscle of the human colon—slow waves and fast activity.

3.1. Slow Waves

Cyclical changes in the electrical potential in the colon are not recorded all the time in distinction to the findings in the small gut and the stomach. Some groups of workers would not agree with this statement, claiming that with effective filtering and spectral analysis, waves can be detected during all recording time. However, there is agreement that the slow wave frequency can vary at the site of recording. Two frequency bands have been distinguished—a low-frequency band 2 to 6 cpm (0.033 to 0.1 Hz; Figure 2) and a high-frequency band at 6 to

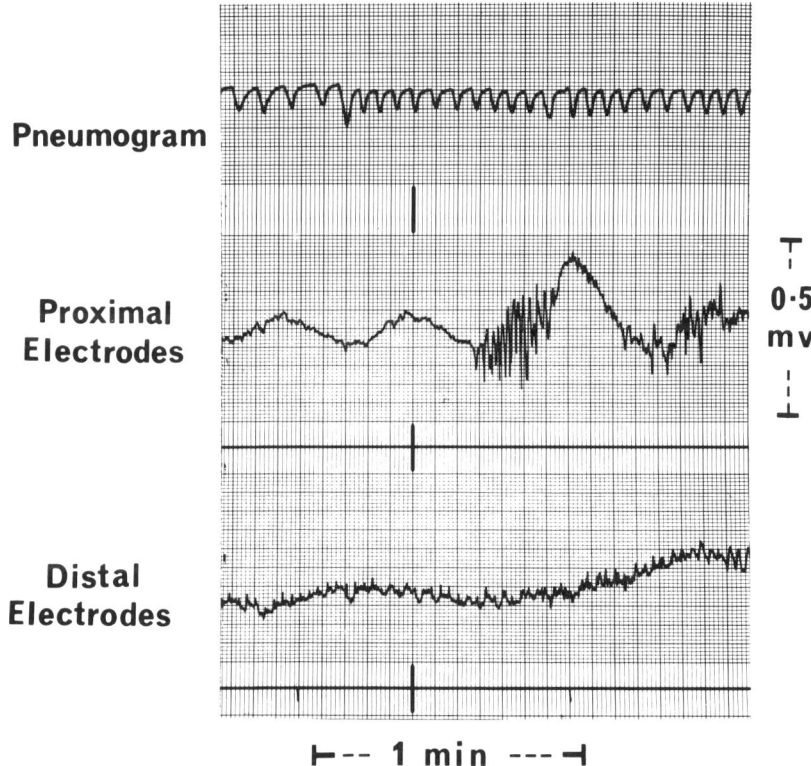

Figure 2. Tracings from bipolar implanted electrodes in the transverse colon showing low-frequency band slow wave electrical activity on the proximal electrodes together with a long spike burst lasting 18 sec.

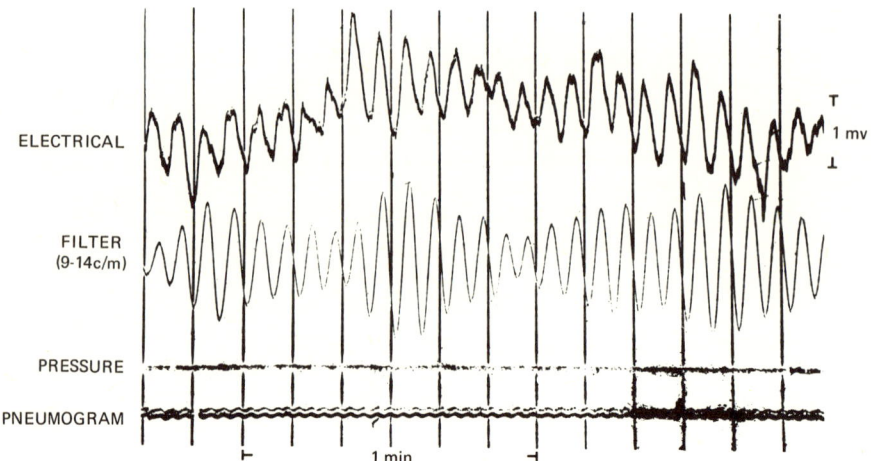

Figure 3. Tracing from a suction electrode placed in the ascending colon through a colostomy showing high-frequency band slow wave electrical activity.

12 cpm (0.1 to 0.2 Hz; Figure 3). The precise cutoff points in these two bands also show some difference from one author to another (Table 1).

The relative incidence of the two frequency bands has also been a matter for some discussion. The high-frequency band has been recorded for the majority of the time by several groups (Duthie, 1975; Snape et al., 1976; Taylor et al., 1975) but another group who have produced some admirable tracings from their subjects find the opposite, namely, that the low-frequency band predominates (Sarna, Latimer, Campbell, & Waterfall, 1980). As might be expected from this, no complete agreement exists on the exact findings from the different parts of the colon, particularly on which is the predominant frequency band (Table 2). Sarna's group has developed the concept that proximal, middle, and distal segment

Table 1
Colonic Slow Electrical Waves in Normal Subjects

Author	Low-frequency	High-frequency
Duthie[a]	2–6	7–13
Sarna[b]	2–9	9–13
Snape[c]	2.5–4.5	6–12
Taylor[d]	2–4	6–10

[a]1979.
[b]Sarna, Latimer, Campbell, and Waterfall (1982).
[c]Snape et al. (1976).
[d]Taylor, Darby, and Hammond (1978).

Table 2
Colonic Electrical Slow Waves (Percentage Incidence on Computer Analysis)

Author	Low-frequency band	High-frequency band
Right colon		
Sarna[a]	94	57
Stoddard[b]	27	19
Transverse colon		
Sarna[a]	45	92
Stoddard[b]	50	37
Left colon		
Sarna[a]	93	47
Sullivan[b]	11	87
Taylor[c]	49	78

[a]Sarna et al. (1982).
[b]Stoddard et al. (1979).
[c]Taylor, Darby, and Hammond (1978).

of the human colon have different patterns of slow wave activity on the basis of studies with multiple implanted electrodes and on-line spectral analysis. They use the concept of dominant frequency. This was found in the low-frequency band in the proximal and distal segments and in the high-frequency band in the middle segment, mainly the transverse colon (Sarna, Bardakjian, Waterfall, Lind, & Daniel, 1980). The lack of agreement between groups of workers may be explained in part by methodological differences in recording and analysis (Stoddard, Duthie, Smallwood, & Linkens, 1979).

When records are made from several sets of electrodes, the slow waves on some occasions can be seen to be of a similar frequency at more than one recording site and have been related either by describing them as being conducted along the bowel if one is looking on the colon as a cable or by calling them "locked-on" if one is using relaxation oscillator theory. In this concept, individual groups of muscle cells are looked upon as relaxation oscillators, and their interconnections with other adjacent groups give rise to the wave patterns recorded. It is possible to use either electronic or computer programmed models of these relaxation oscillators to derive patterns of activity which are similar to the patterns recorded from the intact subject (Bardakjian & Sarna, 1980; Linkens, Taylor, & Duthie, 1976).

3.2. Fast Activity

Unlike recordings from the small bowel it is possible to have a clean record from the colon showing pressure activity in time with slow wave electrical activity and not see any action potentials or spike bursts. It could be said that there is some defect in the recording arrangement, but the same equipment on another occasion may show spike activity associated with muscle contraction. Three main patterns of fast activity have been observed, short spike bursts which last 2–3 sec (Couturier, Rose, Couturier-Turpin, & Debray, 1969); long spike bursts (Figure 2) lasting 10–20 sec, and rapid oscillations in which waves at 30–40 cpm are observed for 1–3 min. In some instances the long spike bursts appear to be propagated in the transverse colon either orad or caudad (Figure 4). Short spike bursts have been associated more with segmental contractions in the high-frequency band and long spike bursts with slower, longer contractions in the low-frequency band which has been suggested to represent more propulsive activity (Sarna, Waterfall, Bardakjian, & Lind, 1980).

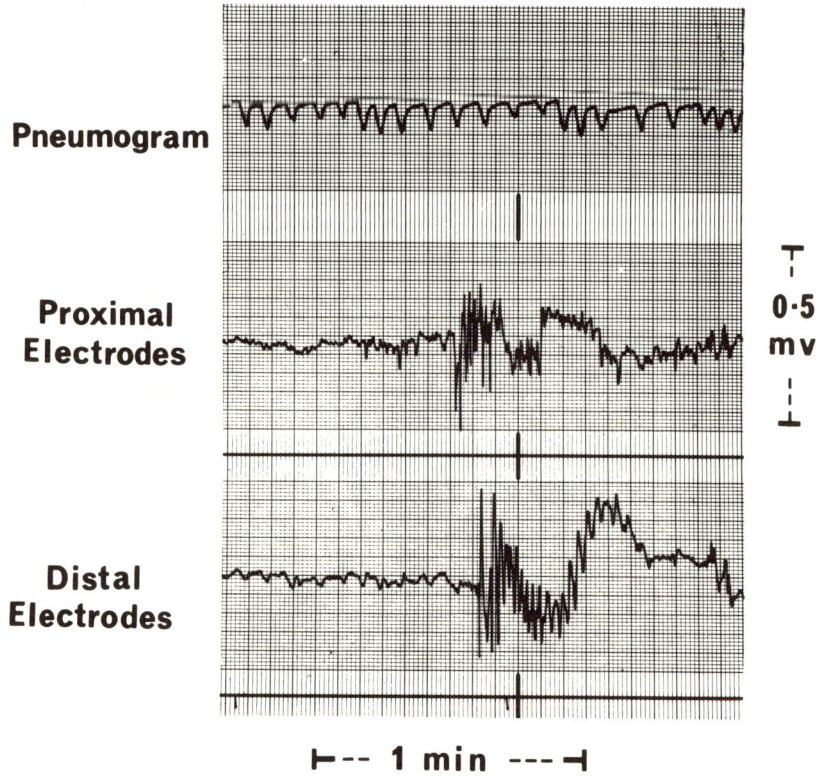

Figure 4. Tracing from bipolar implanted electrodes on the transverse colon showing apparent propagation of a long spike burst from proximal to distal pairs of electrodes which are 5 cm apart.

4. Normal Electrical Patterns *in Vitro*

4.1. Longitudinal Muscle

Studies using intracellular electrodes on strips of human taenia coli obtained from resected specimens show a transmembrane potential of minus 50 mV and a regular spontaneous spiking discharge in most strips at a mean frequency of about 20 cycles/min (Van Merwyk & Duthie, 1980). However, most of the information available in humans is from extracellular recording. The extracellular potential is quite small at 1 mV but the frequency of the spikes is identical with that from a subjacent intracellular electrode (Duthie & Kirk, 1978). The spikes can be associated with a tetanic muscle contraction. In 25% of the strips a prepotential or slow wave is seen which builds up to a level at which spike potentials appear (Figure 5). Continuous spiking occurs in most specimens but intermittent activity is also observed with quiescent periods of about 1 min followed by active periods of about the same duration. Some intrinsic nervous activity seems to maintain the continuous pattern because it is converted to the intermittent pattern by tetrodotoxin which blocks nerve conduction.

4.2. Circular Muscle

Quite a different pattern of spike activity is seen in the circular muscle of the human colon. Groups of 2 to 6 spikes are found together with quiescent periods between. The groups occur at about 3 to 6 per min (0.1 Hz). They are associated with muscle contraction of a phasic type (Figure 6). It is noticeable that *in vitro* studies show a higher frequency of activity than those done *in vivo*. It is possible that the interactions of the two frequencies found in the two muscle coats *in vitro* could form the basis of the changing frequency of slow waves so often recorded from the intact colon.

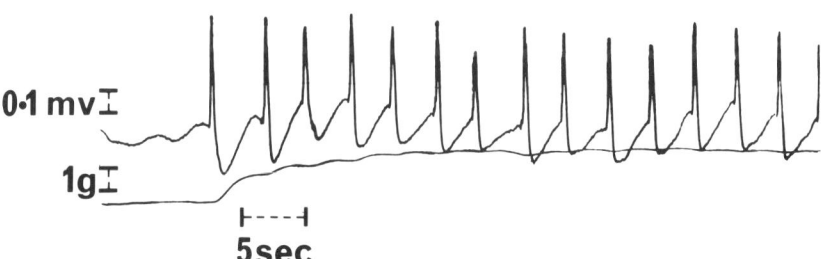

Figure 5. Extracellular recording from a strip of human taenia coli *in vitro* showing slow waves and action potentials at 20 per min (0.33 Hz).

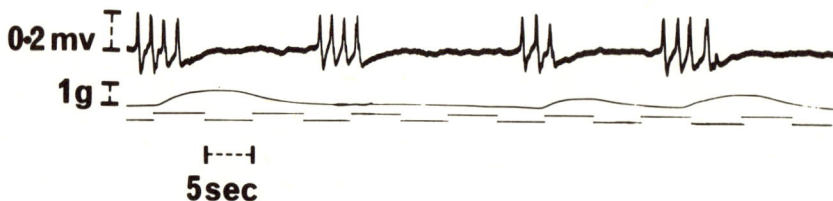

Figure 6. Extracellular recording from a strip of human circular colonic muscle showing groups of spikes at 3 per min (0.05 Hz).

5. Abnormal Electrical Patterns

Abnormal patterns of electrical activity have been observed in patients with diverticular disease, in patients with the irritable bowel syndrome, and in other functional bowel disorders.

5.1. Diverticular Disease

In addition to the tendency seen in measurements of motor activity for the sigmoid colon to be hyperactive in patients with diverticular disease, a typical rhythm of electrical slow waves has been detected in 80% of subjects with active diverticular disease. It is in the range 16–18 cpm. After treatment with bran tablets the symptoms resolve and the electrical rhythm reverts to normal in most cases. After nine months, 16% of subjects still showed the abnormal rhythm (Taylor & Duthie, 1976). In a later study 50% of the patients showed the abnormal activity and a year later it persisted in 20% (Flynn, Hyland, Hammond, Darby, & Taylor, 1980). The fact that the electrical pattern can return to normal would seem to indicate that there is no fundamental abnormality in the smooth muscle of the colon but rather that it shows the pattern in response to the stress of having a small amount of intraluminal content.

5.2. Irritable Bowel Syndrome

Two groups of workers (Table 3) have found an increase in the incidence of the low-frequency band slow waves in patients with the irritable bowel syndrome (defined as patients with colicky abdominal pain, either constipation or diarrhea, and no organic cause found on full gastrointestinal investigation) (Snape, Carlson, Matarazzo, & Cohen, 1977; Taylor, Darby, Hammond, & Basu, 1978). No typical findings were observed to distinguish those with constipation from those with diarrhea. A similar preponderance of low-frequency band activity in the sigmoid has been detected in normal subjects after giving pentagastrin (Taylor,

Table 3
Colonic Slow Electrical Waves in Irritable Bowel Syndrome (IBS) Compared with Normal (N)

Author	Low-frequency band percentage incidence		High-frequency band percentage incidence	
	N	IBS	N	IBS
Sarna[a]	92	95	8	5
Sullivan[b]	11	46	78	54
Taylor[c]	49	76	78	36

[a]Sarna et al. (1982).
[b]Sullivan et al. (1978).
[c]Taylor, Darby, and Hammond (1978).

Duthie, Smallwood, Brown, & Linkens, 1974). In contradistinction to the disappearance of the abnormal rhythm in diverticular disease, the preponderance of the low-frequency band of slow wave activity does not change when the patients become symptomatic, so there may be an underlying abnormality which renders them susceptible to symptoms (Taylor, Darby, & Hammond, 1978). When measurements were made after the patient ate a meal an increase of colonic spiking activity was observed compared with normal subjects (Sullivan, Cohen, & Snape, 1978).

Another group who have studied the electrical activity of the colon in patients with the irritable bowel syndrome have been unable to detect any difference from a matched set of controls (Sarna, Latimer, Campbell, & Waterfall, 1980). In both the patients and the controls, low-frequency band slow waves were observed more frequently than slow waves of the high-frequency band (Table 3). These discrepancies can in part be explained by different techniques of spectral analysis and by the type of electrodes used.

5.3. Other Functional Disorders

In a recent study of myoelectrical activity of the colon in healthy subjects and patients with functional disorders, no group differences were observed in the pattern of slow wave activity. However, the frequency of spike bursts was altered (Bueno et al., 1980). The three groups of "patients did not present well-defined clinical symptoms of functional colonic disorders" (p. 484). In one group, short spike bursts were much increased; in the second there was a marked reduction in the incidence of long spike bursts and an absence of short spike bursts; and in the third a subnormal spiking pattern was found associated with a lack of postprandial response.

6. Summary

This review has been confined to data obtained in humans either from *in vivo* or *in vitro* recordings and has demonstrated the great improvement in recording techniques and in analysis utilizing computer facilities. General agreement has yet to be obtained on the precise relationships of the frequency bands of the electrical slow waves and the mechanical correlates of the different types of fast activity. Nonetheless, it is clear that the electrical activity of the human colon exhibits a highly individual property of having quite widely changing frequencies of slow electrical waves at the one recording point and that these may be present simultaneously.

7. References

Bardakjian, B. L., & Sarna, J. A computer model of human colonic electrical control activity (ECA). *IEEE Transactions on Biomedical Engineering*, 1980, 27, 193–202.

Bueno, L., Fioramonti, J., Ruckebusch, Y., Frexinos, J., & Coulom, P. Evaluation of colonic myoelectrical activity in health and funcional disorders. *Gut*, 1980, 21, 480–485.

Couturier, D., Rose, C., Couturier-Turpin, M. H., & Debray, C. Electromyography of the colon in situ. *Gastroenterology*, 1969, 56, 317–332.

Duthie, H. L. Colonic motility in man. *Mayo Clinic Proceedings*, 1975, 50, 519–522.

Duthie, H. L. Links between basic and clinical studies of gastrointestinal smooth muscle. *British Medical Bulletin*, 1979, 35, 301–303.

Duthie, H. L., & Kirk, D. Electrical activity of human colonic smooth muscle in vitro. *Journal of Physiology*, 1978, 283, 319–330.

Flynn, M., Hyland, J., Hammond, P., Darby, C., & Taylor, I. Faecal bile acid excretion in diverticular disease. *British Journal of Surgery*, 1980, 67, 629–632.

Linkens, D. A. Methods of analysing rhythmic electrical potentials in the gastrointestinal tract. In H. L. Duthie (Ed.), *Gastrointestinal motility in health and disease*. Lancaster, England: M.T.P. Press, 1978.

Latimer, P. R., Campbell, D., Latimer, M. R., Waterfall, W. E., & Daniel, E. E. Colonic motor and electrical activity: A comparative study of normal subjects, psychoneurotic patients and patients with irritable bowel syndrome (IBS). *Gastroenterology*, 1981, 80, 893–901.

Linkens, D., Taylor, I., & Duthie, H. L. Mathematical modelling of the colorectal myoelectrical activity in humans. *IEEE Transactions of Biomedical Engineering*, 1976, 23, 101–110.

Sarna, S. K., Bardakjian, B. L., Waterfall, W. E., Lind, J. F., & Daniel, E. E. The organisation of human colonic electrical control activity. In J. Christensen (Ed.), *Gastrointestinal motility*. New York: Raven Press, 1980.

Sarna, S. K., Latimer, P., Campbell, D., & Waterfall, W. E. Electrical and contractile activities of human rectosigmoid. *Gut*, 1982, 23, 698–705.

Snape, W. J., Carlson, G. M., & Cohen, S. Colonic myoelectric activity in the irritable bowel syndrome. *Gastroenterology*, 1976, 70, 326–330.

Snape, W. J., Carlson, G. M., Matarazzo, S. A., & Cohen, S. Evidence that abnormal myoelectrical activity produces colonic motor dysfunction in the irritable bowel syndrome. *Gastroenterology*, 1977, 72, 383–387.

Stoddard, C. S., Duthie, H. L., Smallwood, R. H., & Linkens, D. A. Colonic myoelectrical activity in man: Comparison of recording techniques and methods of analysis. *Gut*, 1979, 20, 476–483.

Sullivan, M. A., Cohen, S., & Snape, W. J. Colonic myoelectrical activity in irritable bowel syndrome: Effect of eating and anticholinergics. *New England Journal of Medicine,* 1978, *298,* 878–883.

Taylor, I., & Duthie, H. L. Bran tablets and diverticular disease. *British Medical Journal,* 1976, *1,* 988–990.

Taylor, I., Duthie, H. L., Smallwood, R., Brown, B. H., & Linkens, D. A. The effect of stimulation on the myoelectrical activity of the rectosigmoid in man. *Gut,* 1974, *15,* 599–607.

Taylor, I., Duthie, H. L., Smallwood, R., & Linkens, D. Large bowel myoelectrical activity in man. *Gut,* 1975, *16,* 808–814.

Taylor, I., Darby, C., & Hammond, P. Comparison of rectosigmoid myoelectrical activity in the irritable colon syndrome during relapses and remissions. *Gut,* 1978, *19,* 923–929.

Taylor, I., Darby, C., Hammond, P., & Basu, P. Is there a myoelectrical abnormality in the irritable colon syndrome? *Gut,* 1978, *19,* 391–395.

Van Merwyk, A. J., & Duthie, H. L. Characteristics of human colonic smooth muscle in vitro. In. J. Christensen (Ed.), *Gastrointestinal motility.* New York: Raven Press, 1980.

13

COLONIC PSYCHOPHYSIOLOGY
Implications for Functional Bowel Disorders
PAUL R. LATIMER

1. Introduction

1.1. Early Observations on Gastrointestinal Responsiveness

That the gastrointestinal tract is responsive to a variety of phenomena in day-to-day experience is no longer seriously questioned. In the early part of the 19th century William Beaumont (1833) observed that changes in mood and behavior were associated with changes in the gastric mucosa of his famous fistula patient, Alexis St. Martin. Numerous subsequent observations on both animals (Bidder & Schmidt, 1852; Pavlov, 1910) and humans (Hornborg, 1904; Richet, 1878) demonstrated that the mere sight and smells of agreeable food could start the flow of salivary and gastric juices. It was, of course, Pavlov (1910) who made these observations the subject of precise and systematic science. He showed that auditory, visual, and tactile symbols associated with foods could elicit copious secretion of saliva in his experimental dogs and other meaningful experiences could interfere with this effect. Dogs which salivated copiously to conditional stimuli in the lab frequently failed to do so when called upon for a demonstration before an audience. Similarly, Pavlov observed that "psychic" secretion of gastric juice in dogs could be inhibited for a relatively long time after terrifying events such as the famous flood in his kennels. He inferred that meaningful experiences must compete in their effects on an end organ and, if in opposition, one or the other may predominate (Wolf & Welsh, 1972).

PAUL R. LATIMER • Behavior Therapy and Research Unit, Temple University Medical School, Philadelphia, Pennsylvania 19129.

Cannon (1929) replicated and extended these observations in several animal species using X rays to study intestinal contractions, and he emphasized especially the important role of emotions in altering normal digestive processes. For example, he found that the usual secretion and peristalsis following food were inhibited if the food was unappetizing, if the subject was not hungry, or if other strong emotions, such as fear, were present. He found that fear inhibited contractions at all levels of the gastrointestinal tract and cited human examples of delayed gastric emptying which seemed to result from strong emotions inhibiting the normal contractile activity.

1.2. Early Observations on Colonic Responsiveness

The colon, like the rest of the gastrointestinal tract, is responsive to environmental events, although it has much less frequently been the object of study than has the stomach. White and Jones (1938), observing the rectal mucosa through a sigmoidoscope, noted transient engorgement of the mucous membrane in a subject who became "embarrassed" during the procedure. Friedman and Snape (1946), observing the colostomies of children, recorded the occurrence of blanching during noxious stimulation. Weeks (1946), observing several segments of intestine in an Arab soldier who had received extensive perforating wounds of the abdomen, found a marked acceleration of peristaltic activity in both the large and small intestine during the "excitement" caused by the admission of several other injured and noisy Arabs to his ward. Thus, there are many early observations indicating that emotions alter gastrointestinal physiology in general and colonic activity in particular.

2. Colonic Psychophysiology

2.1. Pioneering Experiments

Thomas Almy was among the first to systematically study the relationship between environmental events, emotional experiences, and colonic responses. Almy and his colleagues embarked upon a series of investigations (Almy & Tulin, 1947; Almy, Hinkle, Berle, & Kern, 1949; Almy, Kern, & Tulin, 1949) which make interesting contemporary reading because of the similarity in the questions being asked and in the conclusions reached. Essentially these investigators wanted to know the following:

1. Whether changes in the function of the colon, of the sort we have already been discussing above, could occur consistently as accompaniments of emotional experiences in healthy individuals;
2. Whether or not these changes, when experimentally induced, would differ in kind or in degree from those seen in patients with irritable bowel syndrome (IBS).

In these studies healthy subjects (frequently medical students) and patients chosen partly because of a clear relationship between bowel symptoms and stressful environmental circumstances were studied by continuous proctoscopic examination of the lower sigmoid colon and by a continuous kymographic recording of pressure changes in the sigmoid colon as measured by a balloon. The subjects were exposed to immersion of the hand in ice water at 0°C for 5 min or longer; compression of the head with an adjustable steel band, which produces a severe headache; hypoglycemia induced by intravenous insulin, and the unsympathetic discussion of the stressful life situations which were associated with the bowel symptoms. The colonic effects produced by these stressors were increased motor activity, engorgement of the mucosa, and in some cases increased secretion. Nausea was frequently associated with spasm of the sigmoid. These colonic responses were accompanied by hypertension, sweating, sighing, and pallor of the skin indicating a generalized reaction.

Almy, Hinkle, Berle, and Kern (1949) concluded that:

> In both (the patients with spastic constipation and healthy subjects), the pattern of the colonic reaction was the same with all the experimental stimuli. In both groups the colonic changes occurred only in association with other bodily changes or with evident emotional reactions which indicated that the subject was under stress.
>
> Thus both healthy persons and patients with spastic constipation have been seen to develop the same colonic changes under stress. Yet only in the patient does clinically significant dysfunction of the colon occur. We infer that this dysfunction is not due to a specific "abnormal" pattern but rather to greater intensity and greater duration of the same reactions seen in healthy persons. The exaggeration of these functional changes is probably due to the occurrence of more prolonged stress in the patient than in the average healthy individual. Occasionally, stress in these patients takes the form of unusually severe and sustained physical hardship or personal tragedy which is obvious to the medical observer. More often the patient is under stress, in spite of a reasonably favorable life situation, because his neurotic traits lead him to see in that situation something which threatens his security. These individuals may be considered as almost constantly reacting to the changes they and they alone perceive in their environment. . . . This concept is at variance with previous ideas concerning this disorder, crystallized in such names as "unstable colon" or "colonic neurosis." These terms are unsatisfactory in that they locate the fundamental disturbance in the bowel, and suggest that the disorder is limited to the bowel. Yet most patients exhibit other clinical manifestations of bodily disorder, such as sweating of the hands, headaches, nasal discharge and hypertension. These and other bodily changes were observed in our experiments as concomitants of sigmoid spasm. . . . Whatever the neural and humoral mechanisms by which they are produced, we believe that these reactions of the colon are part of a "normal" and generalized bodily reaction to stress. (pp. 447–448)

However accurate these conclusions may eventually prove to be, the experiments on which they were based had several serious shortcomings. The technology used in recording pressure changes was primitive and the data were not presented in a quantitative manner; none of the statements was, therefore, supported statistically. The lack of a neurotic control group is crucial; perhaps there are equally neurotic individuals who do not have IBS. How is this to be explained? The conclusions of this study, therefore, went beyond the data presented.

2.2. Hyper- versus Hypomotor Responsiveness

Following up on this work Grace, Wolf, and Wolff (1949) focused on the fact that although numerous previous authors had reported changes in colonic physiology in response to stress and changing emotions, there was a divergence in the nature of the response reported. For example, Almy *et al.* (Almy & Tulin, 1947; Almy, Hinkle, Berle, & Kern, 1949; Almy, Kern, & Tulin, 1949) had reported hyperemia, hypermotility, and hypersecretion, consistent with earlier observations by Weeks (1946) and by White and Jones (1938). Cannon (1929), on the other hand, had reported general hypomotility throughout the gastrointestinal tract in animals during pain and fright, and this was consistent with the reports of Pavlov (1910) and Friedman and Snape (1946). Grace *et al.* (1949) undertook a series of experiments on two fistulous patients to attempt to reconcile these apparently divergent findings. Subject A was a 26-yr-old man with a 6-yr history of ulcerative colitis who had an ileostomy and a large prolapse of ascending colon and cecum onto the surface of the abdomen. Subject B was a 54-yr-old man who had a large prolapse of descending and sigmoid colon through a colostomy incision on the left side. The colostomy had been performed because of a rectal stricture due to lymphogranuloma venereum.

Motor activity was observed and photographed by still and motion pictures. Pressure changes were recorded in the unprolapsed segments using the methods of Almy (Almy & Tulin, 1947; Almy, Hinkle, Berle, & Kern, 1949; Almy, Kern, & Tulin, 1949). Mucosal vascularity was recorded by comparing the color of mucosa to an appropriately graded color scale, and quantity of secretion was rated on a four-point scale. Naturalistic observations were made together with experimental manipulations modeled closely after those previously used by Almy (Almy & Tulin, 1947; Almy, Hinkle, Berle, & Kern, 1949; Almy, Kern, & Tulin, 1949).

In response to the relatively standardized noxious stimuli of hand immersion in ice water and tightening of a head screw the two subjects responded in opposite ways. Subject A exhibited hypervascularity and hypercontractility while Subject B had the reverse. After the experiment Subject A was described as ambivalent about future repetitions of the experiments, wanting on the one hand to please the investigators and on the other hand to avoid pain. Subject B refused outright to participate in any repetition and was fearful that permanent damage might have been produced by the ice water and the head screw.

Later Subject A experienced a period of depression of one month's duration. During this period there was little motor activity and reduced vascularity. Attempts to stimulate changes in vascularity or motor activity were singularly unsuccessful. The usual increases in vascularity, secretion, and motor activity which follow eating (the gastrocolic reflex) were also absent during this period.

Daily observations of Subject A further indicated that his colon was more hyperemic, engorged, and hypermotile on days marked by anger, hostility, and resentment. Furthermore, it was observed that emotive interviews had a much greater effect on days when the subject felt angry and resentful as opposed to days when he felt relaxed and secure. It was also observed that a given emotive topic had less effect with repeated discussion.

Subject B was also later observed to exhibit hyperemia and hypermotility when he was angry. Nevertheless, Subject A was in this state more than 50% of the time observed while Subject B was seen this way only once. Similar observations were later made in an additional two subjects (Grace et al., 1951).

Following this work Almy, Abbot, and Hinkle (1950) reported that although the most frequently observed effects in their experiments were hyperemia, hypermotility, and hypersecretion of the sigmoid colon, the opposite responses were occasionally observed. Like Grace et al. (1949) they observed that these episodes seemed to be associated with a change in a patient's attitude to one of hopelessness, personal inadequacy, or self-reproach. Such an episode of hypomotility was frequently associated with weeping and in reviewing their records they could find only one example in which the phenomena did not occur when a patient wept. They hypothesized that these changes (decreased contractions, vascularity, and secretion) might be functionally related to diarrhea, and that shifting attitudes could account for the frequently observed alternating diarrhea and constipation in some patients.

On the basis of these and other observations Grace et al. (1951; Wolf & Welsh, 1972) proposed that there are three distinct patterns of colonic behavior which may be elicited under differing circumstances. These include the following:

1. *Transport activity* (the gastrocolic reflex) characterized by peristalsis on the right side and a sustained shortening and narrowing on the left which results from the sustained contraction of longitudinal and circular muscles and is typically associated with sudden fear;
2. *Desiccating activity* characterized by persistent, nonpropulsive segmental contractions which result in delayed transport and in small, hard, dry stools and which is typically associated with mild depression and an attitude of grim persistence;

3. *Inactivity* characterized by muscular relaxation, dilatation and redundancy of the entire colon, which is typically associated with severe depression.

While the studies discussed so far were pioneering and demonstrated that different patterns of motility existed, that these occurred at different times in the same individual, and that they were susceptible to the effects of changes in emotions and day-to-day activities, the conclusions concerning the patterns of activity possible and the nature of their relations to changes in attitude were probably an oversimplification (Cohen, Long, & Snape, 1979; Latimer, 1979a).

3. Implications for Functional Bowel Disorders

3.1. Five Hypotheses

The relevance of the observed changes in colonic motility to the functional bowel disorders is by no means proven by these studies and has in fact become a topic of increasing interest, particularly since the studies by Almy. Several possibilities exist: (1) IBS patients may have a distinctively abnormal colonic response based either on a physiological or learned predisposition; (2) they may have a normal colonic response to particular stimuli and differ from asymptomatic individuals only in the extent of their exposure to the relevant stimuli; (3) they may experience normal colonic responsiveness as abnormal and therefore behave symptomatically in what they say and do; (4) the illness behavior (i.e., the reports of symptoms and the nonverbal observable behavior related to these reports) may be partially or completely uncoupled to colonic events; (5) each of these possibilities may apply to some individuals among the patient population or even to the same individual at different times, that is, there may be both within and between subject heterogeneity with respect to these possibilities. In the remainder of this chapter I will review the available evidence with respect to these possibilities for one of the functional bowel disorders—irritable bowel syndrome. This is a common disorder characterized by abdominal pain and change in bowel habit (either constipation, diarrhea, or both) in the absence of any abnormalities detected by the usual medical investigations for these symptoms.

3.2. Abnormal Colonic Responsiveness Hypothesis

Following Almy's pioneering studies 12 years passed before the next experimental attempt to address the hypothesis that IBS is characterized by abnormal physiological responses. Chaudhary and Truelove (1961), using perfused catheters in a comparative study of normal subjects, patients with ulcerative colitis, and patients with IBS, studied colonic motility during a baseline period, an emotive interview, and following a dose of neostigmine (1 mg i.m.). During base line they found that symptomatic pain-predominant IBS patients had greater colonic activity than the normals as judged by frequency, amplitude, and duration of waves, while asymptomatic patients did not. Patients with diarrhea-predominant IBS had reduced colonic activity when they were symptomatic and a normal pattern when symptom free. All clinical categories of the IBS displayed more colonic activity after neostigmine than normal subjects whether or not they were symptomatic. The response of patients with ulcerative colitis to a standard dose of neostigmine was little, if any, different from that of normal subjects. In response to the emotive interview, subjects in all three groups were said to have shown hyperactivity in relation to certain topics specific to the particular individual. The possibility of hypoactivity as a response does not seem to have been considered. There was said to be no difference among the three clinical groups in the proportion of subjects showing such a positive colonic response to an emotionally charged interview. In the absence of any data or any attempt at a quantitative analysis of the emotive interview data, it is difficult to know how much reliance to place on these findings.

Wangel and Deller (1965), using perfused catheters, investigated the motility of the large intestine in patients with IBS and in patients with miscellaneous organic disorders capable of causing constipation or diarrhea. IBS patients were again subdivided into pain-predominant and diarrhea-predominant groups. In addition, results were compared with those from a previous study of the motility of the colon in normal subjects. Compared with normal subjects, patients with the pain-predominant IBS had high levels of activity and patients with diarrhea-predominant IBS had low levels of activity. Only the diarrhea-predominant IBS patients were significantly different from the normals, and then only during the rest phase. Emotion, food, and neostigmine enhanced colonic motility in normals and in both groups of patients with the IBS, although patients with diarrhea-predominant IBS had significantly less motility than pain-predominant IBS throughout the experiments. Hypermotility in response to the emotive interview occurred with similar frequency in IBS patients and in both control groups. Moreover, a clinical history of aggravation of the symptoms by emotional factors was elicited in patients of all groups.

Connell, Jones, and Rowlands (1965) likewise used perfused catheters to compare sigmoid colonic motility in three groups of patients—those with duodenal ulcers in remission, spastic colon, and those with intermittent attacks of postprandial abdominal pain with negative investigations. Motility was recorded before and after ingestion of a meal. No differences were found between the duodenal ulcer patients and the spastic colon group. All of the patients chosen because they experienced postprandial abdominal pain, not surprisingly, experienced postprandial abdominal pain. In this group the resting level of motility was doubled after eating. The postprandial motility index for 7 of these 12 patients, however, fell within the range of the other two groups. Three of them actually experienced a decrease in the motility index. It is therefore unclear why these patients experienced symptoms. It is also not clear how this postprandial pain group relates to IBS patients in general.

Murrell and Deller (1967), using a similar methodology to the two preceding studies, compared sigmoid motility in four groups (normal subjects, patients with diarrhea, constipation, and IBS) during rest and following intravenous bradykinin. Although statistical analysis was not provided, it does not appear that the groups differed in percentage activity or motility index either during rest or following bradykinin.

Taking their lead from the studies by Chaudhary and Truelove (1961) and Wangel and Deller (1965), Kopel, Kim, and Barbero (1967) evaluated rectosigmoid motility (using perfused catheters), in 18 children with recurrent abdominal pain (RAP), in 10 children with ulcerative colitis, and in 18 normal children. (RAP is a childhood equivalent of IBS.) The degree of activity during the basal period was not statistically significantly different between normals and IBS, but ulcerative colitis patients had significantly less activity. In response to neostigmine all groups showed an increase in activity, and the IBS group had a significantly heightened response.

Bloom, LoPresti, and Farrar (1968) reported on the use of an ingestible radio telemanometer to compare colonic motility in normals, ulcerative colitis, IBS, and constipation patients. The IBS patients had significantly less colonic activity than normals with wave forms that were lower in amplitude and shorter in duration. It is difficult to compare these results with those previously reviewed since it is unclear whether these patients were diarrhea or pain predominant. There was no clear relationship between the occurrence of cramps and intraluminal pressure changes. The patients with simple constipation had waves of significantly higher amplitude and shorter durations.

Waller, Misiewicz, and Kiley (1972) used perfused catheters to compare the effect of eating on motility of the pelvic colon in patients with constipation and diarrhea. In several ways this study was an advance over previous studies. The criteria for including subjects were clearly stated, and the recording procedure was standardized with respect to prior use of medication, relationship to last meal, and time of day. The intraluminal pressure records were analyzed by computer. This was a method of known reliability (Misiewicz, Waller, Healy, & Piper, 1968) which eliminated the possibility of subjective bias; the results were statistically analyzed. Unfortunately for our purposes, the results for patients with IBS were not analyzed separately, and there was neither a normal nor a neurotic comparison group. During the basal period, the mean frequency of pressure waves in constipated patients was significantly greater than that in diarrhea patients. In patients with diarrhea, colonic motility increased significantly during the ingestion of the meal, as measured by both intensity and frequency of contractions. Pressure activity in the postmeal period did not differ significantly from that before the meal. In constipated patients there were no consistent changes either during the meal or after it. Increases in activity in the diarrhea group during the meal were significantly greater than in the constipation group, but only in one of three leads. It is not clear whether there were significant differences between the groups in the postmeal period. Among the patients with constipation there were no significant differences between those with pain and those without. The authors make the point that previous studies (Connell et al. 1965; Wangel & Deller, 1965) had only looked at postprandial response while ignoring motility during the meal. It is not clear how this finding of increased sigmoid motility during a meal in the patients with diarrhea relates to the patient's symptoms.

Chowdury et al. (1976), using perfused catheters, studied rectosigmoid motor activity in normals and in patients with functional constipation, colonic diverticulosis (with and without constipation), and IBS. After a baseline period the recording tubes were gradually withdrawn in 0.5–1 cm intervals and motor activity was recorded for 3 min at each level. If a hyperactive segment was observed, responses to various test substances were studied (secretin, cholecystokinin, atropine sulfate, glucagon). The hyperactive segment was characterized by continuous or repetitive waves over a length of 1.5–2 cm at a distance of 9–15 cm from the anal verge and was identified in 18 of the 24 patients with constipation (75%) regardless of diagnosis. It was not persistently present in any normal subjects or in any patients with IBS who had a normal bowel habit or diarrhea at the time of the study. The hyperactive segment was abolished or suppressed by atropine sulfate and glucagon but was unaffected by secretin or cholecystokinin; there were apparently no differences between groups in this respect.

Whitehead, Engel, and Schuster (1980) used rectal balloons to compare the contractile motor responses to rectal distension in normals and diarrhea-predominant and constipation-predominant IBS patients. Both IBS groups had a greater motility index than normals in response to distension; the differences increased with increasing volume of rectal distension and were greatest for the diarrhea-predominant group. The relative occurrence of contractions greater than and less than 15 sec in duration was also calculated for each group, and I will return to these results below.

There are several other papers which involve the measurement of intraluminal colonic pressures in patients with IBS (Champion, 1973; Harvey & Read, 1973a,b; Kirwan & Smith, 1977). Unfortunately the design of these studies, particularly the lack of appropriate control groups, does not permit conclusions about pathophysiological characteristics of IBS.

I have attempted to summarize some of these results in Table 1. This shows the results of studies which involved the measurement of colonic motor activity

Table 1
Summary of Studies of Colonic Motor Activity IBS (Pain-Predominant or Mixed) versus Normal

Investigator	Baseline[a]	Emotive interview	Meal	Neostigmine	Other
Almy et al. (1949)[c]	−	−			−
Chaudhary and Truelove (1961)	+	−		+	
Wangel and Deller (1965)	−	−	−	−	
Murrell and Deller (1967)	−				−
Snape et al. (1976)	−				
Chowdhury et al. (1976)	+				−
Snape et al. (1977)	−				−[b] +
Whitehead et al. (1980	−				+
Latimer et al. (1981)	+	−	−	−	

[a] "+" indicates study concluded there was a difference between groups.
[b] No difference in motility index; difference in frequency.
[c] Includes Almy, Kern, and Tulin (1949), and Almy, Hinkle, Berle, and Tulin (1949).

in at least a normal and an IBS group; painless diarrhea or diarrhea-predominant IBS groups are excluded. The experimental conditions are listed across the top. A "+" sign indicates that the investigator concluded that there was a difference between the groups in response to a given situation; a "−" sign indicates the opposite. The table demonstrates the inconsistent results of studies to date and that differences between diagnostic groups have most often not been found.

Snape, Carlson, and Cohen (1976) were the first to publish results of colonic myoelectrical recordings in IBS. Myoelectrical recordings were made using a bipolar clip electrode in the upper rectum and simultaneous intraluminal pressure recordings were made using perfused catheters. IBS patients were compared to normal subjects; there was no differentiation between diarrhea-predominant and pain-predominant patients. They placed major emphasis on describing the electrical control activity (ECA) and reported that each individual had two frequencies of ECA–6 and 3 cpm. The major distinction in ECA between groups was in the percentage of time occupied by each frequency. The slower frequency (3 cpm) was recorded for a significantly greater proportion of the total recording time in patients with IBS. Motor activity was no different between groups or between the two ECA frequencies. There were also no differences in myoelectrical activity among patients with different types of symptoms. The authors speculated on the basis of a previous report (Taylor, Duthie, Smallwood, Brown, & Linkens, 1974) that in the presence of a 3 cpm ECA the colon is more susceptible to respond to additional stimulation, either hormonal or emotional. This hypothesis found support in a second similar study (Snape, Carlson, Matarazzo, &

Cohen, 1977) in which they added an injection of cholecystokinin and pentagastrin to the protocol. Both normal subjects and patients with IBS had *quantitatively* similar responses to the administration of either cholecystokinin or pentagastrin, but patients with IBS had a greater proportion of 3 cpm contractions than did normals. The increase in motor activity among the normal subjects was composed of isolated or 6 cpm contractions.

Taylor, Darby, and Hammond (1978) also studied IBS patients and normal subjects. Myoelectrical activity was recorded from intraluminal suction electrodes, and changes in intraluminal pressure were measured by open-ended perfused tubes. Among the IBS patients comparisons were also made between symptomatic and asymptomatic periods. The frequency contents of the myoelectrical recordings were analyzed by means of a frequency spectrum analyzer. A peak was found in the mean incidence of slow wave rhythms at 3 cpm and a minimal incidence at 8 cpm among the IBS patients. In normal subjects there were peaks at both these frequencies. There was no statistically significant difference in the mean frequency or mean incidence of each slow wave rhythm in those patients with constipation as compared to those with diarrhea. There were no significant differences in the incidence of slow wave rhythms between symptomatic and asymptomatic periods. Patients with constipation had a significantly higher percentage motility value than those with diarrhea; normals fell in between. Although the authors made much of the similarities between their findings and those of Snape, there are notable differences. Snape *et al.* (1976, 1977) claimed there was either 3 cpm, 6 cpm, or isoelectric activity in their records—the proportions of these added up to 100%. Taylor *et al.* (1978), on the other hand, found a continuous spectrum of frequencies within the range examined and more than one frequency present at a time. Even the two peak frequencies were apparently present simultaneously and no account was taken of the contributions of harmonic frequencies; all frequencies present above a certain threshold value were included in the computations. A comparison of the proportions of time that the 3 cpm activity was present in the two studies (Snape *et al.* [1976, 1977] versus Taylor *et al.* [1978]) also highlights the differences: in IBS patients 40% versus 70% and in normal subjects 10% versus 50%. Thus, although differences between groups were clearly found by Taylor *et al.* (1978), their significance and origin are unclear. No information was provided on their relationship to frequency of contractions, and no convincing model was provided of how the observed differences could have accounted for the clinical features. (See also Chapters 5 and 6 for a detailed discussion of problems inherent in the interpretation of spectral data.)

In the most recent study of this type, I, together with several colleagues (Latimer, 1980; Latimer, Campbell, Latimer, Sarna, Daniel, & Waterfall, 1979) compared both colonic electrical activity (ECA) and motor activity in IBS patients to that found in patients who were equally psychologically disturbed but without bowel symptoms and to that found in normal subjects. The rationale for the psychoneurotic control group was that patients with IBS are, on average, psychologically disturbed (see Section 3.3. Abnormal Stimulation Hypothesis), and as we have already seen, there is evidence that psychological factors are associated with changes in colonic physiology. To show definitively that there is a colonic abnormality peculiar to IBS, such a control group is essential. Psychiatric interview and psychometric inventories were used with all the subjects. Activity in the rectosigmoid colon was measured during base line, a neutral interview, a stressful interview, and following a meal or neostigmine (0.5 mg i.m.). Myoelectrical activity was recorded from two intraluminal bipolar suction electrodes (4 cm apart); motor activity was recorded from two intraluminal strain gauges at the same sites. The number and duration of contractions per minute were determined by inspection of the motor activity record; the frequency content of both the motor and myoelectrical records was determined using a fast Fourier transform (FFT) computer-assisted method. Patient selection was successful in producing two groups of subjects psychologically similar to each other and both more disturbed than normal subjects. The IBS group did not differ significantly from the neurotic group on any measure of colonic activity; during a period of baseline recording the IBS group had a greater number and duration of contractions than the normals at one recording site only (see Figure 1). These results do not agree with the previous reports that IBS patients have unique colonic motor and myoelectrical characteristics.

As an aside, it can be seen in Figure 2 that there was considerable heterogeneity of response to the various conditions of the experiment in all three

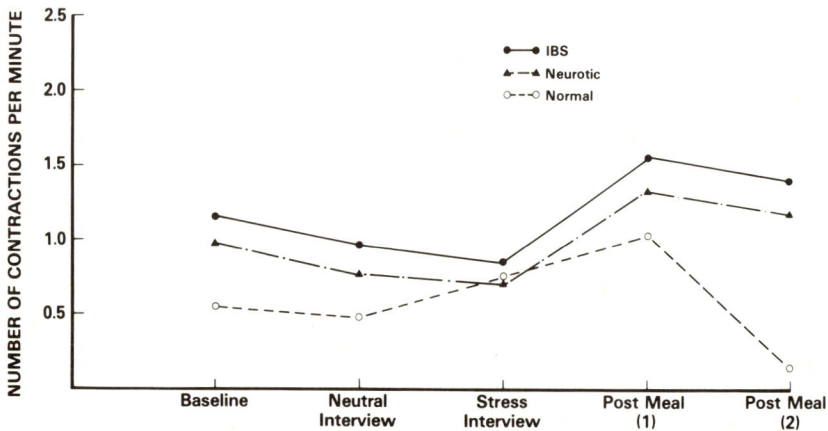

Figure 1. The mean number of contractions per minute in each experimental condition for each group—IBS, neurotic, normal. These data were recorded at the most proximal of two recording sites.

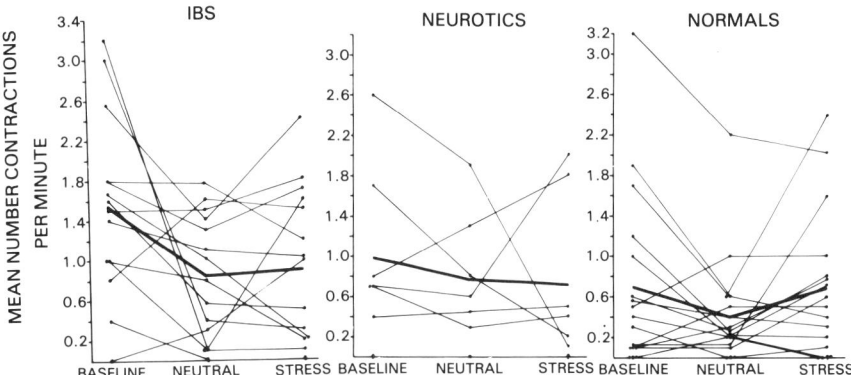

Figure 2. The mean number of contractions per minute in each of the first three experimental conditions—baseline, neutral interview, stressful interview. The results for each subject are shown for each of the three groups—IBS, neurotic, normal. These data were recorded at the most proximal of two recording sites.

groups. There were both increases and decreases in motor activity in response to the discussion of upsetting material, even within a single subject. Although these changes may have occurred in response to the sort of changes in attitude described earlier, this was not obvious.

Discrepancies between this study and those previously described that report an abnormality of ECA, cannot be attributed to psychological factors because the ECA of our IBS group did not differ from *either* control group. There are many methodological differences between these studies which *may* account for the different outcomes: subject selection, method of bowel preparation, the recording site, the recording device, and the methods of data analysis. At present the data available are insufficient to indicate the effect of each of these differences.

Whitehead *et al.* (1980) interpreted their motor activity results as being consistent with the abnormal ECA hypothesis. They found a greater preponderance of slow contractions (≥ 15 sec in duration) in both their IBS groups as compared to normals and more fast contractions (<15 sec in duration) in the diarrhea-predominant group than in either of the other groups. This interpretation notwithstanding, their results do not really test the hypothesis. We too had a greater number of slow contractions in the IBS group; this is not, however, the same as saying that in the face of an identical motility index they had a greater proportion of slow contractions than did normals. They also interpreted their results as being inconsistent with ours because there was no correlation between psychometric test scores and either symptom severity or amount of colonic motility. The use of correlation coefficients in this manner cannot replace the use of an appropriate control group. We selected a control group who seemed to have psychological and behavioral problems similar to those of patients with IBS but who, at the same time, did not have bowel symptoms. Since we were interested in comparing two groups with equally severe psychological and behavioral problems we used a battery of psychometric measures, a global assessment scale, and psychiatric diagnosis as crude ways of describing them. It is possible for such a group to have, on average, more colonic contractions without those being significantly correlated with any particular psychometric test score. Phenylketonuria may provide a useful analogy: phenylalanemia is not correlated with IQ scores although the mean levels of blood phenylalanine and IQ differ significantly between patients and normals. It is well known that not every IBS patient has elevated scores on psychometric tests and conversely that many people with elevated scores do not have IBS. These are the very facts which make the relations between psychological, behavioral, and physiological observations so complex.

The methods employed in these many studies have not been uniform and any evaluation of their results must consider their differences. In Table 2, I have prepared a simple summary of some of the methodological characteristics of these studies. The features are listed across the top; a "+" sign indicates its presence, a "−" sign its absence and a "?" that it is not mentioned in the published report. A few words about each of the headings will facilitate interpretation of Table 2. A "+" sign means that

1. Operational selection criteria—the criteria are stated in a relatively unambiguous way so that the same criteria could be applied by an independent investigator.
2. Psychological control—a group to control for the effects of psychological characteristics was included in the design—as discussed above.
3. Bowel preparation—enemas or other measures were used to evacuate the bowel.
4. Standard procedures—the physiological recordings were made under identical circumstances for all subjects including such factors as time of day, time since last meal, and last bowel movement.
5. Statistical analysis—a statistical analysis was done irrespective of how appropriate the method used.
6. Blind data scoring—the person scoring the motility records was unaware of the individual or group identity of the records at the time of scoring.
7. Reliable data—two independent scorers achieved similar results scoring the same records independently.

Before leaving these results one other observation is in order. It would be impossible to discriminate the three patterns of motility described by Grace, Wolf, and Wolff (1951; see Section 2.2. Hyper- versus Hypomotor Responsiveness) using any of the measures of colonic physiology described above; with the

Table 2
Summary of Methodological Characteristics of Colonic Motility Studies

Investigator	Operational selection criteria	Psychological control	Bowel preparation	Standard procedures	Statistical analysis	Blind data scoring	Reliable data
Almy et al. (1949)[a]	−	−	+	−	−	−	−
Chaudhary and Truelove (1961)	−	−	−	−	−	−	−
Wangel and Deller (1965)	−	−	?	?	+	?	?
Connell et al. (1965)	−	−	?	?	−	?	?
Murrell and Deller (1967)	−	−	?	?	−	−	−
Kopel et al. (1967)	−	−	?	?	+	?	?
Bloom et al. (1968)	−	−	?	?	+	?	+
Waller et al. (1972)	−	−	?	+	+	+	?
Snape et al. (1976)	+	−	−	?	+	+	?
Chowdury et al. (1976)	−	−	+	?	+	?	?
Snape et al. (1977)	+	−	−	?	+	+	?
Taylor et al. (1978)	−	−	?	?	+	?	?
Whitehead et al. (1980)	+	−	?	?	+	?	?
Latimer et al. (1981)	+	+	+	+	+	+	+

[a]Includes Almy, Kern, and Tulin (1949), and Almy, Hinkle, Berle, and Kern (1949).

exception of the Bloom *et al.* (1968) study, in each case measurements were made in the rectosigmoid colon only. Under these circumstances pattern (1)—transport activity—and pattern (3)—inactivity—would presumably appear identical, that is, one would observe reduced nonpropulsive segmental contractions in the rectosigmoid colon. That two distinct motility patterns resulting in changes in bowel habit at the opposite ends of the spectrum cannot be discriminated on the physiological measures, reflects the limitations of colonic motility measures in current use.

In summary, it can only be said that the evaluation of these studies with their many methodological differences is extremely difficult. At the very least, however, I think it can be said that this review of the existing studies supports the view that the importance of a unique pattern of altered colonic motility in IBS is not proven.

3.3. Abnormal Stimulation Hypothesis

What, then, about the second possibility, that is, that patients with IBS have a normal colonic response to particular stimuli and differ from asymptomatic individuals only in the extent of their exposure to the relevant stimuli? This is essentially the conclusion reached years ago by Almy (Almy, Hinkle, Berle, & Kern, 1949). It is supported as well by the many studies of the psychological characteristics of these patients. Since psychological problems, conflicts, stress, and the stimuli for them are frequently considered to be relevant, this possibility would be supported by finding that patients with IBS differ from individuals without IBS with respect to the occurrence of these phenomena in their lives.

There have been three systematic studies involving psychiatric assessment (leaving aside numerous uncontrolled examinations). Hislop (1971) found symptoms of an affective disorder in 64 of 67 patients with IBS, and this was significantly greater than that found in a control group matched for age and sex. It is not clear from this report how the IBS patients were selected, nor are the details of the methodology of the psychological assessment given, but the author concluded that IBS was a concomitant of an affective disorder. Liss, Alpers, and Woodruff (1973) improved on the previous study by including all IBS patients referred to a particular gastroenterology clinic over a specified period and by using specific research diagnostic criteria in the assessment of psychiatric state. They also differentiated pain-predominant from diarrhea-predominant IBS. They made a psychiatric diagnosis in 92% of the patients seen; Young, Alpers, Norland, and Woodruff (1976) repeated the Liss *et al.* (1973) study in a sample of private internal medicine patients (as opposed to patients from a university gastroenterology clinic) and used a control group of consecutive outpatients without IBS seen by one gastroenterologist. Only 18% of controls had a psychiatric disorder as defined by their research criteria as against 75% of the IBS patients.

These studies make several observations possible. First, in every study a remarkably high percentage of the IBS patients received a psychiatric diagnosis; second, a large proportion of these diagnoses go unrecognized by the attending physician; third, from the psychiatric perspective the patients formed a heterogeneous group; and fourth, the studies involving patients at teaching hospitals as opposed to private practice found more psychiatric disorder.

In addition to these studies involving a direct psychiatric assessment of IBS patients, there have been a number of investigations using other methods to assess psychological characteristics. West (1970) assessed personality using the Minnesota Multiphasic Personality Inventory (MMPI) and compared patients with IBS, ulcerative colitis, dermatological conditions, upper gastrointestinal disorders, muscle tension, headache, and asthma. The MMPI profiles for these groups were quite similar although there were significant differences in degree of psychological disturbance. Patients with IBS were among the most disturbed while those with ulcerative colitis were the least disturbed. These data supported the view that these groups differ psychologically from normals but argue against the assumption of a specific personality profile for each specific disorder. Esler and Goulston (1973) assessed anxiety by the Institute for Personality and Ability Testing anxiety scale questionnaire and the urinary excretion of epinephrine under stressful conditions. They compared IBS patients with ulcerative colitis and general medical patients. The mean anxiety score as measured by the questionnaire, in patients with the diarrhea-predominant IBS was significantly higher than that in all other groups including the pain-predominant group. Urinary epinephrine excretion was significantly higher in the diarrhea-predominant IBS group than in the others; urinary norepinephrine excretion was similar in all groups. Increased excretion of the catecholamine metabolite vanilyl mandelic acid in patients with "nervous diarrhea" has been reported by Wright and Das (1969). Palmer, Stonehill, Crisp, Waller, and Misiewicz (1974) measured forearm blood flow in IBS patients and compared their results with those previously published (Kelly & Walter, 1969). The average basal forearm blood flow in the IBS group was significantly higher than in the normal population. It was significantly lower than that observed in patients with chronic anxiety states, similar to that in patients with agitated depression and schizophrenia, and higher than that found in most other psychiatric groups. Palmer et al. (1974) also administered the Eysenck Personality Inventory to a group of IBS patients and to a group of psychoneurotic patients who were matched with IBS patients for sex, age, social class, marital status, and race. There were selection factors involved because his patients were referred to a hospital clinic and because a fairly high proportion of these were not included for a variety of reasons; he also included both diarrhea-predominant and pain-predominant cases. No mention is made of the role of gastrointestinal complaints in selecting the psychoneurotic group. The information included concerning bowel habits and laxative use, however, indicates that many of the psychoneurotic group had symptoms similar to those of the IBS group. There was, for example, no significant difference in the number of laxative takers between the two groups. Esler and Goulston (1973) also used the Eysenck Personality Inventory in assessing a consecutive series of IBS patients who were categorized into pain-predominant and diarrhea-predominant groups. Despite the difficulties in making comparisons between these studies, both studies found patients with IBS to be significantly more neurotic and less extraverted than the normal population. The one study which reported data for the lie score, a measure of a social desirability response set, found the scores for IBS patients to be significantly higher than the normal population; I made the same observation (Latimer, 1980).

Two methodologically poor studies using the "life-stress score" approach have found the IBS frequently preceded by events generally regarded as undesirable and involving losses from the social field (Fava & Pavan, 1977; Mendeloff, Monk, Siegel, & Lilienfield, 1970).

In summary, the evidence shows that patients with IBS are psychologically disturbed when compared with both the general population and patients suffering from other medical conditions. There is little evidence that IBS patients have a distinctive personality "profile"; they fall somewhere between normals and neurotics with respect to their neuroticism and extraversion scores on the Eysenck Personality Inventory (EPI), and they are more anxious than normals or general medical patients as judged by a variety of methods. On the basis of standardized psychiatric interviews a high percentage of IBS patients may be assigned a psychiatric diagnosis; diagnoses of hysteria and depression are common.

As compelling as this evidence is in support of this second possibility (see above), it does not take account of the fact that there may be many equally neurotic, anxious, or depressed patients who have no bowel disturbances.

3.4. Abnormal Interoception Hypothesis

The third possibility proposed was that these patients may experience normal colonic responsiveness as abnormal and therefore behave symptomatically in what they say and do. There is relatively little direct evidence on this point. This possibility is suggested by (a) the studies in which colonic responsiveness in IBS patients cannot be distinguished from normals and (b) certain clinical cases.

Consider the case outlined in Figure 3 as an example. For this patient (a middle-aged business executive) increasing responsibility, cessation of smoking, and a hectic work schedule initially gave rise to changes in physiological activity (1) which in turn gave rise to symptoms of IBS (3). The symptoms themselves (interoceptive stimuli), however, were a source of fear (4) because of previous experience with serious illness in others (5) and because the medical examina-

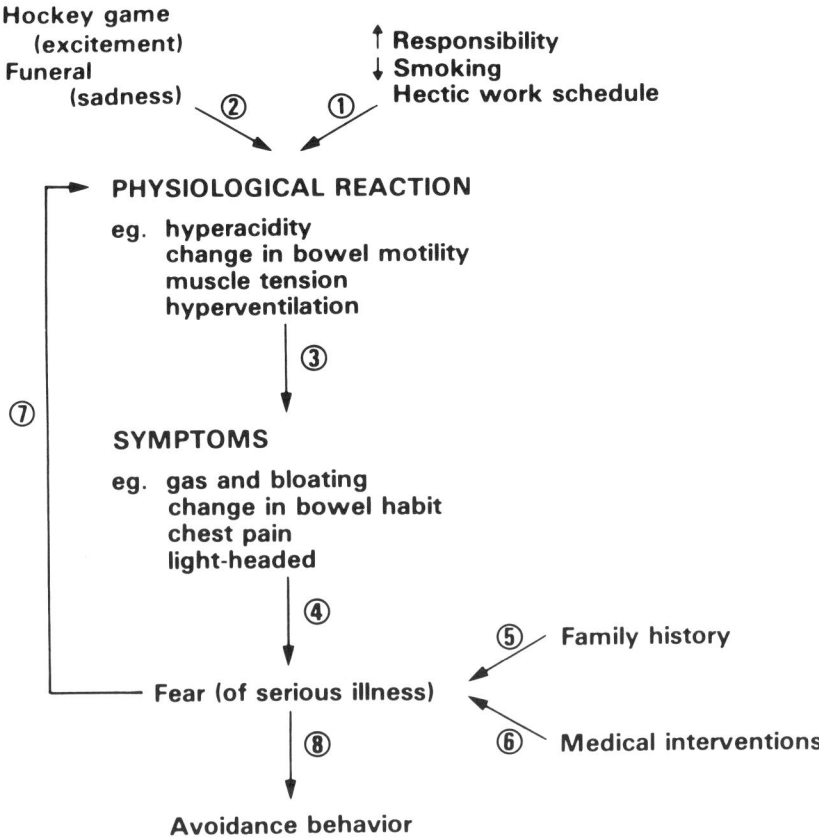

Figure 3. This is a schematic representation of the factors contributing to the symptoms of IBS in the case example.

tions and explanations he had had seemed at best only partially correct (6). A vicious circle was thus established (7) in which changes in physiological activity which could also be appropriate responses to everyday occurrences (2) had become phobic stimuli; the avoidance (8) of circumstances leading to the feared symptoms was the natural, if disabling, outcome.

When this happens, an intestinal disturbance from any source, however ordinary, is perceived by the patient as something alarming and to be avoided. In these patients stress too may lead to the sensations that are the source of concern but they are only one of many such causes which may also include such everyday phenomena as food, exercise, excitement, and changes in emotion. When such individuals attempt to avoid the interoceptive stimulus, which may be a normal and necessary change in intestinal activity, their lives become restricted; they are, of course, ultimately unsuccessful since they are trying to do the impossible. It is easy to see in this situation that most traditional approaches to therapy are doomed to failure. It is as unrealistic for the physician to try to eliminate the occurrence of the offending interoceptive stimulus using diet or anticholinergics as it is for the patient, and attempts to reduce stress only address a portion of the problem. It is also evident, however, why each of these methods leads to some improvement as the physicians collude in the avoidance behavior.

The colonic hyperalgesia hypothesis may also be construed as relevant to this point. Ritchie (1973) proposed that patients with IBS had a greater propensity than normals to report pain in response to a standard distension (60 cm^3; 35 cm from the anal margin) of the sigmoid colon. In his study among the 16 "normal and constipated" subjects 6% reported pain, while in contrast, among the IBS patients 55% reported pain. Latimer, Campbell, Latimer, Sarna, Daniel, and Waterfall (1981), however, found no difference in the proportion of normals (68%), IBS patients (58%), and psychoneurotics (80%) who experienced pain in response to a similar standard distension (50 cm^3; 25 cm from the anal margin). Recently, Whitehead et al. (1980) extended these findings by using a forced-choice method of assessing perception and demonstrated that both normal subjects and IBS patients were able to detect the addition of 5 cm^3 of air to a rectal balloon which already contained 10 cm^3 of air; there were no differences between groups. In the same experiment they reported that a greater proportion of IBS patients than normal subjects reported pain to rectal distension. The differences between their results and ours (Latimer, Campbell, Latimer, Sarna, Daniel, & Waterfall, 1979) may be due to different procedures. They used a cumulative distension, increasing the stimulus by 20 cm^3 every 2 min, whereas Latimer et al. (1979) used successive inflations and deflations alternating at 1-min intervals. IBS patients may differ from normals in their tolerance of pain rather than in their threshold for pain. Such a possibility might reconcile these conflicting results, since the Whitehead et al. (1980) procedure is probably more sensitive to differences in pain tolerance. The possibility cannot be ruled out that among those patients with abdominal pain individuals exist who experience pain in response to normal colonic distension. Clearly, however, more research is needed.

3.5. Illness Behavior Hypothesis

The fourth possibility, that is, that of uncoupling between symptom related behaviors and colonic events, is one which I have discussed previously (Latimer & Campbell, 1980). It is suggested by studies which fail to demonstrate distinctive physiological characteristics for IBS since one is then apparently faced with two or more groups of patients who, in the presence of similar colonic events, engage in different symptomatic behavior. This possibility is also suggested by recent findings from other psychophysiological research. That symptom reports, nonverbal observable symptomatic behavior, and physiological responses may be relatively independent under some circumstances has become rather widely accepted. To put it another way, there may be little concordance between what a patient says about his symptoms, what he may be seen to do by an independent observer, and how he responds physiologically in those measures most relevant to his symptoms. The origin of this notion may be traced to the classical experiments of Schachter and Singer (1962), in which identical injections of epinephrine elicited different emotions depending on the social context in which they occurred. To put it differently, quite diverse verbal and other observable emotional behaviors were elicited in the presence of identical physiological responses.

A similar point has been made about anxiety, insomnia, and tension headaches. A patient may report fear and yet show no signs of physiological arousal or even behavioral avoidance (Lang, 1968; Rachman, 1978), he/she may report sleep onset insomnia and yet have a normal latency to EGG-determined sleep onset (Borkovec, 1979), and he/she may have "tension" headaches, the occurrence and severity of which bear no relation to the EMG potentials measured in the apparently offending muscle (Haynes, 1981). This observation is of fundamental importance in both the study and treatment of such problems; unless behavior at the three levels is measured independently, there is no way to know how the populations selected by different investigators compare in this respect. It is possible that a considerable amount of the variance between all the studies on IBS can be accounted for in this way. This distinction is also likely to be relevant for treatment. It is quite possible that a different treatment will be required for someone who complains of abdominal pain and an ability to have a spontaneous bowel movement in the absence of any other objective evidence of disordered function than for someone with the same complaints, but concordantly disturbed colonic segmental contractions and bowel movements. Although both these patients may say the same thing, and by so doing be given the same diagnosis, the only behavior they have in common is what they say.

3.6. Heterogeneity Hypothesis

Finally, and most importantly, is the possibility that the group of patients being discussed is quite heterogeneous. Each of the above possibilities may apply to some patients. It is clear that all currently used selection criteria for IBS, relying, as they do, on self-report and the exclusion of other diseases, yield a mixed bag of patients. One need only look at the variety of psychiatric disorders found in those studies using operational psychiatric diagnostic criteria, at the variety of other nongastrointestinal symptoms exhibited, or at the variance in the various physiological measures used to record colonic responses. It is this heterogeneity which has led me to call for a moratorium on further comparative studies until standardized methods of three-systems behavioral assessment are developed (Latimer, 1979b).

3.7. Treatment Implications

What are the implications of these psychophysiological findings for the treatment of IBS? The available evidence suggests that apart from their presenting complaints, patients with IBS do not differ from neurotic psychiatric outpatients. They have similar age and sex distributions, similar psychological characteristics, and cannot be distinguished by their colonic responses (Latimer, 1980). It is therefore reasonable to expect the methods of behavior therapy, which have proven so effective in the treatment of neurotic disorders, to be effective; likewise, no single treatment will apply to all. I have tentatively suggested (Latimer, 1981) the following guidelines for the choice of behavioral techniques for patients with IBS:

1. *Maladaptive verbal behavior.* For some patients, the symptom reports themselves turn out to be the major identifiable problem, rather than pointing the way to a significant physiological disturbance. These cases frequently arise for one of two reasons: (a) misconceptions about some aspect of toileting behavior or digestive functioning and (b) inappropriate reinforcement of the symptom reports. A complaint of pain, for example, may elicit attention and concern from otherwise undemonstrative friends and relatives. The first situation calls for identification and correction of the relevant misconceptions—cognitive therapy; the second requires rearranging the social contingencies so that attention and concern are received for more appropriate behavior—operant procedures, contingency contracting.

2. *Maladaptive nonverbal behavior.* Patients for whom nonverbal symtomatic behavior is prominent (e.g., grimacing, taking medication) are frequently being reinforced by the consequences of such behavior, and operant conditioning procedures are indicated as described above. Obsessional patients also frequently fall into this category; although they may have diarrhea, for example, the most prominent symptoms may be their avoidance of situations leading to diarrhea or their avoidance of any situation which does not allow easy access to a toilet. In these cases, exposure and response prevention is the treatment of choice. The patient is asked to engage in the behaviors and situations which they fear and to do nothing to avoid the feared consequences. The individual afraid of incontinence is taken into a public place and encouraged not to escape to a toilet no matter how strong his urge to defecate. Likewise the individual afraid of vomiting is asked to eat in public and not to avail themselves of a receptacle or private place in which to vomit. Gradually the urgency declines

and with each successive session the urge to avoid the feared situation diminishes.

3. *Maladaptive physiological behavior*. This is the group most consistent with the traditional conception of IBS; these individuals actually have an identifiable colonic correlate of their symptoms. As discussed earlier, their behavior may be a qualitatively normal response which is occurring excessively in response to identifiable environmental stimuli. Such a situation could result in a multitude of ways, as for example, in association with a marital problem, difficulties at work, interpersonal conflicts, and phobias. In each case treatment necessitates identifying the problematic stimuli and either problem solving (e.g., marital therapy and assertive training) to remove the stimuli or changing the individual's response to the stimuli (e.g., systematic desensitization and exposure). In cases where the excessive response is not associated with identifiable stimuli relaxation training alone may be indicated. Biofeedback of specific colonic responses would only seem logical in cases where a distinctive colonic characteristic is identified.

Many and perhaps most cases will be mixed and require combinations of methods dictated by the behavioral analysis.

4. Conclusion

Although the responsiveness of the human colon to the vicissitudes of everyday life is now well established, the role of such responses in functional bowel disorders is by no means settled. The task of unraveling the complex interrelations between behaviors at several levels of organization is complicated by the ill-defined nature of the syndromes in question. The hope for the future may lie in the integration of the traditional biomedical focus on the development of valid physiological measures and the traditional behavioral scientific focus on the objective and reliable measurement of observable behavior. Only with a greater emphasis on a tripartite assessment of behavior which samples concurrently the domains of what a patient says (symptom reports), what he does (nonverbal symptomatic behavior), and how he responds physiologically (colonic motility), can we transform this task into a scientific exercise. Effective treatment should not be far behind.

5. References

Almy, T. P., & Tulin, M. Alterations in colonic function in man under stress: Experimental production of changes simulating the "irritable colon." *Gastroenterology*, 1947, *8*, 616–626.

Almy, T. P., Kern, F., & Tulin, M. Alterations in colonic function in man under stress. II. Experimental production of sigmoid spasm in healthy persons. *Gastroenterology*, 1949, *12*, 425–436.

Almy, T. P., Hinkle, L. E., Berle, B., & Kern, F. Alteration in colonic function in man under stress. III. Experimental production of sigmoid spasm in patients with spastic constipation. *Gastroenterology*, 1949, *12*, 437–449.

Almy, T. P., Abbot, F. K., & Hinkle, L. E. Alterations in colonic function in man under stress. IV. Hypomotility of the sigmoid colon and its relationship to the mechanism of functional diarrhea. *Gastroenterology*, 1950, *15*, 95–103.

Beaumont, W. *Experiments and observations on the gastric juice and the physiology of digestion.* Plattsburg, New York: F. P. Allen, 1833.

Bidder & Schmidt. *Die Verdauungssafte und der Stoffwechsel.* Leipzig, 1852. (Quoted in W. B. Cannon, 1929.)

Bloom, A. A., LoPresti, P.,& Farrar, J. T. Motility of the intact human colon. *Gastroenterology*, 1968, *54*, 232–240.

Borkovec, T. D. Pseudo (experiental) insomnia and idiopathic (objective) insomnia: Theoretical and therapeutic issues. *Advances in Behavior Research and Therapy*, 1979, *2*, 27–55.

Cannon, W. B. *Bodily changes in pain, hunger, fear and rage* (2nd ed.). New York: Appleton-Century-Crofts, 1929.

Champion, P. Some cases of the irritable bowel syndrome studied by intraluminal pressure recordings. *Digestion*, 1973, *9*, 21–29.

Chaudhary, N. A., & Truelove, S. C. Human colonic motility: A comparative study of normal subjects, patients with ulcerative colitis and patients with the irritable colon syndrome. *Gastroenterology*, 1961, *40*, 1–36.

Chowdhury, A. R., Dinoso, V. P., & Lorber, S. H. Characterization of a hyperactive segment at the rectosigmoid junction. *Gastroenterology*, 1976, *71*, 584–588.

Christensen, J. Myoelectrical control of the colon. *Gastroenterology*, 1975, *68*, 601–609.

Cohen, S., Long, W. B., & Snape, W. J. Gastrointestinal motility. In R. K. Crane (Ed.), *International Review of Physiology and Gastrointestinal Physiology III* (Vol. 19). Baltimore: University Park Press, 1979.

Connell, A. M., Jones, F. A., & Rowlands, E. N. Motility of the pelvic colon. Part IV. Abdominal pain associated with colonic hypermotility after meals. *Gut*, 1965, *6*, 105–112.

Esler, M. D., & Goulston, K. J. Levels of anxiety in colonic disorders. *New England Journal of Medicine*, 1973, *288*, 16–20.

Fava, G. A., & Pavan, L. Large bowel disorders. Illness configuration and life events. *Psychotherapy and Psychosomatics*, 1977, *27*, 93–99.

Friedman, M. H. F., & Snape, W. J. Color changes in the mucosa of the colon in children as affected by food and psychic stimuli. *American Physiological Society, Federation Proceedings*, 1946, *5*, 30–31.

Grace, W. J., Wolf, S., & Wolff, H. G. Life situations, emotions and colonic function. *Gastroenterology*, 1949, *14*, 93–108,

Grace, W. J., Wolf, S., & Wolff, H. G. *The human colon.* New York: Paul B. Hoeber, 1951.

Harvey, R. F., & Read, A. E. Effect of cholecystokinin on colonic motility and symptoms in patients with irritable bowel syndrome. *Lancet*, 1973, *1*, 1–3. (a)

Harvey, R. F., & Read, A. E. Effect of oral magnesium sulphate on colonic motility in patients with irritable bowel syndrome. *Gut*, 1973, *14*, 983–987. (b)

Haynes, S. N. Muscle-contraction headache: A psychophysiological perspective of etiology and treatment. In S. N. Haynes & L. R. Gannon (Eds.), *Psychosomatic disorders: A psychophysiological approach to etiology and treatment.* New York: Holt, Rinehart & Winston, 1981.

Hislop, I. G. Psychological significance of the irritable colon syndrome. *Gut*, 1971, *12*, 452–457.

Hornborg. Skandinavisches Archiv für Physiologie (XV). 1904. (Quoted in W. B. Cannon, 1929.)

Kelly, D. H. W., & Walter, C. J. S. The relationship between clinical diagnosis and anxiety,

assessed by forearm blood flow and other measurements. *British Journal of Psychiatry,* 1969, *114,* 611–626.
Kirwan, W. O., & Smith, A. N. Colonic propulsion in diverticular disease, idiopathic constipation and the irritable colon syndrome. *Scandinavian Journal of Gastroenterology,* 1977, *12,* 331–335.
Kopel, F. B., Kim, I. C., & Barbero, G. J. Comparison of rectosigmoid motility in normal children, children with recurrent abdominal pain and children with ulcerative colitis. *Pediatrics,* 1967, *39,* 539–545.
Lang, P. J. Fear reduction and fear behavior: Problems in treating a construct. In T. M. Shlien (Ed.), *Research in psychotherapy* (Vol. 3). Washington, D.C.: American Psychological Association, 1968.
Latimer, P. R. Psychophysiologic disorders: A critical appraisal of concept and theory illustrated with reference to the irritable bowel syndrome (IBS). *Psychological Medicine,* 1979, *9,* 71–80. (a)
Latimer, P. R. *Behavior analysis: Its importance in therapy and its implications for future research.* NIAMDD Workshop on Functional Disorders of the G.I. Tract, Washington, D.C., October 25–27, 1979. (b)
Latimer, P. R. *Irritable bowel syndrome: A psychophysiological study.* Unpublished doctoral thesis, McMaster University, 1980.
Latimer, P. R. Behavior therapy, biofeedback and the gastrointestinal tract. *Journal of Psychotherapy and Psychosomatics,* 1981, *36,* 200–212.
Latimer, P. R., & Campbell, D. Behavioral medicine and the functional bowel disorders. *International Journal of Mental Health,* 1980, *9,* 111–128.
Latimer, P. R., Campbell, D., Latimer, M., Sarna, S. K., Daniel, E. E., & Waterfall, W. E. Irritable bowel syndrome: A test of the colonic hyperalgesia hypothesis. *Journal of Behavioral Medicine,* 1979, *2,* 285–295.
Latimer, P. R., Sarna, S. K., Campbell, D., Latimer, M. R., Waterfall, W. E., & Daniel, E. E. Colonic motor and myoelectrical activity: A comparative study of normal subjects, psychoneurotic patients and patients with irritable bowel syndrome (IBS). *Gastroenterology,* 1981, *80,* 893–901.
Liss, J. L., Alpers, D., & Woodruff, R. A. The irritable colon syndrome and psychiatric illness. *Diseases of the Nervous System,* 1973, *34,* 151–157.
Mendeloff, A. I., Monk, M., Siegel, C. I., & Lilienfield, A. Illness experience and life stress in patients with irritable colon and with ulcerative colitis. *New England Journal of Medicine,* 1970, *282,* 14–17.
Misiewicz, J. J., Waller, S. L., Healy, M. J. J., & Piper, E. A. Computer analysis of intraluminal pressure records. *Gut,* 1968, *9,* 232–236.
Murrell, T. G. C., & Deller, D. J. Intestinal motility in man: The effects of bradykinin on the motility of the distal colon. *American Journal of Digestive Diseases,* 1967, *12,* 568–576.
Palmer, R. L., Stonehill, E., Crisp, A. H., Waller, S. L., & Misiewicz, J. J. Psychological characteristics of patients with irritable bowel syndrome. *Postgraduate Medical Journal,* 1974, *50,* 416–419.
Pavlov, I. *The work of the digestive glands* (W. H. Thompson,Trans.). London: Griffin, 1910.
Rachman, S. J. *Fear and courage.* San Francisco: W. H. Freeman, 1978.
Richet, C. Des Propriétés chimiques et physiologiques du suc gastrique chez l'homme et les animaux. Appendix A. *Journal d' Anatomie et Physiologie,* 1878, *14,* 170–333. (Quoted in W. B. Cannon, 1929.)
Ritchie, J. Pain from distension of the pelvic colon by inflating a balloon in the irritable colon syndrome. *Gut,* 1973, *14,* 125–132.

Schacter, S., & Singer, J. E. Cognitive, social and physiological determinants of emotional state. *Psychological Review*, 1962, *69*, 379–399.

Snape, W. J., Carlson, G. M., & Cohen, S. Colonic myoelectric activity in the irritable bowel syndrome. *Gastroenterology*, 1976, *70*, 326–330.

Snape, W. J., Carlson, G. M., Matarazzo, S. A., & Cohen, S. Evidence that abnormal myoelectrical activity produces colonic motor dysfunction in the irritable bowl syndrome. *Gastroenterology*, 1977, *72*, 383–387.

Taylor, I., Darby, C., & Hammond, P. Comparison of rectosigmoid myoelectrical activity in the irritable colon syndrome during relapses and remissions. *Gut*, 1978, *19*, 923–929.

Taylor, I., Duthie, H. L., Smallwood, R., Brown, B. H., & Linkens, D. The effect of stimulation on the myoelectric activity of the rectosigmoid in man. *Gut*, 1974, *15*, 599–607.

Waller, S. L., Misiewicz, J. J., & Kiley, N. Effect of eating on motility of the pelvic colon in constipation and diarrhea. *Gut*, 1972, *13*, 805–811.

Wangel, A. G., & Deller, D. J. Intestinal motility in man. III. Mechansims of constipation and diarrhea with particular reference to the irritable bowel syndrome. *Gastroenterology*, 1965, *48*, 69–84.

Weeks, D. M. Observations of small and large bowel motility in man. *Gastroenterology*, 1946, *6*, 185–190.

West, K. L. MMPI correlates of ulcerative colitis. *Journal of Clinical Psychology*, 1970, *26*, 214–219.

White, B. V., Jr., & Jones, C. M. Effect of irritants and drugs affecting autonomic nervous system upon the mucosa of the normal rectum and rectosigmoid, with especial reference to "mucous colitis." *New England Journal of Medicine*, 1938, *218*, 791–797.

Whitehead, W. E., Engel, B. T., & Schuster, M. M. Irritable bowel syndrome: Physiological and psychological differences between diarrhea-predominant and constipation-predominant patients. *Digestive Diseases and Sciences*, 1980, *25*, 404–413.

Wolf, S., & Welsh, J. D. The gastrointestinal tract as a responsive system. In N. S. Greenfield & R. A. Sternback (Eds.), *Handbook of psychophysiology*. New York: Holt, Rinehart & Winston, 1972.

Wright, J. T., & Das, A. K. Excretion of 4-hydroxy-3 methoxy mandelic acid in cases of ulcerative colitis and diarrhea of nervous origin. *Gut*, 1969, *10*, 628–630.

Young, S. J., Alpers, D. H., Norland, C. C., & Woodruff, R. A. Psychiatric illness and the irritable bowel syndrome. *Gastroenterology*, 1976, *70*, 162–166.

14

IRRITABLE BOWEL SYNDROME
Applications of Psychophysiological Methods to Treatment
MARVIN M. SCHUSTER

1. Introduction

A study of the patient population which appeared at a busy gastrointestinal clinic in New Orleans (McHardy, Browne, McHardy, Welch, & Ward, 1962) makes several important points about functional bowel disorders. Approximately half of the patients had an organic diagnosis, and the other half were functional. Over the 13-yr follow-up, only 6% of the patients in the functional category received a different, organic diagnosis. This emphasizes that the diagnosis of irritable bowel syndrome, which is the major functional bowel disorder represented here, can be made with a reasonable degree of accuracy and reliability in one or two sessions with the patient. It also makes the point that further diagnostic evaluation or further discoveries will separate out a small group who have specific organic disorders. One of the best examples are patients who have a lactase deficiency resulting in lactose intolerance, with symptoms identical to those of the irritable bowel syndrome. At the time of the McHardy *et al.* study (1962) such patients would have been included in the functional bowel group. With time we will discover other hormonal, biochemical, and electrophysiological disorders which carry specific indications for therapy, but it is also likely that there will remain a large core which will continue to be identified as irritable bowel syndrome.

MARVIN M. SCHUSTER • The Johns Hopkins School of Medicine and the Division of Digestive Diseases, Baltimore City Hospital, Baltimore, Maryland 21224.

2. Diagnostic Criteria for Irritable Bowel Syndrome

The definition of irritable bowel syndrome is something about which gastroenterologists are approaching a consensus. The criteria are abdominal pain, altered bowel habits (meaning either constipation or diarrhea or more often an alternation between constipation and diarrhea), and no detectable organic disease. Abdominal pain is an important criterion. Painless diarrhea is a different disorder, not the irritable bowel syndrome. It is nervous diarrhea—the kind of diarrhea that a medical student gets before he takes an exam, or that a speaker gets before he discusses the irritable bowel syndrome. And that, by definition, is perfectly normal.

The diagnosis of irritable bowel syndrome is not simply a diagnosis of exclusion; it can be made positively. If I were permitted to ask only one question to determine whether the patient had functional bowel disease, the question would be "Does the pain awaken you at night?" Rarely, is the patient awakened at night when the pain is functional. If the pain regularly awakens the subject at night, one can almost always discover some organic etiology. There is no weight loss in irritable bowel syndrome unless there is an associated serious depression. Things like milk intolerance (lactase deficiency) have to be ruled out. One can find a palpable, tender sigmoid in most instances. On sigmoidoscopy, the patient complains of tenderness, and spasm is seen by the examiner. These are positive findings.

There are many different names by which this entity, *the irritable bowel syndrome*, is known. The major plea which I would make is that we not call it *itis*—neither mucous col*itis*, nervous col*itis*, nor adaptive col*itis*. There are two reasons for not using this term: It is physiologically and anatomically incorrect because there is no inflammation. The second reason is that every patient who has this diagnosis applied to him knows someone who has had ulcerative colitis and who may have had a colostomy or may have died. The last thing a person with irritable bowel syndrome needs to worry about is whether he has colitis. We must, therefore, avoid the term colitis.

The disorder involves a heterogenous group of people, and investigators will have to learn to separate some from the others. The work of Taylor, Duthie, Smallwood, Brown, and Linkens (1974) and Snape and Cohen (1979) has raised the possibility that there is a group of people labeled as having irritable bowel syndrome who have a predominant frequency of electrical rhythm that is different from a normal group. This may permit us to select out a group of people who are responsive to a particular type of treatment. Our task is to be splitters as much as possible before we become lumpers.

3. Psychophysiology of Irritable Bowel Syndrome

Connell's (1962) concept of paradoxical motility suggested that in constipation one finds an augmentation of haustral contractions whereas in diarrhea one finds an absence or a diminution of haustral contractions. In normal subjects, one occasionally sees small, impeding contractions of the haustral segmentation of the colon. In patients with constipation, there are exaggerated haustral contractions, and in patients with diarrhea, diminished contractions are found.

These contractions are sometimes associated with pain, very much like diffuse esophageal spasm (see Chapter 3). Very often pain is associated with simultaneous, high-amplitude contractions which appear over a large area of the colon. However, contractions are not always associated with pain, and we cannot always record colonic motor activity when the patient is reporting pain. This may be related to many factors, including the possibility that we are recording in the wrong area. We can only measure from a very limited area of the colon.

3.1. Effects of Meals

It has been demonstrated that meals are one of the stimuli to which people with irritable bowel syndrome are hypersensitive; they may experience postprandial pains associated with increases in motor activity. This can be mimicked by cholinergic agents such as Prostigmine. One can either use a meal stimulus to elicit these contractions or one can use a pharmacologic agent which is a neurotransmitter. This activity can also be reproduced by administering gastrointestinal hormones such as cholecystokinine, a hormone which is released when food or acid reaches the duodenum. This is one of the hormones believed to be involved in the gastroileocolic reflex, which results in the urge to defecate following a meal. There seem to be a subset of people with irritable bowel who are hypersensitive to meals. Not all people with irritable bowel claim that a meal sets off their syndrome, but those who do may also be hypersensitive to cholecystokinine. Figure 1 (from a study by Harvey & Read, 1973) demonstrates that patients who are sensitive to meals are also sensitive to cholecystokinine. Of those people who had postprandial complaints (dotted lines in Figure 1), most also had an increase in motility, whereas people who did not have postprandial complaints (solid lines) did not have increased motility following the injection of cholecystokinine.

Snape and Cohen (1979) have shown that patients with irritable bowel syndrome exhibit an increase in motility which is delayed in its onset following a standard meal and also prolonged in duration compared to normal subjects. Figure 2 illustrates this. In normal subjects there is an increase in activity which declines 40 or 50 min after a meal, whereas subjects with irritable bowel syndrome seem to have a delayed onset of activity, and this corresponds frequently to the onset of pain.

Clindinium, an anticholinergic drug, supresses the baseline activity as well as the postprandial activity. That in itself looks encouraging. Discouraging, however, is the fact that clinical trials show that anticholinergics are not very

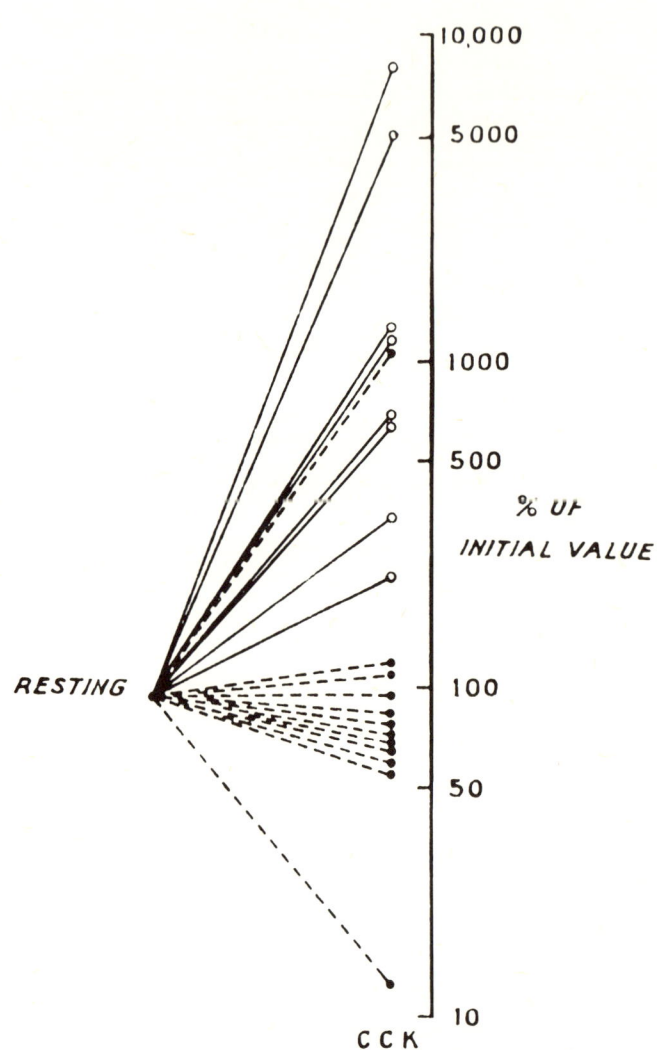

Figure 1. Motility changes induced by injection of cholecystokinin (CCK) in patients with (dotted lines) and without (solid lines) a history of food-induced pain. (Reprinted from Read & Hartley, 1973, with permission.)

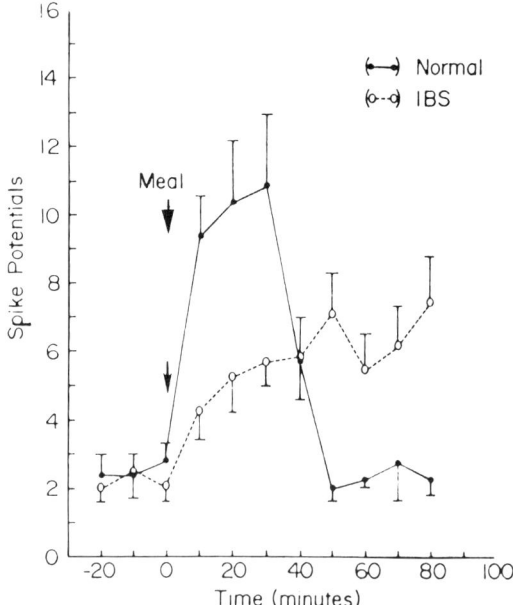

Figure 2. Meal induced motor activity in normal subjects and patients with irritable bowel syndrome (IBS). (Reprinted from Snape & Cohen, 1979, with permission.)

effective therapeutically. There is an objective response without a clinical response.

3.2. Psychological Characteristics of Patients with Irritable Bowel Syndrome

The classic studies of Almy (e.g., Almy & Tulin, 1947) are described and critically evaluated by Latimer (Chapter 13, this volume). Almy made the appropriate point that different affects (emotions) are associated with different types of motility; the topic of conversation might be the same (in both instances the subject was talking about her stepdaughter), but the affect and associated behavior were different. But as Latimer points out, this is not specific to patients with irritable bowel syndrome; it occurs in normal subjects as well. Perhaps Hans Selye was right when he said, "It is not what happens to you that matters, but how you take it."

There have been a number of studies on this point which demonstrate that patients with irritable bowel syndrome have a higher incidence of phenomena associated with depression than do others. They are more frequently fatigued and more frequently diagnosed and reported to have anorexia, insomnia, and weeping. A very few are suicidal. Hislop (1971) demonstrated that an antidepressive drug is more effective in producing a symptom-free status than a tranquilizing drug in comparing tricyclics and phenothiazines.

Young (1979) demonstrated that not only do a large percentage of irritable bowel patients have psychiatric symptoms, but also that the psychiatric symptoms antedate the gastrointestinal symptoms in 65% of patients; and in 85% of patients they antidated or were simultaneous with the onset of gastrointestinal symptoms. However, despite the high frequency of an association of psychiatric illness with the diagnosis of irritable bowel syndrome, the psychiatric diagnosis was made correctly by the internist in only 28% of patients. A high proportion of patients reported by Young had neither anxiety nor depression as a primary symptom, but had ill-defined psychiatric symptoms.

Whitehead, Winget, Fedoravicius, Wooley, and Blackwell (1982) found that, compared to normals, irritable bowel patients were more preoccupied with their somatic symptoms, more sensitive to them, or they had more somatic symptoms than normal subjects. Many of the patients with irritable bowel syndrome reported more colds than did other people. They reported more serious colds, they went to the doctor more often, they sought medical attention more frequently for their colds, they had more sick days for their colds, and they had been hospitalized in the past year for complaints other than irritable bowel syndrome more frequently than people without irritable bowel syndrome. These were complaints which were presumably unrelated to the irritable bowel syndrome, showing again that there is something about this population which may speak to heightened sensitivity, heightened reportability, or heightened labeling.

Some of the psychiatric symptoms which have been known to be associated with irritable bowel symptoms are depression, anxiety, preoccupation with illness, and cancer phobia. This is a major preoccupation in very many patients; they have a disorder and are worried that they may have cancer, especially if the doctor has told them that what they have is mucous colitis or nervous colitis. They may know that there is a fairly substantial increase in the incidence of cancer in ulcerative colitis. As new symptoms appear, they begin to wonder if what they have is developing into cancer. A very important part of the physician's approach is to deal effectively with this particular misconception.

Whitehead and Schuster (1979) have emphasized that there are several critical questions which need to be asked when evaluating the irritable bowel patient: (1) Is the patient depressed? (2) Are the symptoms aggravated by stress or tension? (If so, what stress or tensions, and how can one alter these?) (3) Are the symptoms maintained by social reinforcement? Is the patient getting attention because of the complaints, perhaps from childhood and, later on, is there a reenactment of the childhood situation? (4) Does the patient have irrational beliefs about the cause of his symptoms? Is he concerned that he will end up with a colostomy or that he will die of cancer?

3.3. Pain from Gas

One symptom frequently associated with irritable bowel syndrome is the *splenic flexure syndrome*. Patients with irritable bowel complain that they have a large volume of gas. The differential diagnosis may need to distinguish between coronary pain and gas pain because the splenic flexure sits up high under the diaphragm, and the gas, seeking its highest level, elevates the diaphragm. The splenic flexure is the highest portion of the gastrointestinal tract within the abdomen except for the stomach, so the gas rises there, distends the colon, and the patient thinks he has a heart attack. However, this is the kind of heart attack that is relieved by passing gas.

Both Ritchie (1979) and Lasser, Bond, and Levitt (1975) have shown that, although patients with irritable bowel complain of excess gas, they do not have excess gas. Lasser *et al.* infused radioactive helium into the bowel and were able to wash out gas and demonstrate how much gas was present. Patients who complained of excess gas did not have excess gas, but they were exquisitely sensitive to distension of the bowel. More patients with the irritable bowel syndrome complain of pain when the bowel is distended with 60 ml of air than do normal subjects, and the same thing is true when a larger volume of air is instilled (Figure 3) (Richie, 1973; Whitehead, Engel, & Schuster, 1980).

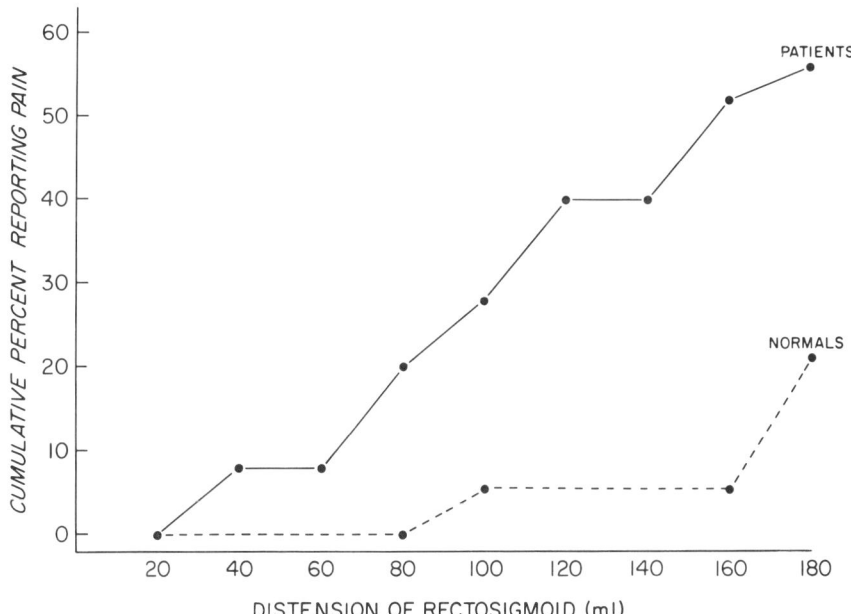

Figure 3. Pain threshold during incremental rectosigmoid distension in normal subjects and patients with IBS. (Reprinted from Whitehead, Engel, & Schuster, 1980, with permission.)

4. Fiber in the Treatment of Functional Bowel Disorders

Increased fiber in the diet has been proposed for the treatment of diverticular disease and in the treatment of irritable bowel syndrome. This is in part due to the fact that some of the motor disturbances which are found in diverticular disease are also found in irritable bowel syndrome (which may be due to the limited repertoire of the colon; the colon can only respond by contracting or relaxing, or by contracting in a peculiar fashion). The fact that irritable bowel syndrome and diverticular disease have common motor abnormalities in no way implies a common etiology. However, most people do receive fiber as treatment when the diagnosis of irritable bowel syndrome is made, and fiber has been demonstrated to specifically increase stool weight. In patients who have rapid transit, fiber tends to slow transit, and in patients who have slow transit, fiber tends to speed up the transit. Also, intracolonic pressures are diminished, and an engineering principle (Laplace's law) relating tension, pressure, and radius states that the pressure is inversely related to the radius, so that the higher the radius the lower the pressures. Therefore, if you can increase the radius, you will decrease the pressure. This is one of the theoretical reasons for the efficacy of bran in the treatment of diverticular disease. There are many different types of fiber, and this fact is often overlooked. Bran seems to be the fiber that is most effective in diverticular disease.

5. Biofeedback Training to Decrease Colonic Motility

The biofeedback technique for treatment of irritable bowel syndrome uses the technique of stepwise distension of the rectosigmoid to elicit colonic spasm as described in Chapter 16. The examination table is elevated so that the patient is able to look down to the recording. The instructions to the patient are to use whatever internal means he can to suppress the variability in the recorded pressure as the spasm is occurring. He is told to do this without using his skeletal muscles. At the end of a training session, which lasts about 1½ hr, there is suppression of the spastic activity, which can persist for at least 8 weeks. This finding has more theoretical significance than it has clinical interest because it shows that a person can influence autonomically innervated smooth muscle, even in a pathologic state. We do not know at this stage what this would mean clinically. We are trying to evaluate the clinical implications of this training.

There are theoretical considerations as to why this procedure might not be a satisfactory clinical tool. One reason is that the irritable bowel syndrome involves not simply an irritable rectosigmoid but an irritable bowel, and if the same degree of specificity is being achieved in the colon as has been demonstrated in temperature self-regulation (in which the temperature of one finger can be changed to the exclusion of the other nine fingers), we would not be effecting a reduction in the motility in other parts of the colon. If there is some extension of these learning phenomena to other areas of the colon and of the gastrointestinal tract, then perhaps there will be some amelioration in the symptoms. This is an area which is under investigation.

Treatment of irritable bowel syndrome, at present, has to be a multifaceted approach attacking all of the aspects that we believe to be important, and at the same time establishing a very close therapeutic relationship with the patient. Biofeedback and other behavioral treatment procedures are important ingredients of such a treatment program.

6. References

Almy, T. P., & Tulin, M. Alterations in colonic function in man under stress: Experimental production of changes simulating the "irritable colon." *Gastroenterology,* 1947, *8,* 616–626.

Connell, A. M. The motility of the pelvic colon. II. Paradoxical motility in diarrhea and constipation. *Gut,* 1962, *3,* 342–348.

Harvey, R. F., & Read, A. E. Effect of cholocystokinin on colonic motility and symptoms in patients with irritable bowel syndrome. *Lancet,* 1973, *1,* 1–3.

Hislop, I. G. Psychological significance of the irritable colon syndrome. *Gut,* 1971, *12,* 452–457.

Lasser, R. B., Bond, J. H., & Levitt, M. D. The role of intestinal gas in functional abdominal pain. *New England Journal of Medicine,* 1975, *293,* 524–526.

McHardy, G., Browne, D. C., McHardy, R. J., Welch, G. E., & Ward, S. S. Psychophysiologic gastrointestinal reactions: Therapeutic observations. *Postgraduate Medicine,* 1962, *31,* 346–357.

Ritchie, J. Pain from distension of the pelvic colon by inflating a balloon in the irritable colon syndrome. *Gut,* 1973, *14,* 125–132.

Ritchie, J. Pain in irritable bowel syndrome. *Practical Gastroenterology,* 1979, *3*(4), 16–23.

Snape, W. J., Jr., & Cohen, S. How colonic motility differs in normal subjects and patients with IBS. *Practical Gastroenterology,* 1979, *3*(3), 21–25.

Taylor, I., Duthie, H. L., Smallwood, R., Brown, B. H., & Linkens, D. The effect of stimulation on the myoelectrical activity of the rectosigmoid in man. *Gut,* 1974, *15,* 599–607.

Whitehead, W. E., Engel, B. T., & Schuster, M. M. Irritable bowel syndrome: Physiological and psychological differences between diarrhea-predominant and constipation-predominant patients. *Digestive Diseases and Sciences,* 1980, *25,* 404–413.

Whitehead, W. E., & Schuster, M. M. Psychological management of the irritable bowel syndrome. *Practical Gastroenterology,* 1979, *3*(6), 32–43.

Whitehead, W. E., Winget, C., Fedoravicius, A. S., Wooley, S., & Blackwell, B. Learned illness behavior in patients with irritable bowel syndrome and peptic ulcer. *Digestive Diseases and Sciences,* 1982, *27,* 202–208.

Young, S. J. Psychiatric considerations in irritable bowel syndrome. *Practical Gastroenterology,* 1979, *3*(4), 29–34.

PART IV

ANAL CANAL AND RECTUM
WILLIAM E. WHITEHEAD

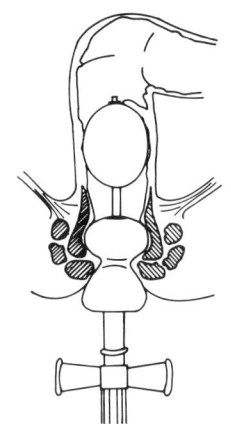

The study of the anal canal and rectum provides many opportunities for psychophysiologists to make both scientific and clinical contributions. It is an area which is readily accessible to noninvasive measurement techniques, and what we know of it so far suggests that behavioral concepts such as stimulus control, motivation, and operant and classical conditioning are essential to an understanding of its physiology. Smooth muscle, striated muscle, and visceral afferent sensation all participate in an elegant physiological function which coordinates a homeostatic process to the demands of the social environment.

Fecal incontinence, moreover, is a common and serious clinical problem. Defined as defecation in socially inappropriate situations at least once a month after the age of 4 years (Parker & Whitehead, 1982), fecal incontinence occurs in about 0.1% of the population (Milne, 1976). It is unequally distributed, occurring primarily in children and in persons over 65. There are, however, many young and middle-aged adults with fecal incontinence secondary to abdominal surgery, connective tissue disease, diabetes, ulcerative colitis, and disorders of the spinal cord. For example, at least 40% of children born with meningomyelocele are fecally incontinent (Lorber, 1971).

Fecal incontinence involves few medical risks, but it is a tremendous social handicap. In a study which compared fecal incontinence to urinary incontinence in adults with meningomyelocele, Evans, Hickman, and Carter (1974) found that only 31% of fecally incontinent adults had ever worked compared to 78% of those with urinary incontinence, and none of the fecally incontinent group had married compared to 21% of those with urinary incontinence. Incontinence is a nearly insurmountable obstacle to keeping a child in school (Welbourn, 1975), and it is the second most common cause for institutionalizing an elderly person (ranking above mental incompetence). Fortunately, biofeedback and other behaviorally based treatment procedures have made it possible to reestablish continence in many of these patients. In this section, Engel discusses the diagnosis and treatment of incontinence (Chapter 15) and stresses the importance of a behavioral and a psychophysiological analysis. In Chapter 16, Whitehead and Schuster describe the psychophysiological assessment techniques in current use and summarize the biofeedback training procedures which are based on these assessment techniques.

References

Evans, K., Hickman, V., & Carter, C. D. Handicap and social status of adults with spina bifida systica. *British Journal of Preventive Social Medicine,* 1974, *28,* 85–92.

Lorber, J. Results of treatment of meningomyelocele: An analysis of 524 unselected cases, with special reference to possible selection for treatment. *Developmental Medicine and Child Neurology,* 1971, *13,* 279–303.

Milne, J. S. Prevalence of incontinence in the elderly age groups. In E. L. Willington (Ed.), *Incontinence in the elderly.* London: Academic Press, 1976.

Parker, L., & Whitehead, W. E. Treatment of urinary and fecal incontinence in children. In D. C. Russo & J. W. Varni (Eds.), *Behavioral pediatrics: Research and practice.* New York: Plenum Press, 1982.

Welbourn, H. Spina bifida children attending ordinary schools. *British Medical Journal,* 1975, *1,* 142–145.

15

FECAL INCONTINENCE AND ENCOPRESIS
A Psychophysiological Analysis
BERNARD T. ENGEL

1. Introduction

There are three logical elements in any clinical program. Furthermore, these elements are equally operative whether the program is medical or behavioral. The elements are (1) *diagnosis,* (2) *mechanism or process,* and (3) *intervention. Diagnosis* means the determination of the signs and symptoms by which one assigns a probability that a specific clinical state is present, or that it is likely to occur. Diagnostic indices have two attributes: sensitivity and specificity. Sensitivity means that the index is an attribute of the disease—that is, the index is a positive sign; and specificity means that the index discriminates the absence of the disease from the presence of the disease—that is, the index also is a negative sign. Most indices meet one or the other criterion but not both. *Mechanism or process* refers to the factors which are responsible for the etiology or course of the disease. Clearly, the mechanisms associated with the etiology of a disease need not be the same as the mechanisms which mediate its course. For example, the mechanisms associated with the etiology of diverticulosis (herniation of the colonic mucosa between the fibers of the inner, circular muscles) undoubtedly are different from those which mediate the natural history of that disorder (elaboration of the diverticula, often accompanied by inflammation and occasional rupture of a diverticulum). Finally, *intervention* refers to the process by which one tries to disrupt the natural history of the disease. Interventions could be preventive, therapeutic, or rehabilitative.

BERNARD T. ENGEL • Gerontology Research Center (Baltimore), National Institute on Aging, National Institutes of Health, P.H.S., U.S. Department of Health and Human Services, Bethesda, and the Baltimore City Hospital, Baltimore, Maryland 21224.

In this chapter, I will consider the diagnostic, mechanistic, and therapeutic processes that are relevant to the assessment and control of fecal incontinence. However, my focus throughout this chapter will be on psychophysiological factors. By psychophysiological, I mean not only behavioral and physiological factors, but also the interaction of these factors. It is my thesis that the separation of mind and body is artificial and that the distinction even has led to a number of judgments about diagnosis, mechanism, and intervention which probably have been detrimental to the best interests of patients.

2. Diagnosis

Table 1 is an outline of the major data that would be collected during the diagnostic evaluation of an incontinent patient. The first step in the assessment is a clinical history. That history would be carried out either directly with the patient or, if that was not possible, with a relative or a guardian. The history would attempt to elicit data that would enable the interviewer to characterize the symptoms with particular emphasis on their development and severity to determine the role of trauma or disease in the disorder and to identify any special features about the patient or his family which might either exacerbate the symptoms or interfere with or facilitate treatment. Note the extent to which the clinical interview focuses on the elicitation of behavioral data.

After the clinical history is completed, a physical examination would follow. The examination would have a reasonably circumscribed course that would be modulated by clues obtained during the clinical history, by the physician's knowledge about the alternative diagnoses, and by the special characteristics of the patient that might rule out specific kinds of examinations. Finally, samples of blood, urine, or stool might be taken to permit specific laboratory tests.

After these initial studies had been completed, a number of diagnostic studies would be prescribed. The rules for selecting these studies would be in part rational and in part fortuitous. For example, specific analyses carried out on the blood, urine, or stool samples would be rational and would be designed to determine the presence or absence of specific bacteria, parasites, or secondary signs (e.g., bleeding) which might be either complications or mediators of the underlying disorder. Other procedures which might be prescribed are proctosigmoidoscopy, barium enemas, rectal biopsy, or anorectal manometry. What would almost certainly not be prescribed, but what might be exceptionally useful, is a behavioral analysis.

The reasons that a behavioral analysis would not be prescribed are: (1) that the physician either does not have the ability to conduct the assessment, or does not know anyone who could carry out such an evaluation, or does not even know that such an assessment is possible; (2) the physician does not know what behavior to study, and the behavior analyst also does not know what behavior to

Table 1
Diagnostic Assessment of Patient[a]

1. Clinical history

Symptom features	Medical history	Patient characteristics	Family history
Onset characteristics	Injuries	Age	
Progression	Surgeries	*Mental ability*	
Current status	Other illnesses	*Affective status*	
Specific features			
Duration			
Frequency			
Quality			

2. Physical examination

Structural abnormalities *Motor and sensory ability*

3. Specific tests

[a] Italics indicate areas where behavioral analysis could be helpful.

assess. The physician might not know because he is unaware of what possibilities exist in the assessment of behavior, and the behavior analyst might not know because he has not been trained in the diagnostic assessment of medical patients. In fact, the behavioral analysis could provide useful data which would help to determine (1) whether the patient (or his advocate) had described the quality, intensity, duration, or frequency of the symptoms accurately; (2) whether the intuitive judgments about the patient's mental ability or affective status were valid; and (3) if we include anorectal manometry as a behavioral procedure, then the behavior analysis could characterize various sensory and motor aspects of the anus and rectum such as their absolute and differential thresholds to specific stimuli, and such as their capacity to habituate, become sensitized (or desensitized), or their ability to be modified.

A behavioral analysis is a technique which is designed to obtain specific and objective, behavioral data. These data are intended to provide information about the responses which are the basis for the patient's symptoms, to identify the antecedent conditions which may be responsible either for eliciting or signaling the aberrant responses, and to characterize the environmental consequences of the symptoms. It often is the case that consequential events—for example, family reactions to the aberrant behavior of the patient—maintain the behavior by rewarding it. Because of the wide range of patients who can become incontinent and the variety of causes of incontinence, it is not possible *in vivo* to provide a specific model for conducting a behavioral analysis of fecal incontinence. A behavioral analysis, like any diagnostic assessment, proceeds in stages from the generation of hypotheses about the causes of the incontinence to the collection of data which would confirm or disconfirm those hypotheses. The hypotheses which are generated during the initial interview dictate the kinds of data which would be appropriate. Of course, if the hypotheses are disconfirmed, the process must be repeated. However, it is possible to identify the general principles of such an analysis.

Given the nature of fecal incontinence—for example, its relative infrequency (the unit of measure probably would be episodes/week)—much of the behavioral analysis of this disorder would need to be carried out in the field. However, as I will indicate later, some important data can be obtained in the clinic. The source of the field data would depend upon the particular patient: It could be the patient, a parent or spouse, or a caretaker. In any case, this analysis would require quantifiable data which would facilitate the assessment of the disorder and of the antecedent or consequent events which might mediate the symptoms.

Table 2 is an outline of a field analysis. The first set of data that needs to be collected characterizes the disorder. On a daily basis specific data should be obtained which will enable the therapist to determine the frequency and nature of the incontinence. Probably the most important questions to answer are (1) is the patient always incontinent or does he toilet occasionally; (2) is the patient incontinent when asleep as well as when awake; (3) does the patient have bowel movements at least every two days; (4) are the stools well formed or does the patient show evidence either of diarrhea or constipation?

The second set of questions is designed to determine in some detail the antecedent conditions which might mediate the probability that the patient will be incontinent. The most important questions to ask are those which identify (1) the relationship of an incontinent episode to a meal (note also the prevalence of continence in this context); (2) the availability of a toilet; (3) the latency between the sense of urgency and the incontinence; and (4) the relationship of the incontinence to medication. The last set of data is that which will enable the therapist to judge whether the incontinence reflects an interpersonal problem or whether other factors such as faulty knowledge or habit are primary determinants of the incontinence. The most important questions to answer here are (1) whether the incontinence is more or less likely in a social context; (2) whether specific individuals are more likely to be in the vicinity at the time when the patient is incontinent; (3) whether the patient tried to toilet; (4) whether the patient knows how to toilet (there are instances where parents have failed to train their children to toilet; these are most likely to occur in cases where the child has been judged to be "organically impaired" and, therefore, untrainable); (5) how the episode was treated.

In addition to field studies, there also should be laboratory studies using anorectal manometry. The purpose of these studies is to determine whether the patient's problem reflects a sensory defect, abnormal motor responsivity, a lack of integration between the sphincters, or whether the sensory-motor aspects of

Table 2
Outline of a Behavioral Analysis to Be Carried Out Daily

Characteristics of the problem	Antecedent factors	Contingent factors
Number of bowel movements for the day	Latency of sense of urgency to time of incontinence	Social context at time of incontinence
Number of incontinent episodes	Less than 30 sec 30 sec to 2 min Greater than 2 min	Alone Others in vicinity (specify)
Loss of solid stool Staining of clothes only	No sense of urgency	Patient's behavior during episode
Time of day incontinence observed	Availability of a toilet None available within latent period Available but not used	Stopped activity Sought aid Tried to reach toilet
Less than 1 hr after a meal Greater than 1 hr after a meal Within 30 min after waking Time of day	Medication Drug Amount taken Time of day drug taken	Behavior after episode Continued activity Reported episode Tried to hide episode (explain)
Nature of stool Small and hard Formed, soft Liquid or "loose"	Specific events Exercise Emotional arousal (specify) Other (specify)	Toileting behavior None Undresses appropriately Sits on toilet Wipes appropriately
		Response to episode Patient punished (explain) Patient cleaned self Patient cleaned by another (identify) Episode ignored (How long? How was episode resolved?)

retention are normal. In Chapter 16, Whitehead and Schuster report that in children with spina bifida, sensation in the rectum is normal; however, the sphincters are hyporeactive and poorly integrated. This knowledge has proved useful in designing a training procedure which has enabled Whitehead and his colleagues to teach a number of these children to be continent.

3. Analysis of Mechanism

The distinction between a diagnostic judgement and a specific mechanism has become regrettably dulled. Nowhere is this more prominent than in the diagnosis of encopresis where one frequently can find the phrase "functional disorder" coupled with a diagnosis. Thus, the patient is encopretic *and* the disease is psychogenic. In fact, except for a good deal of clinical experience, there are almost no data which show that mental processes can cause incontinence. The few, almost trivial exceptions are in the cases of patients who either intentionally soil themselves or who are indifferent to their soiling. However, there are no sound experimental data that any case of overflow incontinence is caused by a "psychic" process. In fact, many of the putative psychic processes are themselves of questionable validity.

In the contemporary language of the philosophy of science, a mechanism is either a necessary or a sufficient condition. A necessary condition is one which must be present if an event is to occur; a sufficient condition is one which assures that the event will occur if it is present, but does not assure that the event will not occur in its absence. Stool in the rectum is a necessary condition for fecal incontinence; scleroderma is a sufficient condition for incontinence. Table 3 presents what I believe is an exhaustive list of the mechanisms underlying fecal incontinence. I do not mean to imply that all of the specific mechanisms are known. However, as Table 3 indicates, the classes of mechanisms are known. There are two necessary conditions which must be met if a patient is to be incontinent. He must have a patent anal tube so that stool can be excreted, and he must have stool in his rectum. Obviously, neither of these necessary conditions is sufficient to cause incontinence. However, in the absence of either, no patient could be incontinent. Colostomy is a therapeutic procedure which is directed at these necessary conditions.

Table 3
Psychophysiological Mechanisms Which
Mediate Fecal Incontinence

Necessary conditions
  Patent anal tube
  Stool in rectum
Sufficient conditions
  Organic
    Endocrine
    Muscle or connective
    Neural
  Behavioral
    Learning
    Motivation
  Physiological
    Dietary
    Inflammatory
    Pharmacological

The sufficient conditions are divided into three broad categories—organic, behavioral, and physiological. However, it should be clear that these classes are not intended to be mutually exclusive. As anyone who treats patients is aware, an anatomic defect in a patient commonly is associated with both physiological and behavioral problems, and these require adjustments which can either compensate for the structurally induced problem or can add to the difficulties of the problem. Likewise, any so-called primary mechanism can increase the likelihood that so-called secondary mechanisms can become operative; and these secondary mechanisms can operate even when the primary defect has been corrected. Although the presence of such interactions makes an analysis of a given patient difficult, the analysis is still an essential ingredient in a rational approach to treatment and in an understanding of the significance and relevance of diagnostic signs and symptoms.

Among the organic factors, I have identified three major organ systems which have been shown to be causal in some forms of incontinence. Patients with hyperparathyroidism or hypothyroidism can be constipated and can suffer from overflow incontinence. There are a great number of muscle or connective tissue disorders associated with incontinence, and the incontinence itself could be present with or without fecal retention. Some of the muscle or connective tissue or neural defects could be iatrogenic—for example, postsurgical—but most are associated either with genetic defects or with other diseases such as anal or rectal fissures or stenosis. Various defects in the muscles of the abdominal wall or floor also could contribute to stool retention and consequently to overflow incontinence. Finally, there are a variety of neurological disorders which include fecal incontinence as one of their sequellae. These could be congenital, such as Hirschsprung's disease or spina bifida; or acquired, such as diabetes, scleroderma, multiple sclerosis, or stroke (Liebman, 1979; Schuster, 1977).

Table 3 lists two primary behavioral defects which can be associated with fecal incontinence. One is a defect in learning, and the other is a defect in motivation. Some patients may never have learned how to defecate. For example, Whitehead and his colleagues (Whitehead, Parker, Masek, Cataldo, & Freeman, 1981) are finding that many children with spina bifida can be trained to become continent. However, the training must be highly specialized and cannot follow the strategy used with normal children. Likewise, Engel, Nikoomanesh, and Schuster (1974) showed several years ago that adults with incontinence secondary to surgical trauma or neurological defects could be trained to become continent again. There are many kinds of patients who will present with fecal incontinence secondary to motivational disorders. Included among these patients are those diagnosed as having amentia or dementia. Foxx and Azrin (1973) have demonstrated that many of these patients also can be treated.

There are a variety of physiological mechanisms which can be associated with fecal incontinence with or without stool retention. Dietary factors, primarily the lack of bulk in the diet, can cause constipation; inflammatory bowel disorders can mediate either constipation or diarrhea; and there are a host of pharmacological factors which can be associated with constipation, diarrhea, and incontinence—for example, chronic lead poisoning in children, chronic phenothiazine therapy (usually in schizophrenic patients), and misuse of laxatives, which can operate in conjunction with faulty learning (or more likely, faulty training) to produce constipation and consequent overflow incontinence.

I would like to present what I regard as an interesting sidelight on the analysis of mechanism. As I already indicated, we have been able to show that it is possible to train or to retrain patients to become continent. In our training procedure we utilized a method which Schuster and his colleagues had developed to diagnose anal sphincter function (see Chapter 16). The technique is based on the observation that in the normal, continent subject brief rectal distension elicits phasic, internal anal sphincter relaxation and phasic, external anal spincter contraction. A diagnostic sign of fecal incontinence is an absent or weak external sphincter contraction. Our studies showed that we could operantly condition patients to produce this contraction. This clinical finding created a dilemma which has only recently been resolved. The dilemma is that there was a contradiction between what was regarded as a neurological mechanism and what is regarded as a behavioral mechanism.

The neurological inference was that the phasic contraction of the external anal sphincter is a reflex which was elicited by rectal distension, the behavioral fact is that this response was operantly conditioned, and the dilemma is that reflexes cannot be operantly conditioned. Therefore only two interpretations are possible. Either we did not operantly condition the sphincter, but rather conditioned another, unknown response which then reflexly elicited the sphincter contraction; or the phasic, external anal sphincter contraction is not a reflex. The first interpretation is difficult to support since in many patients the diagnostic studies indicated that rectal distension did not elicit the putative reflex. Thus, it was difficult to see how chaining of a response sequence could produce a reflex when a primary stimulus could not. However, the notion that a reflex is not a reflex is heretical: neurological concepts have high face validity. Finally, there now are data which seem to solve this dilemma conclusively: the reflex is not a reflex. On the basis of a series of experiments carried out by Whitehead in our laboratory and by Orr in his laboratory (Whitehead, Orr, Engel, & Schuster, 1982), it now seems very clear that the phasic contraction of the external anal sphincter is a highly overlearned response which probably operates in a similar way as do the muscles which act to maintain posture. Thus, these experiments have shown both the importance of analyses of mechanism and the scientific value of an integrative psychophysiological approach over separate, isolated psychological and physiological approaches.

4. Intervention

It should be clear by now that the central thesis of this chapter is psychophysiological, not psychological and not physiological (i.e., not behavioral therapy and not medical therapy but behavioral/medical therapy). In taking this position I am not arguing against specialization. In fact, I see no alternative to specialization. What I am proposing is medical and behavioral cooperation and integration, not a blurring of special skills but an interdigitation of them. I have already spoken about how such an integration would improve diagnosis and the analysis of mechanism. I want now to carry this model to a consideration of intervention. As I noted at the beginning of this chapter, intervention can occur in three different ways. Intervention can be preventive, therapeutic, or rehabilitative. All of the behavioral applications to incontinence have been therapeutic or rehabilitative. Yet, it is very clear that there also is a great need for prevention.

It is possible that a number of patients with fecal incontinence are suffering from what has been called a functional, nonspecific, psychogenic disorder. It seems very clear that we need to be able to identify the children who may be at risk for these problems, we need to understand the mechanisms underlying their problems, and we need to prevent the problems from ever occurring. We need formal programs which will train parents how to toilet train their children, and we need to put these programs in a format that would enable every pediatrician and preschool teacher to utilize them. There is more we can do in the way of prevention. Any retarded child is a candidate for incontinence. Even if one allows that Foxx and Azrin's (1973) methods are highly successful (although they treat fecal incontinence as an epiphenomenon, and urinary incontinence as a primary disorder), we still do not know at what age to begin bowel training in these children. Furthermore, at the other end of the age scale where fecal incontinence becomes a serious problem, we need to develop liaison programs that will train nursing home staff how best to deal with their elderly patients. Even though such programs may only be temporal rather than preventive or therapeutic, at least they will optimize patient care.

In clinical practice, it is usually impossible to separate treatment from diagnosis. That is as much the case for behavioral therapy as it is for medical therapy. Thus, in discussing behavioral interventions I again emphasize that a behavioral analysis must be implemented. It now seems clear that behavioral treatment is a major modality of treatment of fecal incontinence secondary to any of a variety of different causes. Biofeedback is effective in treating children with spina bifida (Whitehead, Parker, Masek, Cataldo, & Freeman, 1981) and in treating adults with fecal incontinence secondary to a number of postsurgical or neurological defects (Cerulli, Nikoomanesh, & Schuster, 1979). It even may be the case that many elderly patients with fecal incontinence can be rehabilitated by the use of biofeedback. However, there are a number of other behavioral treatments possible for incontinent patients. For example, Young (1973) used a classical conditioning model based on the elicitation of the gastrocolic reflex to treat a series of 19 children diagnosed as "encopretic," and Rovetto (1979) used a similar technique to train chronically constipated (but not incontinent) women to normalize their bowel movements. There are other patients who need to be trained to adopt better dietary practices. There are still other patients for whom habit-training procedures are needed. And finally, there are patients who are incontinent because they have any of a variety of possible motivational problems. Clearly, each of these different classes of patients poses a different set of therapeutic challenges. Only a proper diagnostic workup—namely, a behavioral history and a behavioral analysis—will enable one to sort out the variables that underlie the incontinence in a given patient, and only such a workup will allow the therapist to implement an appropriate therapeutic program that will be based on a rational understanding of mediating mechanisms.

5. References

Cerulli, M. A., Nikoomanesh, P., & Schuster, M. M. Progress in biofeedback conditioning for fecal incontinence. *Gastroenterology,* 1979, *76,* 742–746.

Engel, B. T., Nikoomanesh, P., & Schuster, M. M. Operant conditioning of rectosphincteric responses in the treatment of fecal incontinence. *New England Journal Of Medicine,* 1974, *290,* 646–649.

Foxx, R. M., & Azrin, N. H. *Toilet training in the retarded.* Champaign, Ill.: Research Press, 1973.

Liebman, W. M. Disorders of defecation in children. *Postgraduate Medicine,* 1979, *66*(2), 105–110.

Rovetto, F. Treatment of chronic constipation by classical conditioning techniques. *Journal of Behavioral Therapy and Experimental Psychiatry,* 1979, *10,* 143–146.

Schuster, M. M. Constipation and anorectal disorders. *Clinics in Gastroenterology,* 1977, *6,* 643–657.

Whitehead, W. E., Parker, L. H., Masek, B. J., Cataldo, M. F., & Freeman, J. M. Biofeedback treatment of fecal incontinence in patients with meningomyelocele. *Developmental Medicine and Child Neurology,* 1981, *23,* 313–322.

Whitehead, W. E., Orr, W. C., Engel, B. T., & Schuster, M. M. External anal sphincter response to rectal distention: Learned response or reflex. *Psychophysiology,* 1981, *19,* 57–62.

Young, G. C. The treatment of childhood encopresis by conditioned gastroileal reflex training. *Behavioral Research and Therapy,* 1973, *11,* 499–503.

16

MANOMETRIC AND ELECTROMYOGRAPHIC TECHNIQUES FOR ASSESSMENT OF THE ANORECTAL MECHANISM FOR CONTINENCE AND DEFECATION

WILLIAM E. WHITEHEAD and MARVIN M. SCHUSTER

1. Introduction

There are several reasons for concerning oneself with the accurate measurement of physiological responses in the anal canal and rectum. The anorectal area provides a critical interface between the external, social, and physical environment and the internal, biological environment. Society places considerable importance on the self-control of defecation, and the assessment and treatment of incontinence is therefore important. In addition, this part of the gastrointestinal tract is well supplied with visceral afferent nerves which give rise to subjective and reflex control: This provides a unique opportunity to study the mechanism by which self-regulation of a visceral response is achieved. This chapter will summarize what is known of the anatomy and physiology of the anorectal area and will describe the advantages and disadvantages of various measurement techniques.

WILLIAM E. WHITEHEAD • Department of Psychiatry, the Johns Hopkins School of Medicine, and Department of Medicine, Baltimore City Hospital, Baltimore, Maryland 21224. MARVIN M. SCHUSTER • The Johns Hopkins School of Medicine and the Division of Digestive Diseases, Baltimore City Hospital, Baltimore, Maryland 21224. Preparation of this chapter was supported by Research Scientist Development Award 5 K01 MH00133 from the National Institute of Mental Health and by Grant 1 R01 NS15781 from the National Institute of Neurological and Communication Disorders and Stroke.

2. Anatomy and Physiology

The anatomy of the anal canal and rectum is shown in Figure 1. The rectum is a specialized segment of bowel approximately 7 cm in length. One of its unique characteristics is that it easily expands to accommodate increased volume. However, the rectum is not a passive receptacle; it contracts along with the distal colon in response to a variety of stimuli. The functional significance of rectal contractions is not known. Another important characteristic of the rectum is its sensibility. So sensitive is the rectum to distension and to the osmolarity of its contents that most normal subjects can distinguish whether their rectum is filled with solid, liquid, or gas. The rectum is classically thought to be innervated by S2 and S3 sympathetic fibers. However, evidence which is reviewed below suggests that there are other fiber tracts supplying afferent innervation to the rectum.

The anal canal is a narrow passage approximately 4 cm long which is guarded by two sphincter muscles. One is the internal anal sphincter which is

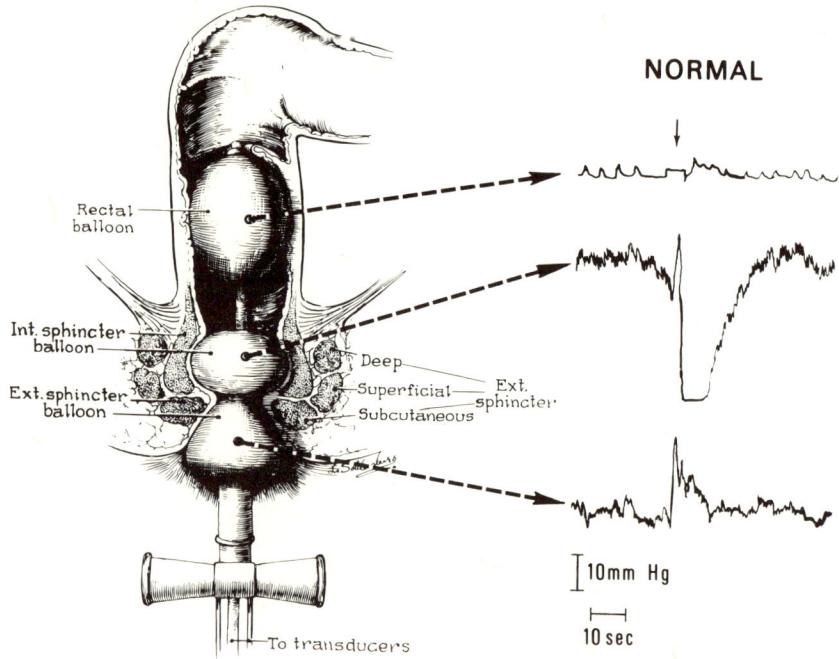

Figure 1. Anatomy of the anal canal and the balloon device used for assessment. The highest balloon is 5 cm long and is used to transiently distend the rectum in order to assess rectal sensation and to stimulate the reflex inhibition of the internal anal sphincter. The middle balloon is partially surrounded by the internal anal sphincter (smooth muscle) and the lowest balloon is partially surrounded by the external anal sphincter (striated muscle). Manometric recordings on the right show the normal response of the sphincters to rectal distension. (From Engel, 1978, with permission.)

composed of smooth muscles. It is actually a specialized segment of bowel and shares some of the same characteristics as other gastrointestinal sphincters such as the lower esophageal sphincter. It is ordinarily kept tightly closed, but distension of the bowel (rectum) above the sphincter or a strong contraction of the distal bowel causes a reflex inhibition of the internal anal sphincter lasting approximately 30–45 sec. The internal anal sphincter is supplied by afferent nerves from S2 and S3 of the spinal cord as well as being innervated by the myenteric plexus (Schuster, 1968).

The external anal sphincter is composed of striated, skeletal muscle innervated by the pudendal nerves. The external sphincter partially surrounds the internal anal sphincter and is composed of three bundles. The deep bundle, called the puborectalis, can be felt on digital examination at the proximal edge of the anal canal. There is also a middle bundle of the external sphincter which overlies the internal sphincter, and a superficial bundle of fibers at the distal end of the anal canal. The superficial bundle can be felt to contract with a fingertip, or it can be seen to contract. The external anal sphincter is unlike most other skeletal muscles in that it has a relatively high resting tone which keeps it closed. Mild distension of the rectum is usually associated with a further brief contraction of the external anal sphincter (Alva, Mendeloff, & Schuster, 1967; Ustach, Tobon, Hambrecht, Bass, & Schuster, 1970). However, distension of the rectum with larger volumes elicits reflex inhibition of the external anal sphincter below resting levels (Bishop, 1959).

The pattern of physiological events which together constitute the continence mechanism are shown in Figure 1. Also shown is the type of recording device usually used to assess these physiological events. The measuring device consists of three balloons. The highest balloon is located in the rectum and is used to distend the rectum to mimic the effects of stool or gas entering the rectum. When the rectal balloon is transiently distended, this elicits reflex inhibition of the internal anal sphincter, which is measured as a decrease in pressure inside the middle balloon. Rectal distension usually also leads to contraction of the external anal sphincter, which is recorded as an increase in the pressure in the third and lowest balloon. The amount of inhibition of the internal anal sphincter is directly proportional to the amount of rectal distension, but the amplitude of external sphincter contraction is variable. Under natural conditions, it is critical that the external sphincter contract during the period of internal sphincter inhibition to prevent the accidental loss of gas or stool.

3. Measurement Techniques

3.1. External Anal Sphincter Contraction

The method which was first developed by Schuster and his colleagues (Alva et al., 1967) to assess anorectal motility utilized the tube shown in Figure 1. In comparing normally continent subjects to patients with fecal incontinence, they observed that most of their incontinent patients showed no contraction of the external sphincter following rectal distension or only a weak contraction. They interpreted their data as suggesting that the external sphincter contraction is a reflex response which is elicited by rectal distension, and they proposed that the cause of incontinence for many patients is a disruption of this reflex arc.

Subsequent observations in the same laboratory suggested, however, that the external sphincter response to rectal distension is not a reflex but a voluntary response which is cued by the perception of rectal distension (Whitehead, Orr, Engel, & Schuster, 1981). The observation which first led us to this conclusion was the fact that half of the chronically constipated patients whom we evaluated did not show an external anal sphincter contraction following rectal distension although they were neurologically intact. We concluded that chronically constipated patients do not show this response because it is a voluntary response which they have little motivation to practice. These inferences were confirmed by subsequent observations which showed that normal subjects were able to omit the external sphincter contraction after little or no practice when they were instructed to do so. The voluntary response hypothesis also agrees well with observations on spinal cord transected cats (Bishop, 1959) and humans (Rodriquez & Awad, 1979), which show that when the lower spinal cord is separated from the brain, the reflex response to rectal distension is an inhibition of resting tone in the external anal sphincter rather than a contraction.

One purpose in raising the issue of whether external sphincter contraction is a reflex or a voluntary response is to point out the differences which this distinction makes in the diagnostic assessment of incontinent patients. Failure to observe a reflex response provides strong evidence for a physical disruption of the reflex arc, that is, a neurological disorder. However, failure to observe an operant response following the discriminative stimulus which cues it may have many causes: The subject may not have perceived the stimulus, he may be unable to emit the response, he may never have learned what the correct response was, or he may lack motivation to control defecation because of his cognitive or psychological deficiencies. This suggests that the best circumstance in which to test ability to squeeze the external sphincter muscle appropriately is to explicitly instruct the subject to squeeze when he feels the rectal balloon being inflated. It may also be necessary to instruct the subject to emit some other simple behavior to ensure that he understands the instructions.

The protocol which we use for assessing external sphincter muscle strength and control is to instruct the patient to squeeze four times without rectal distension and then to instruct him to squeeze when he feels the rectal balloon distension. The balloon is distended first with 50 ml of air and then with 40, 30, 20, 10, and 5 ml of air. Use of a descending series is preferable to an ascending series because it reduces the patient's confusion about what the sensation is to which he is supposed to respond.

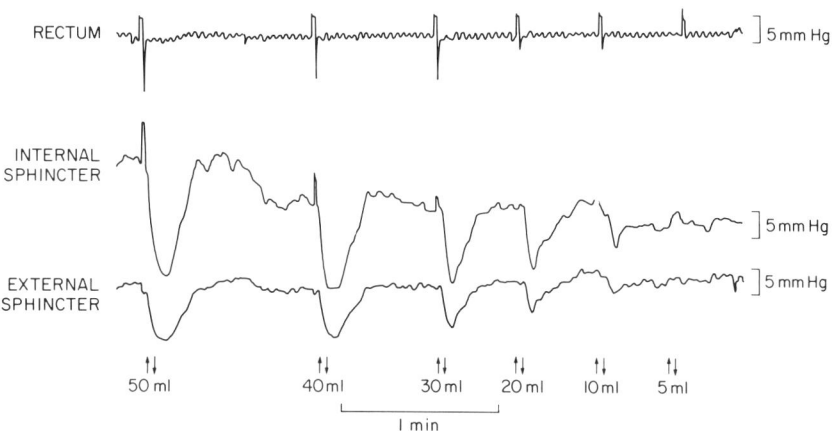

Figure 2. Response of the anal sphincters to rectal distension in a 16-yr-old male with fecal incontinence secondary to meningomyclocele. The balloon device shown in Figure 1 was used to record these responses. Rectal distension produced dilation of the lower anal canal as well as the internal anal sphincter because of weakness in the external anal sphincter. (From Whitehead, Parker, Musek, Cataldo, & Freeman, 1981, with permission.)

When these procedures are used and when a balloon is used to detect external anal sphincter contraction, we find that normals can produce at least a 30-mm Hg pressure response in the balloon, and that the threshold volume of rectal distension to which they respond with such a contraction is 5 ml of air. Incontinent patients vary in their response to this task. Some show a relatively strong contraction to large rectal distensions but cease responding at a high threshold (i.e., when the rectum is distended with small volumes) because they do not feel weak distensions of the rectum. Others, exemplified by the child with meningomyelocele shown in Figure 2, are unable to squeeze the sphincter muscle even with maximum effort.

The use of a balloon to measure external anal sphincter strength has certain limitations: The gluteal muscles can also bring force to bear on the external sphincter balloon making it difficult to determine whether one is measuring the contraction of sphincter muscle or gluteal muscle. Variations in the amount of adipose tissue in the buttocks can influence the resting pressure in the balloon, and the volume of air in the balloon will vary unless care is taken to completely deflate the balloon before inflating it with a measured volume.

A more selective measure of sphincter muscle contraction can be achieved by EMG recordings. The oldest technique is to insert a rigid needle into the muscle which contains two recording wires in the tip of the barrel. This technique is not preferred because the rigid needle left in the muscle causes pain on contraction and may also cause artifacts due to movement of the tissue relative to the rigid tip. A preferable technique is to inject flexible fine wires into the muscle with a small-gauge needle and then withdraw the needle leaving the wires in the muscle (Rodriquez & Awad, 1979). The wires are less irritating and do not produce artifacts because they move with the muscle.

An alternative to needle electromyography, which is better tolerated by patients and which involves fewer medical hazards, is to use skin surface electrodes. The sensors are positioned on opposite sides of the anus but as close to the opening as possible. Because surface electrodes may pick up activity from adjacent large muscles by volume conduction, one should also record the EMG activity in the gluteal muscles to determine the source of the signal.

An example of simultaneous gluteal and external sphincter EMG recordings from a normal subject is shown in Figure 3. Note that instructions to squeeze produce EMG responses which are seen primarily, but not exclusively, in the sphincter recording, whereas instructions to tense the hip produce EMG activity which is recorded primarily in the gluteal electrodes. Thus, a reasonable degree of selectivity is possible with this recording technique.

Use of EMG electrodes does not obviate the need for a rectal tube in assessing and treating incontinence. It is necessary to stimulate the rectum in

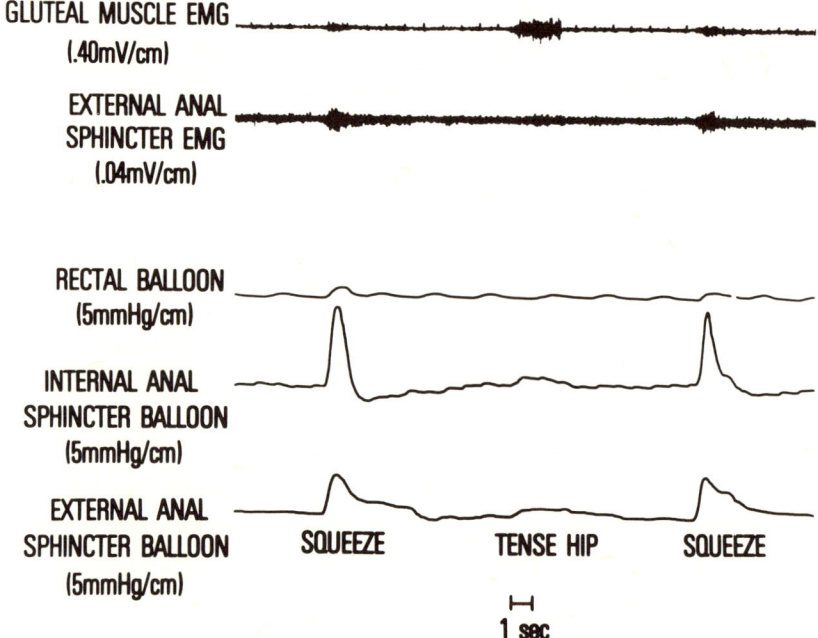

Figure 3. EMG recordings of the external anal sphincter made from skin surface electrodes. Instructions to squeeze the sphincter and tense the hip, shown at the bottom, produce differential activation in the external sphincter and gluteal muscle leads. Balloon responses are shown for comparison.

order to teach the patient to contract the sphincter in response to the appropriate stimulus and at the appropriate time, for example, during internal anal sphincter inhibition.

A perfused catheter can also be used to evaluate the strength of the external anal sphincter. The catheter is first inserted well into the rectum and is then pulled out slowly. Every half cm the investigator stops withdrawing and instructs the patient to squeeze as hard as possible. One records a gradient of high pressure, the peak of which should indicate the strength of external anal sphincter contraction. This technique has the advantage of giving a good estimate of absolute pressure generated in the anal canal by efforts to squeeze. However, it does not differentiate between external sphincter contraction and gluteal muscle contraction. It is possible to use this technique to measure the response of sphincters to rectal distension by inserting a balloon into the rectum and distending the balloon when the perfused catheter is at different locations in the anal canal.

The perfused catheter gives normal values of approximately 155 mm Hg. Read, Harford, Schmulen, Read, Santa Ana, and Fordtran (1979) reported that normal subjects have significantly higher maximum squeeze pressures than do patients with incontinence associated with diarrhea (average–99 mm Hg). However, there was a substantial overlap between the two groups.

Another test which was developed by Read *et al.* (1979) consists of perfusing saline into the rectum at a constant rate (60 ml/min) and measuring the volume which can be infused before the first 10 ml leaks out as well as the volume which is retained when 1500 ml has been infused. This enema-holding volume obviously depends on more than the strength of the external anal sphincter; among other things it is influenced by the compliance of the rectum and descending colon. Despite this, Read *et al.* (1979) found this test to reliably discriminate normal subjects from those who are incontinent. All but 3 of 29 incontinent patients had leaked at least 10 ml before 500 ml had been infused, but only 3 of 37 normals had leaked below 500 ml. None of the incontinent patients retained as much as 1400 ml by the end of the test (total infusion of 1500 ml), whereas all but 4 of the continent controls retained at least 1400 ml by the end of the test.

Read *et al.* (1979) also measured the strength of the external anal sphincter by inserting a cork sphere (1.8 cm in diameter) into the rectum which was attached by means of string to a bottle outside the rectum. With the subject in a seated position, small metal weights were poured into the bottle while the patient squeezed until the cork was pulled out of the rectum. An average of 1,056 grams was required to pull the sphere out of normal subjects, but only 721 grams pulled the cork from incontinent patients. Although these values were significantly different, there was a substantial overlap between groups.

3.2. Sensibility for Rectal Distension

The hypothesis that the external anal sphincter contraction following rectal distension is an operant response under stimulus control rather than a reflex (Whitehead, Engel, & Schuster, 1981) implies that the ability to consciously perceive rectal distension is critical to the preservation of continence. In fact, this seems to be the case. In our clinic, the threshold volume of rectal distension which is required to produce subjective sensation is higher on the average in fecally incontinent patients than it is in normals, although there are many patients who have normal sensation and whose incontinence is due to other causes. In addition, we find that if patients do not acquire an ability to sense distensions as low as 15 ml of air (using the device shown in Figure 1) they do not benefit greatly from biofeedback training even though they can contract the external anal sphincter adequately. Figure 4 illustrates this point. The patient was a 72-yr-old woman with a history of diabetes and hemorrhoidectomy who was incontinent

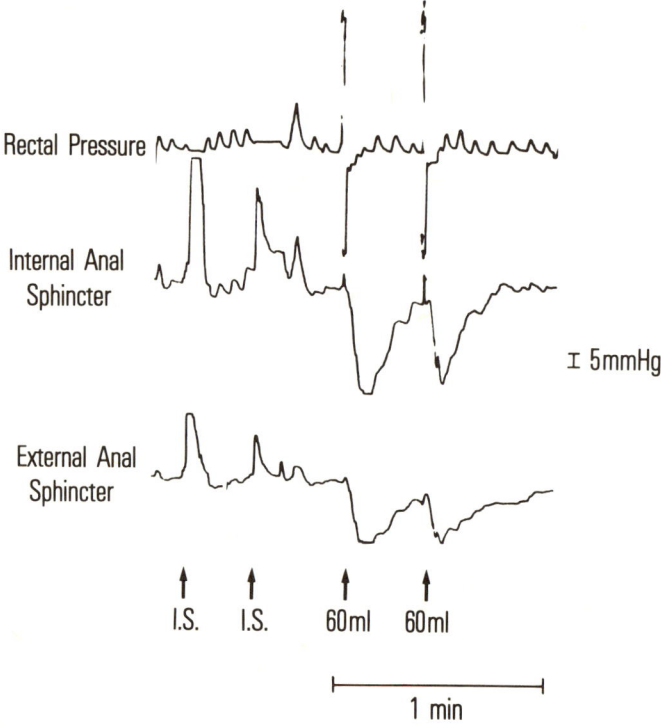

Figure 4. Inability to discriminate rectal distension in a 72-yr-old patient with fecal incontinence. When instructed to squeeze (labeled I.S.) she can contract the external anal sphincter adequately. However, when the rectum is distended with a large 60-ml volume of air, she does not contract the external anal sphincter because she cannot feel the stimulus.

several times daily. The manometric tracing shows that she was able to contract the external sphincter when instructed to do so but she could not detect even large distensions of the rectum. The internal anal sphincter reflex was observed, indicating that stretch receptors were present in the rectal wall, but the afferent information apparently did not get through to the central nervous system.

It has been known for some time that rectal surgeries which excise the rectum and create an artificial rectum by pulling down the colon often result in fecal incontinence (Goligher & Hughes, 1951). This indicates that the afferent receptors in the rectal wall are necessary to preserve continence but does not indicate that conscious perception is important. If external sphincter contraction were a reflex response to rectal distension, conscious perception would not be necessary for continence.

The method we use to assess subjective sensation for rectal distension employs the device shown in Figure 1. The rectal balloon is first rapidly inflated with 50 ml of air and immediately deflated, and the patient is asked to indicate whether he felt it. This is repeated for 40, 30, 20, 10, and 5 ml of air in a descending method of limits. A descending series of stimulus intensities is used to ensure that the patient knows what stimulus he is being asked to discriminate. Otherwise, subjects tend to deny sensation when they are presented with unfamiliar, weak stimuli.

The method of limits described above is only used to obtain an approximate value for the sensory threshold because the method of limits is very susceptible to response bias, that is, the tendency of subjects to give one kind of response rather than another when they are not certain for reasons which have nothing to do with perception. Older subjects are particularly likely to respond conservatively and to deny the perception of ambiguous stimuli. For example, one elderly subject reported that he could not perceive any distension of the rectum below 40 ml, although use of a different perception test (see below) which is less sensitive to response bias revealed that he could perceive stimuli as weak as 5 ml distension.

Once the approximate sensory threshold has been identified by the method of limits, we switch to a forced-choice procedure. This involves presenting the stimulus in one of two time intervals and asking the subject whether it was presented the first or second time. Over a series of such pairs of trials the stimulus is presented randomly in both positions. Since the subject has to choose between two equally likely events, his choice cannot be influenced by response bias unless he refuses to "guess." Consequently, an unbiased estimate of sensory threshold is obtained in a relatively short period of time.

Using the procedure described previously, normal subjects have sensory thresholds of 5 ml or less. The technique does not permit us to measure sensory thresholds lower than 5 ml, and it could be argued that this makes the discrimination test insensitive to individual differences in perceptual sensitivity. However, the addition of 5 ml of air to this 5-cm-long balloon is probably the weakest stimulus which has physiological significance. The test does discriminate continent subjects from many incontinent patients and is predictive of the benefits of biofeedback training (Whitehead, Engel, & Schuster, 1981).

Limitations to the method of measuring perception (see p. 319) include the fact that the rate of inflation is an important determinant of whether the balloon is felt. For safety and convenience, we inflate the balloon with a hand-held syringe, and we attempt to standardize the rate of inflation so that it is rapid and reproducible. However, differences between experimenters may give somewhat different results. This could be resolved by inflating the balloon with a fixed-rate, volume pump. Another problem is that the forced choice procedure is difficult for young children and cognitively impaired subjects to comprehend.

The alternative method of testing rectal sensibility is to gradually fill the rectum (Read et al., 1979) or a rectal balloon with air or water until a first sensation or an urge to defecate is felt. This technique is extremely susceptible to response bias and is not recommended. Estimates of first sensation using this technique are approximately 60 ml with a standard error of 22 ml. This is 12 times the value obtained by the forced-choice procedure.

The neural pathways which mediate subjective sensation for rectal distension are classically thought to be S2–S3. However, we (Whitehead, Parker, Masek, Cataldo, & Freeman, 1981) have observed normal sensation (i.e., a threshold of 5 ml) in many patients with meningomyelocele who have suprasacral lesions believed to be complete. The pathways for this sensation are not known, but they may involve fibers which ascend through the inferior hemorrhoidal and pelvic sympathetic plexuses to enter the cord at the thoracic level or higher.

A surgical procedure which has recently been suggested for treating chronic fecal incontinence is the reconstruction of an external sphincter by transplanting a strip of gracilis or other muscle (Corman, 1979). These procedures often have not succeeded at controlling incontinence even though the patient can squeeze the new sphincter by "intending" to move his leg in certain ways. Biofeedback training should be an effective way of retraining these patients, if they have normal sensation for rectal distension.

One sometimes encounters patients who have a normal sensory threshold but who have become confused about what the stimulus is to which they are supposed to respond (e.g., patients with stroke). Training these patients to discriminate and correctly label rectal distension has often helped them to recover continence.

3.3. Internal Anal Sphincter

The internal anal sphincter is normally kept tightly closed. This provides a passive barrier to the leakage of liquid stool or gas. It must be regarded as a passive barrier because significant distension of the rectum causes reflex inhibition of the internal anal sphincter tone. Nevertheless this resting pressure is important. Read *et al.* (1979) using the perfused catheter technique found the resting pressure in the anal canal to be significantly lower in incontinent patients (41 mm Hg) compared to normals (60 mm Hg).

The resting pressure can only be measured accurately by pulling a perfused catheter through the anal canal. The peak pressure recorded when the subject is not contracting is taken as a measure of internal sphincter pressure. Read *et al.* (1979) report normal values of 60 mm Hg using this procedure.

Read *et al.* (1979) also reported the weight required to pull a cork sphere from the rectum when the patient was not squeezing. Significantly more weight (712 g) was required to pull the cork from normals compared to incontinent patients (519 g).

It is important to be able to measure the active inhibition of the internal anal sphincter following rectal distension. This inhibition is absent in congenital aganglionosis of the bowel (Hirschsprung's disease) and in other neurological and connective tissue disorders (e.g., scleroderma). Failure of the internal sphincter to relax normally is associated with constipation and with leakage of small amounts of liquid stool.

One must distinguish between the failure of a tight sphincter to be inhibited by rectal distension and the apparent absence of inhibition in a lax or patulous sphincter. Visual inspection of the anus (without a proctoscope) and digital examination will indicate whether the sphincter is atonic.

The most practical way to measure inhibition of the internal anal sphincter is by means of a balloon device such as that shown in Figure 1. The amplitude of sphincter inhibition can be measured only in relative terms because of variations in the size and shape of the anal canal. Internal sphincter inhibition can also be measured by placing a perfused catheter in the anal canal and then distending the rectum with a balloon. However, care must be taken to ensure that the patient does not move the catheter out of the sphincter when he squeezes in response to rectal distension. The balloon device in Figure 1 avoids this problem.

A source of error in the measurement of internal sphincter inhibition is that the internal sphincter is surrounded by the external anal sphincter. When the subject squeezes hard, the contraction of the surrounding external sphincter may prevent one from detecting the inhibition in tone of the internal sphincter. This is particularly likely if the patient is anxious about the study and/or if the patient fears that he/she will defecate or that the balloon device will slip out. Consequently, when the investigator fails to see inhibition of the internal sphincter, he/she should always attempt to get the patient to relax and then repeat the rectal distension.

The EMG activity of the internal anal sphincter can be recorded, but only with difficulty. Ustach *et al.* (1970) recorded this signal by attaching sil-

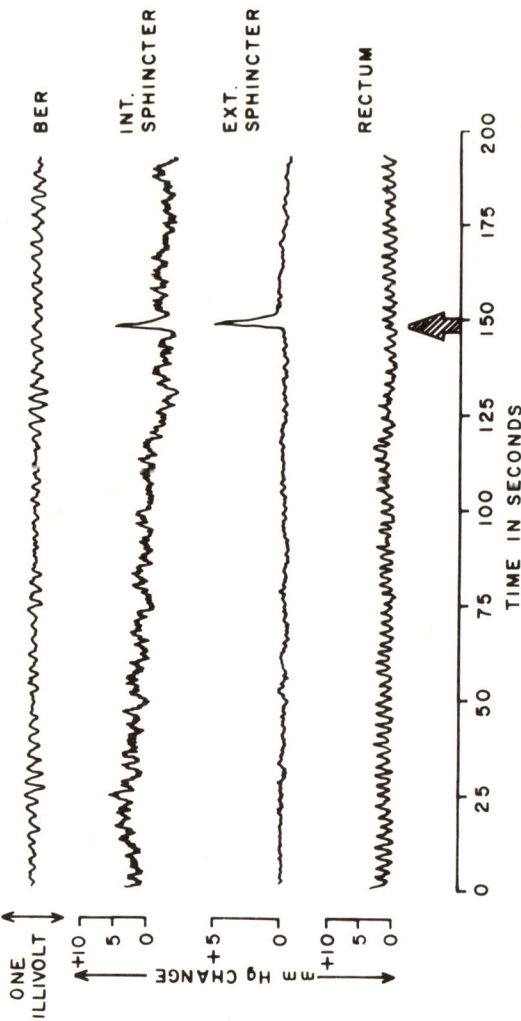

Figure 5. Spindle-shaped slow waves (BER) from the internal sphincter. (From Ustach *et al.*, 1970.)

ver–silver-choloride electrodes to the surface of a balloon, such as that shown in Figure 1, which is held in position in the internal anal sphincter.

In the resting state one can record a constant sinusoidal electrical slow wave, also called basal electrical rhythm or electrical control activity. One does not generally see spikes; this is almost exclusively a slow wave phenomenon. The frequency of the slow wave is quite high, approximately 18 cpm.

In addition to this constant sinusoidal activity one can also record a crescendo and decrescendo pattern, a spindle-shaped rhythm, which can be seen in Figure 5. This pattern can be reproduced in a physical system by simulating two generators, each generating at a different frequency—Generator A generating at 12 cpm and Generator B at 13.5 (Figure 6). These values were selected because they are close to observed frequencies. We conceptualized the individual muscle cells as batteries or oscillators that polarize and depolarize. If you combine two oscillators which oscillate at different frequencies, they alternately will enhance and inhibit each other, reproducing this kind of spindle-shaped pattern.

This basic electrical activity or slow wave in the sphincter is believed to be one of the mechanisms governing the resting tone in the sphincter. To test this hypothesis, we evaluated the slow waves during rectal distension. Figure 7 shows the mechanical activity of the rectum and internal anal sphincter and the electrical activity of the internal sphincter following rectal distension. An inhibition in the basic electrical activity coincides with the relaxation of the internal anal sphincter tone recorded from the balloon, which occurs immediately after transient distension of the rectum. This provides suggestive evidence that the slow wave (basic electrical rhythm) may control the tonus of the sphincter muscle.

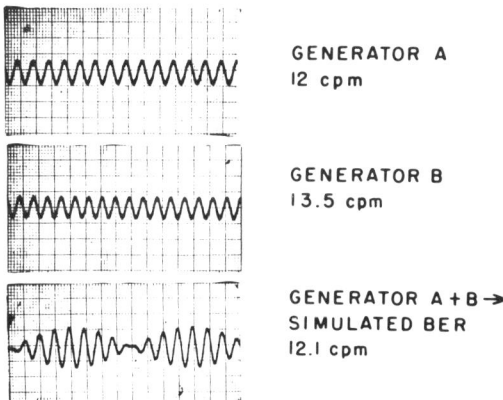

Figure 6. Spindle-shaped waves artificially produced by two generators oscillating at frequencies that alternately inhibit and enhance each other. (From Ustach *et al.*, 1970.)

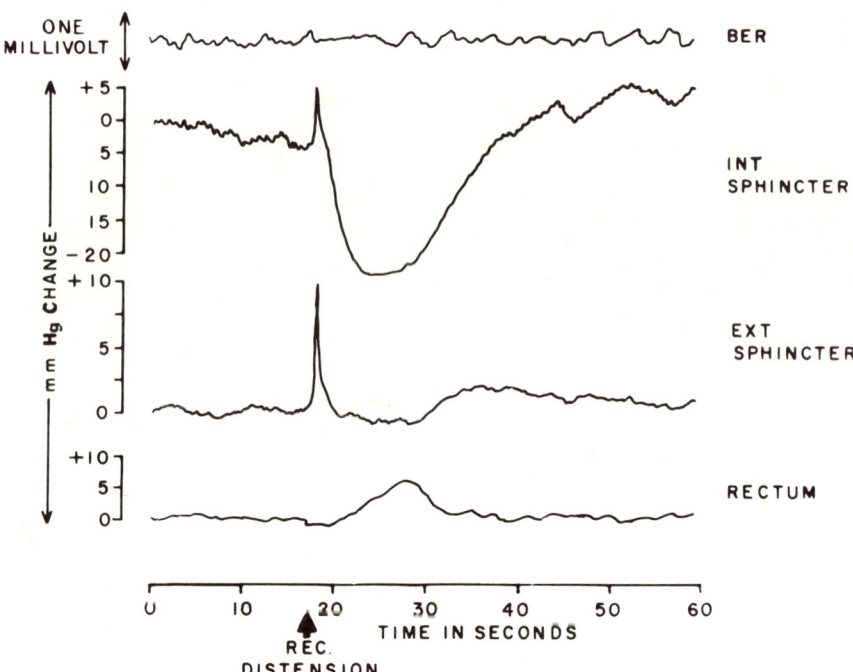

Figure 7. Rectal distension produces inhibition of electrical slow wave (BER) coincident with internal sphincter relaxation. (From Ustach et al., 1968.)

Not all distensions are followed by relaxation, and not all distensions are followed by inhibition of the slow wave; it depends on the strength of the stimulus. There is a thresbold of approximately 10 to 15 ml such that higher volumes of distension result in more complete inhibition of electrical activity. In the *in vivo* situation, when mechanical activity is measured one can also measure a threshold. Decreasing amounts of distension result in decreasing amplitudes of inhibition until one reaches a threshold around 10 ml, after which no detectable inhibition occurs.

There are important experiments that cannot be carried out in humans *in vivo* but which can be done in the *in vitro* situation. We have measured electrical and mechanical activity in muscle strips from both dog and human muscle, both sphincteric and nonsphincteric muscle, from various areas of the gastrointestinal tract from the esophagus to the anus (Bass, Vanasin, Ustach, & Schuster, 1972). We used a chlorided silver electrode held to the muscle strip by suction, and we measured displacement with a displacement tranducer. In the *in vitro* situation very much as in the *in vivo* situation, interruption of the electrical stimulation of human internal sphincter muscle with an external sinusoidal current applied to the muscle strip causes the muscle strip to relax, reproducing the pattern of *in vivo* sphincteric relaxation (Figure 8). Weak electrical stimulation resulted in a

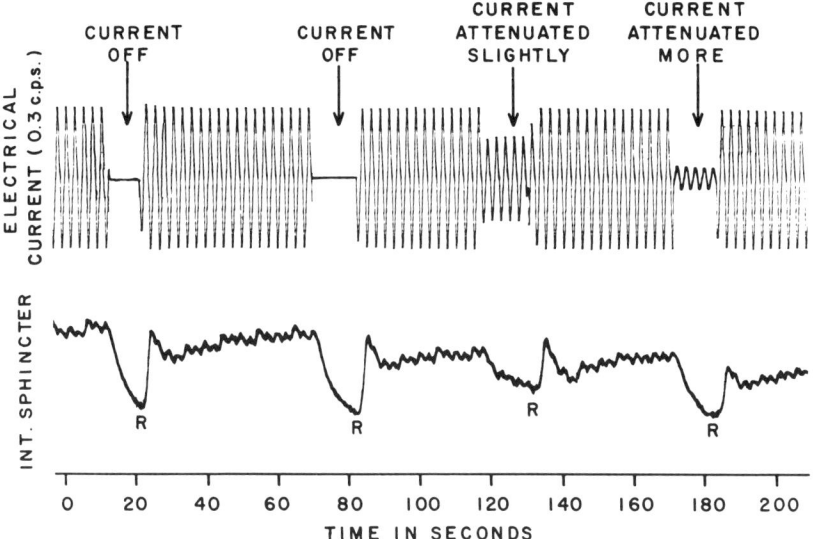

Figure 8. Externally applied electrical sinusoidal current produces contraction of sphincter muscle *in vitro*, while brief interruption of current produces sphincter muscle relaxation. (From Bass *et al.*, 1972.)

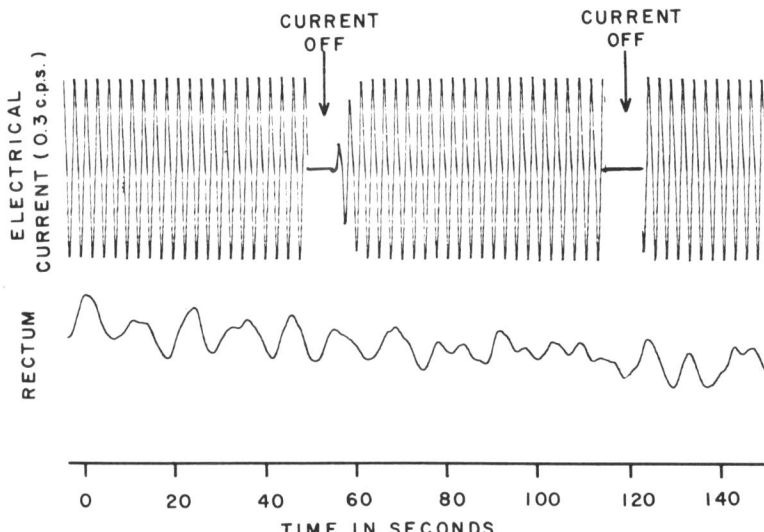

Figure 9. Brief interruption of electrical current fails to result in rectal muscle relaxation. (From Bass *et al.*, 1972.)

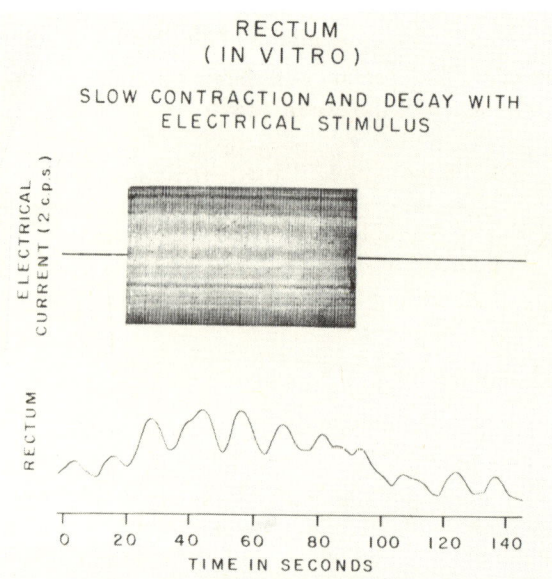

Figure 10. Slow rise and decay of rectal muscle response to electrical stimulation *in vitro*. (From Bass *et al.*, 1972.)

partial sphincter relaxation, and the amplitude of sphincter relaxation was inversely proportional to the intensity of the electrical stimulus. This stimulation *in vitro* mimicked the slow wave or basic electrical rhythm and also the activity of the sphincter muscle *in vivo*.

These characteristics are highly specific for sphincteric muscle as opposed to nonsphincteric muscle. Circular muscle from the rectum immediately proximal to the internal anal sphincter did not reproduce these observations. In addition, inhibition of electrical activity in the rectum does not result in a sharp decrease in tone such as is observed in the internal sphincter (Figure 9). This occurs in part because the circular muscle of the rectum responds to electrical stimulation with a much slower rise and a much slower decay than sphincteric muscle (Figure 10), which behaves in a manner somewhat intermediate between striated muscle and classical, visceral smooth muscle.

4. Applications of Psychophysiological Methods to Treatment of Incontinence

The measurement techniques described above have been incorporated into two highly successful biofeedback training procedures for treating fecal incontinence. Engel, Nikoomanesh, and Schuster (1974) were the first to develop such a procedure. Feedback consisted of having the patient watch a polygraph recording such as that shown at the right side of Figure 1 while the rectal balloon was repeatedly distended. The patient was shown what the response should look like—a brisk contraction of the external anal sphincter immediately after rectal distension—and was given verbal instructions as well as visual feedback during repeated trials. Training began with large, 50-ml distensions of the rectum and progressed to smaller and smaller distensions as the patient began to make appropriate responses. The last stage of training involved witholding the visual feedback so that the patient was forced to respond to the sensation of rectal distension alone and had to judge the strength and timing of the sphincter response without visual feedback. Training sessions were spaced at 4–8 week intervals, and patients were asked to practice squeezing the external sphincter 50 times daily between visits. Usually 2–4 training sessions were sufficient.

Engel et al. (1974) reported that 4 of 6 patients in their initial series were continent and the remaining two were improved following biofeedback training. Subsequently, Cerulli, Nikoomanesh, and Schuster (1979) published a series of 50 patients treated by this technique, and their report provides a more detailed estimate of the outcome of this form of treatment. When all patients were pooled regardless of etiology, 72% were found to be continent or to have at least a 90% reduction in frequency of incontinence. However, outcome did vary as a function of etiology. In the group of patients whose incontinence was secondary to anal or rectal surgery, 88% were successfully treated (at least 90% reduction), whereas the group with incontinence secondary to systemic diseases such as diabetes and scleroderma were less successful; 67% were successfully treated. The poorest outcomes were achieved in patients whose incontinence was secondary to spinal cord injury; only 45% were considered successes.

We (Whitehead, Parker, Masek, Cataldo, & Freeman, 1981) modified the biofeedback training procedures developed by Engel et al. so that they were more successful with spinal cord injured patients. We pointed out that the Engel procedure is primarily a stimulus discrimination training procedure, and in fact many patients with incontinence have an impairment of rectal sensibility (Golligher & Hughes, 1951; Whitehead, Engel, & Schuster, 1981). Our investigations on children with meningomyelocele (a birth defect involving disruption of the lower spinal cord) indicated that they rarely had any sensory impairment for rectal distension and so were unlikely to require discrimination training. Moreover, they had extremely weak external anal sphincter muscles which were passively stretched by the reflex inhibition of the internal anal sphincter when the rectum was distended (Figure 2). This made it impossible to detect weak external sphincter responses with a balloon when the rectum was distended.

These differences led us to redesign the biofeedback training procedure as a response-shaping procedure. We began by teaching the patient to contract the external anal sphincter in the absence of any rectal distension. When he was able to do so reliably, we began to distend the rectum with progressively larger volumes of air. (The protocol we use currently calls for four successive sphincter responses of at least 5 mm Hg amplitude before moving to a larger volume of distension.) As with the old procedure, the patient is asked to do sphincter exercises daily between training sessions. We find that 6–12 biweekly training sessions are required.

Using the altered procedure we were able to improve the outcome in the meningomyelocele group to a level comparable to that achieved in other types of incontinence. In our first series of eight children, five were continent at the end of the training, and one showed an 80% reduction in the frequency of incontinence (Whitehead, Parker, Masek, Cataldo, & Freeman, 1981).

Wald (1981) has also published the results of a series of patients with meningomyelocele whom he treated with biofeedback. He reported that 5 of 14 patients he examined were unable to perceive rectal distension, and a sixth patient showed significant impairment of sensation. He did not attempt to train these patients. In the eight patients who did receive training two became continent and two were significantly improved. The biofeedback training procedure was similar to that which we developed.

These biofeedback training procedures are the treatment of choice for fecal incontinence when the incontinence is attributable to a sensory or a motor deficit in the anorectal area. However, there are other types of incontinence for which biofeedback is not appropriate. These include overflow incontinence secondary to constipation and fecal impaction, which is the commonest cause of incontinence in childhood; and also incontinence which is secondary to social indifference in demented, retarded, or psychotic individuals. Other behavioral and medical treatments are available for such patients (Parker & Whitehead, 1982). A careful psychophysiological assessment can quickly determine which treatments are appropriate.

5. References

Alva, J., Mendeloff, A. I., & Schuster, M. M. Reflex and electromyographic abnormalities associated with fecal incontinence. *Gastroenterology,* 1967, *53,* 101–106.

Bass, D. D., Vanasin, B., Ustach, T. J., & Schuster, M. M. An *in vitro* model demonstrating specificity of sphincteric smooth muscle. *Johns Hopkins Medical Journal,* 1972, *131,* 436–440.

Bishop, B. Reflex activity of external anal sphincter of cat. *Journal of Neurophysiology,* 1959, *22,* 679–692.

Cerulli, M. A., Nikoomanesh, P., & Schuster, M. M. Progress in biofeedback conditioning for fecal incontinence. *Gastroenterology,* 1979, *76,* 742–746.

Corman, M. L. Management of fecal incontinence by gracilis muscle transposition. *Diseases of the Colon and Rectum,* 1979, *22,* 290–292.

Engel, B. T. The treatment of fecal incontinence by operant conditioning. *Automedica,* 1978, *2,* 101–108.

Engel, B. T., Nikoomanesh, P., & Schuster, M. M. Operant conditioning of rectosphincteric responses in the treatment of fecal incontinence. *New England Journal of Medicine,* 1974, *290,* 646–649.

Goligher, J. C., & Hughes, E. S. R. Sensibility of the rectum and colon: Its role in the mechanism of anal continence. *Lancet*, 1951, *1*, 543–548.

Parker, L., & Whitehead, W. E. Treatment of urinary and fecal incontinence in children. In D. C. Russo & J. W. Varni (Eds.), *Behavioral pediatrics: Research and practice*. New York: Plenum Press, 1982.

Read, N. W., Harford, W. V., Schmulen, A. C., Read, M. G., Santa Ana, C., & Fordtran, J. S. A clinical study of patients with fecal incontinence and diarrhea. *Gastroenterology*, 1979, *76*, 747–756.

Rodriquez, A. A., & Awad, E. Detrusor muscle and sphincteric response to anorectal stimulation in spinal cord injury. *Archives of Physical Medicine and Rehabilitation*, 1979, *60*, 296–272.

Schuster, M. M. Motor action of rectum and anal sphincters in continence and defecation. In C. Code & C. L. Prossed (Eds.), *Handbook of physiology. Section 6: Alimentary canal* (Vol IV.) *Motility*. Washington, D.C.: American Physiological Society, 1968.

Ustach, T. J., Tobon, F., Hambrecht, T., Bass, D. D., & Schuster, M. M. Electrophysiological aspects of human sphincter function. *Journal of Clinical Investigations*, 1970, *49*, 41–48.

Wald, A. Use of biofeedback in the treatment of fecal incontinence in patients with meningomyelocele. *Pediatrics*, 1981, *68*, 45–49.

Whitehead, W. E., Engel, B. T., & Schuster, M. M. Perception of rectal distension is necessary to prevent fecal incontinence. In G. Ádám, I. Meszaros, & E. I. Banyai (Eds.), *Advances in Physiological Sciences* (Vol. 17). *Brain and Behavior*. Budapest, Hungary: Akademiai Kiado, 1981.

Whitehead, W. E., Orr, W. C., Engel, B. T., & Schuster, M. M. External anal sphincter response to rectal distension: Learned response or reflex. *Psychophysiology*, 1981, *19*, 57–62.

Whitehead, W. E., Parker, L. H., Masek, B. J., Cataldo, M. F., & Freeman, J. M. Biofeedback treatment of fecal incontinence in meningomyelocele. *Developmental Medicine and Child Neurology*, 1981, *23*, 313–321.

PART V

INTEROCEPTION
WILLIAM E. WHITEHEAD

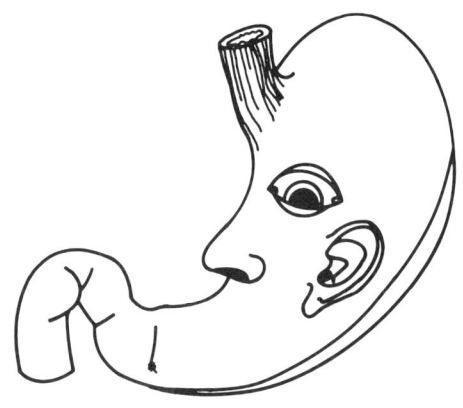

The last section of this book deals with a relatively new field of gastrointestinal psychophysiology—investigation of the role of visceral sensation in behavioral and homeostatic processes. Speculation about the significance of these vague messages from our bodies is of course not new—nearly a century ago James (1884) published a theory of emotion which assigned a primary role to visceral perceptions, and 70 years ago Cannon (1912) proposed a role for such sensations in the regulation of food intake. However, it has been only recently that experimental procedures and physiological transducers have been developed which permit a systematic investigation of this topic.

In Chapter 17, Whitehead describes procedures which have been developed for the investigation of visceral perception in humans. He also summarizes the early observations of Hertz, who in 1911 systematically explored the sensibility of the alimentary tract in humans at the beginning of the century with the methods available at that time. Although many of his methods were primitive, Hertz was able to make some observations which are no longer possible, such as interrogating patients who were undergoing abdominal surgery without anesthesia. Also in Chapter 17, Whitehead describes the five major hypotheses about the significance of visceral perception for human behavior and summarizes the evidence for each. He concludes that visceral sensations which are consciously perceived serve as discriminative stimuli regulating interactions with the environment such as the selection of a socially appropriate time and place for defecation.

Ádám, in Chapter 18, describes his pioneering experiments on visceral perception in animals and humans. It was his work which introduced the study of visceral perception to western scientists. He describes the surgical and other investigative techniques developed in his laboratory and summarizes the experiments which led him to the conclusion that visceral stimuli may have opposite effects depending on their intensity.

It is somewhat puzzling that the study of visceral perception has attracted so few investigators, since visceral perception has been implicated in several major psychological enigmas—the self-attribution of emotion, the regulation of food intake, and the etiology of psychosomatic disorders, among others. Much remains to be learned, and the experimental methods are now available. This is a fertile field for more psychophysiologists to enter.

References

Cannon, W. B., & Washburn, A. L. An explanation of hunger. *American Journal of Physiology*, 1912, *29*, 441–454.

Hertz, A. F. *The sensibility of the alimentary canal*. London: Oxford University Press, 1911.

James, W. What is emotion? *Mind*, 1884, *19*, 188–205.

17

INTEROCEPTION
Awareness of Sensations Arising in the Gastrointestinal Tract

WILLIAM E. WHITEHEAD

1. Introduction

A surprisingly large amount of sensory information comes to the central nervous system from the gut. There are more afferent fibers than efferent fibers in the extrinsic nerves which supply the gastrointestinal tract. Leek (1972) estimates that 80%–90% of fibers in the vagus (parasympathetic) nerves are afferent, more than 50% of fibers in the splanchnic (sympathetic) nerves are afferent, and approximately 30% of the fibers in the pelvic (parasympathetic) nerves are afferent.

The purpose of this chapter is to examine the ways in which this sensory information may influence behavior. The emphasis of the chapter will be on sensory information which reaches or has the potential for reaching subjective awareness. Subjective awareness is defined by verbal behavior (or overt skeletal muscle responses rendered equivalent to verbal responses by instructions) indicative of the accurate discrimination of gastrointestinal stimuli which are either

---

WILLIAM E. WHITEHEAD • Department of Psychiatry, the Johns Hopkins School of Medicine, and Department of Medicine, Baltimore City Hospital, Baltimore, Maryland 21224. Preparation of this chapter was supported by Research Scientist Development Award 5 K01 MH00133 from the National Institute of Mental Health.

produced by the experimenter or, in the case of naturally occurring physiologic events, objectively measured by the experimenter.[1]

Only a small portion of the sensory information which reaches the brain from the gut is available to awareness. This is not a matter of the more intense stimuli being perceived; rather, some types of sensations appear to be selectively represented in awareness.

The best general study of sensory awareness in the alimentary tract was published at the beginning of the century (Hertz, 1911). Hertz used the same investigative techniques which are employed currently with human subjects, namely, the introduction of fluids, balloons, and rods into the gut by mouth, by rectum, or through a gastrostomy, ileostomy, or colostomy. He concluded that the alimentary tract is insensitive to touch from the pharynx to the anal canal, but that touch is appreciated in the anal canal. Distension (stretching) is appreciated throughout the alimentary canal and is interpreted differently in different locations: In the esophagus, distension produces a sensation of fullness, and the subject can accurately point to the location of the balloon. Hertz believed that distension of the stomach produced a sensation of repletion or satiety but that contractions of an empty stomach were interpreted as hunger. Distension of the small or large bowel was felt as fullness and was often attributed to gas. Subjects could not localize the site of the intestinal stimulus. Distension of the rectum produced an urge to defecate. Hertz asserted that overdistension was the only source of pain originating in the gastrointestinal tract.

Hertz investigated other stimuli as well. He found that hot and cold stimuli were perceived in the esophagus down to the gastroesophageal sphincter and in the anal canal. Hertz felt that the evidence for perception of temperature in the colon was equivocal. Acids were not felt when instilled into the stomach or

---

[1]The possibility that there may be discrimination without awareness (as defined by accurate verbal report) has been raised by two groups: Hefferline, Keenan, and Harford (1956) demonstrated that a small EMG response which had been reinforced with escape from or avoidance of aversive noise, increased in frequency even though the subjects could not verbalize the contingency of reinforcement. Although frequently cited as evidence of discrimination without awareness, these data are irrelevant to the issue unless one accepts the assumption that the subject must discriminate the response before he can learn to emit it; this assumption has been challenged by experiments showing that ability to discriminate a response is unrelated to the subject's ability to emit the response or to learn to emit the response (e.g., Whitehead & Drescher, 1980). Secondly, psychodynamic theorists have proposed that subjects may respond to stimuli which they repress from awareness because of threats to self-esteem (e.g., Bruner & Postman, 1947). This is a special case of discrimination without accurate verbal report since the repressed stimuli can be discovered and verbalized through special techniques such as free association and hypnosis. Without denying the potential importance of this special case, this chapter will be concerned only with the general case in which verbal behavior, or a motor response rendered equivalent to a verbal response by instructions, is the indicator of discrimination. Most previous research on visceral perception in humans has followed this convention.

esophagus, but alcohol produced a sensation of warmth or burning when introduced into the stomach. In concentrations of 25%, alcohol also caused a burning sensation in the anal canal, and in concentrations of 50%–90% alcohol produced a sensation of heat in the colon. The anal canal, but not the rectum, was found by Hertz to be sensitive to stimulation by glycerine.

As evidence of the selectivity of perception in the alimentary tract Hertz was able to cite the experience of performing abdominal surgery without anesthesia—a practice more common at the turn of the century than presently. He reported that "the normal stomach, small intestine, colon, and appendix could be touched with cold or hot objects, burnt with a caustic, clipped with forceps, or cut with a knife without producing any sensation" (Hertz, 1911, p. 43). As further evidence of selectivity, Iggo (1957) has shown that there are vagal fibers which respond to acids, alkalies, and touch in the stomach, although these stimuli are not subjectively discriminated.

Hertz (1911) noted at the end of his excellent book that he had observed individual differences in the ability of his subjects to discriminate various stimuli. He found differences both in the threshold amount of intestinal distension required to produce a subjective sensation and differences in whether a thermal stimulus in the colon was perceived at all. Hertz suggested that some form of learning, or sensitization by "neurasthenia" and anemia, might account for such differences. However, experimental methods were not available at that time which would have enabled him to investigate these hypotheses. The next section describes the developments in investigative technique which have enabled the field of visceral perception to advance since the time of Hertz.

2. Methods of Investigating Visceral Perception

2.1. Method of Limits

In studying perception, it is useful to know not only whether a subject can perceive a stimulus, but also how intense the stimulus must be before it is perceived. This threshold is often estimated by progressively increasing the intensity of the stimulus until the subject reports that he perceives it and/or by progressively decreasing stimulus intensity until the subject reports that he can no longer detect it. This procedure, called the method of limits, has a serious limitation, however. It is now known that perceptual judgments are influenced by some nonperceptual variables which are collectively called response bias. An example of response bias would be the tendency of some subjects not to say they see a stimulus until they are absolutely certain because they wish to be seen as conservative, or the tendency of subjects not to report a painful stimulus until it is unbearable because they wish to be seen as strong. Other factors can shift the apparent threshold in the opposite direction; for example, the hunter who shoots at anything that moves because there is a high payoff for a hit and relatively little cost to a "false alarm."

2.2. Signal Detection Analysis

The method of limits does not permit actual perceptual sensitivity to be separated from response bias. However, there are two psychophysical procedures which do permit this separation. The first is based on the theory of signal detection (Swets, 1973). It involves presenting a large number of trials (200–500 trials) on each of which the subject is asked to judge whether or not the stimulus was presented. By examining the ratio of hits to misses and the ratio of false alarms to correct rejections (i.e., saying "no" when the stimulus was not presented), it is possible to obtain independent estimates of perceptual sensitivity and response bias. Stunkard and Fox (1971) and Whitehead and Drescher (1980) have used this technique to assess awareness of stomach contraction in human subjects.

The limitation of the signal detection procedure is that large numbers of trials are required to obtain reliable estimates. This makes the task boring for the subject. Consequently, one may have to pay the subject contingent on his accuracy in order to maintain his attention on the task. Many test sessions may also be required to obtain the necessary 200 trials. For example, Whitehead and Drescher (1980) needed six experimental sessions to obtain 200 trials on a stomach contraction perception test.

2.3. Forced Choice Procedure

An alternative method of estimating perceptual sensitivity which requires fewer trials (approximately 20) is the forced choice procedure (Tanner & Swets, 1954). This involves always presenting the subject with a pair of trials and asking the subject to indicate whether the stimulus was presented in the first or second trial. The subject is told to guess if he is not sure. The stimulus is always presented in one of the two trials. This procedure is insensitive to most sources of response bias, although it will be affected by a strong preference for saying first or second and by a refusal to "guess." The chief limitation of the procedure is that very young children or cognitively impaired adults do not understand the instructions. Whitehead, Engel, and Schuster (1980) used this technique to assess awareness of pressure stimuli in the colon.

2.4. Confounding of Perception and Control

When the goal of an experiment is to assess the subject's perception of a naturally occurring physiologic response such as a stomach contraction rather than his perception of an artificial stimulus such as a balloon inflation, an additional problem arises: One must be able to distinguish between the ability of the subject to voluntarily emit or alter the response and his ability to discriminate occurrence of the response. The importance of this distinction is illustrated by the literature on the discrimination of one's own heart rate. Brener and Jones (1974) developed a procedure for testing heart rate perception by asking the subject to judge whether a sequence of vibratory stimuli were triggered by the R-wave of the EKG or by a machine which produced a train of pulses at a frequency equal to the subject's average heart rate. However, Ross and Brener (1981) subsequently discovered that subjects solved this task by taking a deep breath and observing whether or not this produced a change in the pattern of stimuli. Subjects are less knowledgeable about how to voluntarily control most gastrointestinal responses. However, since these perception tests are often done in the context of biofeedback experiments, one must be careful to make the test of discrimination independent of the subject's ability to control the response.

2.5. Discrimination Training

Another innovation in the study of interoceptive stimuli has been to train discrimination. This is important for two reasons. First, it permits one to estimate the physiological limits of discrimination. Differences between people in their awareness of a gastrointestinal stimulus may represent differences in their learning history or physical differences between them. Discrimination training provides a way of separating these two influences. Stunkard and Fox ((1971) taught human subjects to discriminate stomach contractions which they could not previously discriminate, and Ádám (1967) taught a human subject to discriminate the occurrence of balloon distension of the jejunum at volumes which previously had elicited alpha EEG blocking but no reliable verbal reports.

The second advantage of training discrimination is that it permits one to use animals to study visceral perception. Slucki, Ádám, and Porter (1965) demonstrated that rhythmic inflation of a balloon in an isolated loop of small intestine could be made the discriminative stimulus controlling lever-pressing behavior in the rhesus monkey. They later repeated this using an isolated loop of descending colon as the site of stimulation (Slucki, McCoy, & Porter, 1969). The importance of being able to use animals in the study of visceral perception is that they can be studied over an extended period of time, and the pathways subserving visceral perception can be studied by sectioning.

3. Behavioral Significance of Visceral Perception

In the introduction to this chapter, it was pointed out (1) that people are aware of some events occurring in the gastrointestinal tract, (2) that the types of events which are perceived represent a selected subset of afferent information available to the brain from the gut, (3) that there are individual differences in ability to perceive gastrointestinal stimuli, and (4) that the discriminability of these stimuli improves with training. This combination of circumstances is probably meaningful rather than coincidental, and it suggests that visceral perception plays a role in the organism's behavioral adjustment to its environment. Several hypotheses about what that role is have been advanced, and these hypotheses are reviewed in the next sections.

3.1. Cuing Function in Bowel Control

The most thoroughly investigated and best documented hypothesis is that the perception of rectal distension serves as a cue to the organism to emit certain behaviors which result in (1) the temporary withholding of a bowel movement and (2) the seeking out of an appropriate place in which to defecate. The temporary withholding or postponement of a bowel movement is achieved by a phasic contraction of the external anal sphincter during the period in which the internal anal sphincter is reflexly inhibited by rectal distension. Although this phasic contraction has occasionally been referred to as a reflex (Alva, Mendeloff, & Schuster, 1967), the bulk of evidence suggests that it is a voluntary response (Whitehead, Orr, Engel, & Schuster, 1981). For example, Rodriquez and Awad (1979) have reported that the phasic external anal sphincter contraction does not occur in response to rectal distension in spinal cord transected patients even though reflex inhibition of the internal anal sphincter in response to rectal distension does occur in such patients. Melzak and Porter (1964) reported some years ago that rectal distension did produce external sphincter contraction in spinal cord transected patients. However, their records show very brief electrical potentials which could have been artifactually produced by movement of the tissue relative to their rigid needle electrodes.

Loss of sensation in the rectum as a result of surgery or injury is frequently associated with incontinence of stool (Cerulli, Nikoomanesh, & Schuster, 1979; Goligher & Hughes, 1951). Moreover, in our biofeedback clinic for the treatment of fecal incontinence, we find that patients who are not able to perceive at least 15 ml of air injected into a balloon never achieved continence, whereas most of the patients who can perceive smaller amounts of rectal distension do benefit from biofeedback training (Whitehead, Engel, & Schuster, 1981). The normal threshold of rectal distension which is perceived is 5 ml in our laboratory.

3.2. Hunger and Satiety

Both Hertz (1911) and Cannon and Washburn (1912) stated that contractions of the stomach give rise to sensations of hunger. Hertz based his conclusions on anecdotal evidence, but Cannon and Washburn recorded contractions by means of a large balloon in the stomach and observed that subjects were more likely to report hunger during periods of gastric motility than during its absence.

Stunkard and his co-workers (Griggs & Stunkard, 1964; Stunkard & Koch, 1964; Stunkard & Fox, 1971) were the first to investigate this hypothesis systematically. Their initial studies appeared to confirm the association between hunger and gastric motility in normal subjects, and they generated much excitement by their data which showed that obese subjects gave reports of hunger which were uncorrelated with gastric motility. This suggested that either inability to discriminate gastric contractions or inappropriate labeling of gastric contractions might explain obesity.

Unfortunately, Stunkard's subsequent experiments (Stunkard & Fox, 1971) did not confirm these early impressions. Stunkard found that when subjects were asked to rate the intensity of their hunger rather than to respond "yes" or "no" and when subjects were run for longer period of observation, the association between hunger and gastric motility was weak and inconstant. Only 25% of subjects showed a strong association between hunger ratings and gastric motility, and this association was variable from one occasion of testing to another. Moreover, training subjects to be more accurate discriminators of gastric contractions did not improve the strength of the association between gastric contractions and hunger ratings and did not enable obese subjects to regulate food intake more effectively.

These observations are consistent with the effects of vagotomy (Grossman, Cummins, & Ivy, 1947), which eliminates sensations from the stomach, and gastrectomy (MacDonald, Inglefinger, & Belding, 1947), which eliminates gastric motility. Subjects continue to experience hunger after both types of surgery. Stunkard and Fox (1971) concluded that there is, in fact, an association between subjective hunger and gastric motility, but that variables other than motility are relatively more potent determinants of hunger. They suggest that earlier studies overestimated the strength of this relationship between hunger and motility because they used insensitive measures of hunger; there is a strong tendency for hunger to increase over time from the end of one meal to the beginning of the next, and this tendency may reduce the probability of discovering a lack of association between the two variables.

Whitehead and Drescher (1980) assessed awareness of stomach contractions in 20 normal subjects and asked them to describe all the cues they used to determine when their stomach was contracting. The most common cues mentioned were a tight feeling in the stomach (16/20) and stomach noises (15/20). Only 3 subjects in 20 mentioned hunger sensations, and none of these felt that "hunger pangs" were the most helpful cue for solving the discrimination task.

Sensations arising in the stomach have also been implicated in satiety and the cessation of eating. Hertz (1911) stated that distension of the stomach produced a feeling of fullness which led to the cessation of eating. Deutsch, Young, and Kalogeris (1978) confirmed in an elegant series of experiments that distension of the stomach does play a critical role in regulating the volume of food eaten. They implanted an inflatable cuff around the pylorus of rats to enable them to separate gastric from duodenal stimulation, and they implanted a gastric canula. They were able to show that rats eat a fixed volume of a familiar liquid diet and that withdrawal of part of the stomach contents after the rat has eaten to satiety will cause him to resume eating and to eat enough to replace the amount removed. This quantitative relationship between gastric filling volume and eating behaviors was observed whether or not food was allowed to enter the duodenum.

McHugh (1979) has shown that under normal circumstances gastric distension is a function of gastric emptying rate, and that gastric emptying is a regulated process, the speed of which is determined by the caloric content of the meal. The first part of a meal enters the duodenum where the caloric content of the meal is sensed, and gastric emptying is inhibited proportional to caloric concentration.

This experimental work on the role of gastric distension in eating behavior is supported by clinical observations on gastrectomized patients (MacDonald, Inglefinger, & Belding, 1947). These individuals, in whom stomach distension does not occur or cannot be signaled to the brain, tend to overeat.

Although these observations demonstrate that afferent information from the stomach controls cessation of eating, they do not indicate how this occurs. Hertz (1911) implied that one feels the distension of his stomach directly as fullness and labels it as repletion. However, Garcia, Hankins, and Rusiniak (1974) have suggested that gastric distension controls eating indirectly by modifying the hedonic value of food, that is, whether the taste is preferred. The experimental literature on the reinforcing value of intragastric feeding and on conditioned taste aversions and conditioned taste preferences (see p. 341) supports Garcia's hedonic shift hypothesis.

Several experiments have addressed the question of whether food injected directly into the stomachs of rats will serve as a reinforcer which maintains lever-pressing behavior because this experiment appears to differentiate between drive reduction and hedonic theories of reinforcement. Most of these studies found that intragastric reinforcement would maintain behavior on which it was contingent. However, Holman (1968) demonstrated that intragastric feeding would reinforce lever-pressing behavior only if there was concurrent stimulation of some type to the palate or throat. This oral stimulation could be nothing more than a change in temperature. Holman showed that rats previously trained to press a bar for food would extinguish if they were provided with contingent oral stimulation but no intragastric nutrient, and they would extinguish if provided with contingent intragastric feeding but no oral stimulation. Both cues presented together, however, would maintain the lever-pressing behavior. This outcome is consistent with Garcia's hypothesis that gastrointestinal stimuli exert an influence on behavior which is not mediated by their direct perception but rather is mediated by hedonic shifts in gustatory or related oral stimuli.

Similar conclusions can be drawn from the conditioned taste aversion literature. The general finding is that illness produced by radiation or by lithium chloride ingestion causes the animal to develop conditioned taste aversions to any novel taste which has preceded the illness. Similarly, the animal will develop conditioned taste preferences for any taste which precedes the recovery from illness or recovery from vitamin deficiency. There are several interesting aspects to such conditioning, including the fact that learning occurs even when long delays occur between the gustatory stimulus and the illness, and the fact that the aversion is developed specifically to the taste cue rather than to the place where the food was eaten or to its physical appearance.

Many of the illness-producing agents which Garcia used (e.g., radiation) are not specific to the gastrointestinal tract; he refers to interoceptive stimuli generally as exerting their effects on behavior through shifts in incentive, motivation, or hedonic value.

It is important to note that Garcia's hypothesis does not require that the subject be aware of the interoceptive stimulus or even that he be aware of the hedonic shift in taste for the conditioned taste aversion to develop. Garcia has shown that conditioned taste aversions develop when illness occurs during unconsciousness produced by anesthesia or by chemically-induced cortical depression. This suggests that perception plays little or no role in the effects on eating behavior of afferent information from the gut. Whether actual perception would add anything to the precision of behavioral self-regulation of the internal environment remains to be investigated.

3.3. Labeling of Emotions

The most popular view of the significance of visceral perception is that these sensations represent self-perceptions of emotional arousal. This theory was first formalized by William James (1884) and Lange (1922), and despite empirical data which tended to discredit the theory (Cannon, 1927), the so-called James–Lange theory of emotion continues to attract adherents. It strongly influenced psychoanalytic thinking about psychosomatic etiology. For example, the 1968 edition of the *Diagnostic and Statistical Manual of Mental Disorders* held that psychosomatic symptoms were the normal physiological manifestations of chronic emotional states. The emotions which were said to be associated with gastrointestinal activity included dependency and an angry desire to get revenge in the case of peptic ulcer and hopelessness or humiliation in the case of ulcerative colitis (Alexander, French, & Pollock, 1968; Graham, Lundy, Benjamin, Kabler, Lewis, Kunish, & Graham, 1962).

A modified version of the James–Lange theory of emotion was proposed by Schachter and Singer (1962) and dubbed attribution theory. They argued that awareness of his own autonomic arousal leads the subject to conclude that he is experiencing an emotion, but the subject depends on cognitive cues from the environment such as the behavior of other people or past experience to determine the type of emotion which is occurring.

Attribution theory seems to agree well with most of the available experimental literature. The Schachter and Singer (1962) experiments, which manipulated antonomic arousal by injecting epinephrine and also manipulated cognitive cues, indicated that the injection of epinephrine contributed to the perceived intensity but not to the identity of the emotions which subjects reported. Hohmann's (1966) observations on changes in the emotional experiences of spinal cord transected patients indicated that there is a decrease in the perceived intensity of emotional reactions after injury. The magnitude of the decrease is proportional to the level of the lesion and, therefore, to the amount of decrease in antonomic arousal and sensory feedback about antonomic arousal.

There are few data in the literature which bear directly on the emotional significance which subjects attach to perceptions of gastrointestinal responses. Ádám (1974) has done experiments in animals which suggest that mild stimulation of the gastrointestinal tract dampens negative emotional states and/or induces sleep whereas strong stimulation of the gastrointestinal tract may be perceived as aversive. In our experiments investigating the ability of human subjects to detect spontaneous contractions of their stomachs or distension of a small balloon in their colon, subjects have never described these stimuli in affective terms. Stomach contractions are typically described as a tensing or squeezing sensation in the abdomen, and distension of the colon is described as a feeling like gas distension. However, the experimental setting may have mitigated against subjects' interpreting their perceptions as emotional arousal.

Some incidental observations in our study of stomach contractions are relevant to the hypothesis that perceptions of autonomic responses may contribute to the self-attribution of emotion. We observed a small but statistically significant correlation ($r = .51$) between subjects' ability to perceive stomach contractions and their ability to perceive heart beats. This suggests a generalized tendency to be aware of, or to attend to, internal events, which would appear to be one of the requirements of any theory of emotion which treats self-perceptions as an important determinant. We also observed that men are significantly better than women, on average, at discriminating both stomach contractions and heart beats. The significance of this is unknown.

To summarize the discussion of emotional labeling, it appears that perception of gastrointestinal activity may lead people to attribute emotions to themselves, but this has not been directly verified. It is clear that people do not invariably attribute emotional arousal to their perceptions of gastrointestinal activity; they are capable of attributing these sensations to something they ate, something the investigator did to them, or to disease.

3.4. Acquisition and Retention of Voluntary Control over a Visceral Response

Brener (1974a,b; 1977a,b) proposed a specific role for visceral perception in the acquisition of self-control over a visceral response. He theorized that in order to emit any voluntary act the brain calls up an image of the sensory consequences associated with the response and then executes motor acts until the sensory feedback from the target organ (such as the heart) corresponds to the stored image of what those sensations should be. This theory is derived from William James's (1890) ideomotor theory of voluntary acts. From this, Brener inferred that learning to discriminate the sensory consequences associated with a visceral response is both necessary and sufficient to enable the subject to emit the response on command as a voluntary response. Biofeedback training, according to Brener, is discrimination training in which the subject learns to correctly identify and label the sensations associated with the response he is attempting to learn how to produce.

Brener's theory has a number of practical implications. Not only does it appear to explain biofeedback learning, but it also suggests ways in which biofeedback training might be made more effective. It suggests, for example, that eliciting large-magnitude changes in the visceral response by means of unconditional stimuli while providing feedback would be more effective than the usual procedure of advising the subject to sit quietly and concentrate on the feedback.

Several investigators have reported experimental tests of Brener's theory. Most of these have compared heart beat perception to heart rate control. Some studies have supported the theory (Clemens, 1976; Clemens & MacDonald, 1976; McFarland, 1975), while others have not (Dale & Anderson, 1978; Whitehead, Drescher, Heiman, & Blackwell, 1977).

Whitehead and Drescher (1980) suggested that the inconsistent outcomes in tests of Brener's theory have resulted because heart rate is a poor choice of systems in which to test the theory. We noted that within the normal range of values heart rate is closely linked to respiration, and that this permitted subjects in some experiments to solve the perception task by manipulating their breathing (Ross & Brener, 1981). In other experiments the perception task was insensitive to respiration-induced heart rate changes. A second problem with heart rate is that subjects already know a variety of strategies for altering heart rate prior to biofeedback training. These control strategies include changing respiration, tensing muscles, and using cognitive imagery of stimuli or events which unconditionally elicit heart rate changes. Some of the methods of heart rate control may be related to heart rate perception while others are not. Whitehead and Drescher (1980) suggested that this difficulty can be solved by switching to a new response system, gastric motility, which is not elicited by any known skeletal muscle response and which subjects initially have little ability to control.

In the experiment reported by Whitehead and Drescher (1980) subjects were tested for ability to detect individual contractions of their stomachs. Contractions were recorded as changes in intragastric pressure measured with a perfused catheter. On each of approximately 200 trials, which occurred over six 2-hr sessions, the experimenter turned on a light either at the peak of a stomach contraction or approximately 12 sec following the peak of a contraction. The subject had to indicate on each trial whether he thought the signal light coincided with a stomach contraction. The subject's responses were analyzed by the method of signal detection.

Following the perception test, subjects were asked to increase and decrease their stomach motility prior to feedback training. Then, half the subjects were given biofeedback training to control motility while the other half practiced without feedback. The feedback subjects acquired the ability to increase motility during feedback training but could not reduce motility below resting levels. The no feedback subjects did not acquire control over gastric motility. With respect to Brener's theory, the control of gastric motility was not correlated with individual differences in the ability to perceive gastric contractions either before biofeedback training or at the end of feedback training. This occurred even though half the subjects could perceive stomach contractions at better than chance levels.

Brener's theory of voluntary visceral control is not supported by these data. However, Brener (Ross & Brener, 1981) has recently revised the theory to state that the sensory information which is critical to self-control of a visceral response is not peripheral receptor activity but central efferent monitoring of the brain's motor commands to the viscera. This new formulation of the theory has not been tested experimentally.

In addition to Brener's theory of visceral response acquisition, Weiss and Engel (1971) have proposed that accurate perception of a visceral response learned during biofeedback training may be critical to retention of the response. The reasoning is that if the subject can perceive when he has successfully emitted the response there is secondary reinforcement for the performance, but if the subject cannot perceive the occurrence of the response there will be no reinforcement and the response will extinguish. This plausible hypothesis has not been tested.

3.5. Psychosomatic Etiology

A hypothesis similar to Brener's was advanced by Whitehead, Fedoravicius, Blackwell, and Wooley (1979) to account for the etiology of some types of psychosomatic disorders. This hypothesis owed much to Miller (1977), who had argued that pathophysiological responses underlying many psychosomatic disorders might be inadvertently learned through social reinforcement in the same way that biofeedback training explicitly teaches the subject to modify a physiological response by providing contingent information or rewards. The analogy which Miller used was that a child who is given special attention and allowed to stay home from school when he has a stomachache but not when he has a headache may learn to emit at a greater frequency and a greater amplitude the pathophysiological responses (such as gastric acid secretion) which produced the stomachache. Such a child, Miller proposed, might grow up to have an ulcer.

Whitehead *et al.* (1979) pointed out that this sequence of events could only occur if the subject perceived the pathophysiological response and reported it accurately. Other people in the environment can only reinforce verbal behavior or overt physiological events. If the subject is unaware of when a physiological event is occurring or if he complains at times when it is not occurring, the social reinforcement which he receives contingent on somatic complaints might increase the frequency of complaints but could not reinforce physiological changes. On the other hand, accurate reports of physiological changes could be rewarded in such a way that the reinforcer is temporally close to the physiological change and reinforces it.

This hypothesis led Whitehead *et al.* to make two predictions: (1) Individuals with certain psychosomatic disorders would show greater awareness of the associated physiological response than would individuals without the disorder, and (2) psychosomatic disorders associated with easily perceived pathophysiological responses would be more likely to exhibit a history of control by social reinforcement than would difficult-to-perceive responses.

The first prediction appeared to be supported by Ritchie's (1973) data on irritable bowel syndrome. He found that when he distended the colon with a balloon, patients with irritable bowel syndrome reported pain at a lower threshold of distension than did normal controls. We attempted to replicate this finding and to evaluate the threshold for perceiving any distension in patients with irritable bowel syndrome and in normals (Whitehead, Engel, & Schuster, 1980). We did replicate Ritchie's finding that patients were significantly more likely to report pain with moderate amounts of distension than were normal subjects. However, we were not able to test the hypothesis that the patients could detect weaker stimuli than the normal subjects because we could not find a weak enough stimulus to measure any individual differences. Our apparatus consisted of a flacid balloon 5 cm long which was placed in the rectosigmoid junction. The smallest amount of air which we could reliably inject into this balloon to stimulate the bowel was 5 ml. Nearly all the patients and normal subjects could detect this weak stimulus on 100% of trials. While we could conceivably have made the discrimination test more sensitive by using 2-point discrimination or by inflating the balloon more slowly, we reasoned that any differences between patients and normals which might be discovered in this way were too small to be of physiological or psychological significance. Most subjects appear capable of feeling just about every contraction of their bowel if they attend to it.

We have also found that perceptual sensitivity is excellent in the small intestine. In two patients with ileostomies, we inserted small balloons 5–10 cm into the stoma and found that they could invariably detect the addition of 2.5 ml of air to these balloons.

The second prediction referred to previously was that disorders associated with easily perceived pathophysiological responses should show more evidence of control by social reinforcement than disorders associated with difficult to perceive physiological responses. This question was investigated in an epidemiological survey (Whitehead, Winget, Fedoravicius, Wooley, & Blackwell, 1982) in which we compared patients with irritable bowel syndrome to those with peptic ulcer. Gastric acid secretion, which is the presumed pathophysiological response for peptic ulcer, is very difficult to perceive.

In the epidemiological survey we asked people what illnesses they had and how they treated themselves, and we also asked them whether their parents had rewarded them when they were ill as children. Significantly larger proportions of patients with irritable bowel syndrome as compared to peptic ulcer exhibited chronic illness behavior. They were more likely to report multiple somatic complaints, they believed their colds were more frequent and more serious than those of other people, and they were more likely to go to a doctor for treatment of a cold rather than to treat it themselves. These chronic illness behaviors were shown to be linked to the childhood reinforcement of illness in the form of gifts and special consideration. Patients with irritable bowel syndrome were significantly more likely than people without this disorder to report that their parents rewarded them for illness. This was not true of people with peptic ulcer. These data tend to confirm the prediction that an easily perceived pathophysiological response is more likely to come under the control of social reinforcers than a difficult-to-perceive response.

4. Summary and Conclusions

This review of the behavioral significance of sensations arising in the gastrointestinal tract suggests that these sensations fulfill two very different functional roles. They may serve as discriminative stimuli which are directly perceived and which signal the occasion for behavioral interactions with the social environment. Alternatively, sensory information from the gut may act indirectly on behavior by modifying the incentive value of foods so as to maintain a constant internal environment.

Perhaps the best example of the discriminative stimulus function of gastrointestinal stimuli is the urge to defecate which is produced by rectal distension and which enables the individual to postpone defecation until he can find a socially appropriate place. Another instance of this discriminative stimulus function is when self-perceptions of autonomic arousal lead people to infer that they are emotionally aroused but do not determine what emotion they are feeling; they must apparently depend on prior experience, expectations, and the behavior of others to decide whether they are actually emotionally aroused or just sick and what the emotion is that they are experiencing. The hypothesized role of awareness in psychosomatic etiology can also be grouped under discriminative stimulus functions: The perception of a certain gastrointestinal response is the stimulus in the presence of which a verbal complaint may be reinforced.

It is apparently the case that gastrointestinal sensations which serve as discriminative stimuli must be actually perceived in order for the subject to respond to them. This distinguishes them from the second type of sensation referred to above which may exert its influence on behavior even if the subject is unconscious during the time the stimulus (e.g., illness) occurs. A second distinction is that discriminative stimuli cue behaviors which involve interactions with the external environment but have nothing directly to do with the internal environment. The second category of sensory events, on the other hand, are exclusively concerned with the internal environment.

Perceptual sensitivity for the gastrointestinal sensations which serve as discriminative stimuli can be improved with discrimination training. It is interesting to speculate on just how much awareness of the events in one's gastrointestinal tract could be achieved with such training. There may be additional unsuspected opportunities for these sensations to serve as discriminative stimuli.

The other kind of functional role which gastrointestinal stimuli can serve, namely, the modification of the incentive properties of food, is exemplified by the role of gastric distension in satiety. Garcia argues that satiety and the cessation of eating is mediated exclusively by hedonic shifts in the taste of foods. Other examples are the reinforcing value of food, which seems to depend on a combination of oral stimulation and gastrointestinal stimulation; and the development of conditioned taste aversions and taste preferences.

It appears that perception of gastrointestinal responses is not essential to learning to voluntarily control these responses during biofeedback training. Garcia *et al.* (1974) even suggest that visceral sensations cannot be utilized in the learning of instrumental responses, and indeed biofeedback training of visceral responses almost invariably involves the use of visual or auditory feedback signals to indicate what is happening to a visceral process. Garcia may be right that only such exteroceptive channels of information can be used to establish instrumental responses. This remains to be determined.

A relatively large number of gastrointestinal sensations which we know are discriminable are left with no assigned role by this review and summary. Examples are the sensitivity of the esophagus to temperature and the sensitivity of the stomach and intestines to distension. Since evolutionary selection is rarely so promiscuous as to give an organism sensory modalities which are unrelated to survival, it is likely that gastrointestinal sensations serve important functions in behavioral regulation which are as yet not understood.

The gastrointestinal tract seems to be more richly endowed with sensations that reach awareness than other visceral systems, for example, the cardiovascular system. Perhaps this is because the gastrointestinal tract is actually a body surface like the skin which is in contact with a variable environment. The body may need extrasensory and response capabilities to be able to deal flexibly with the unpredictable environment found in the gut so as to avoid or rapidly eliminate toxins and parasites while maintaining an adequate supply of nutrition.

5. References

Ádám, G. *Interoception and behavior.* Budapest: Akademiai Kiado, 1967.

Ádám, G. Interoceptive stimuli and learning. In *Proceedings of the International Union of Physiological Sciences* (Vol. 10). New Delhi: Core Book Programme of the Government of India, 1974.

Alexander, F., French, T. M., & Pollock, G. *Psychosomatic specificity: Experimental study and results* (Vol. 1). Chicago. University of Chicago Press, 1968.

Alva, J., Mendeloff, A. I., & Schuster, M. M. Reflex and electromyographic abnormalities associated with fecal incontinence. *Gastroenterology,* 1967, *53,* 101–106.

Brener, J. A general model of voluntary control applied to the phenomena of learned cardiovascular change. In P. A. Obrist, A. H. Black, J. Brener, & L. V. DiCara (Eds.), *Cardiovascular psychophysiology.* Chicago: Aldine, 1974. (a)

Brener, J. Factors influencing the specificity of voluntary cardiovascular control. In L. V. DiCara (Ed.), *Limbic and autonomic nervous systems research.* New York: Plenum Press, 1974. (b)

Brener, J. Sensory and perceptual determinants of voluntary visceral control. In G. E. Schwartz & J. Beatty (Eds.), *Biofeedback: Theory and research.* New York: Academic Press, 1977. (a)

Brener, J. Visceral perception. In J. Beatty & H. Legwie (Eds.), *Biofeedback and behavior.* New York: Plenum Press, 1977. (b)

Brener, J., & Jones, J. M. Interoceptive discrimination in intact humans: Detection of cardiac activity. *Physiology and Behavior,* 1974, *13,* 763–767.

Bruner, J. S., & Postman, L. Emotional selectivity in perception and reaction. *Journal of Personality,* 1947, *16,* 69–77.

Cannon, W. B. The James–Lange theory of emotion. *American Journal of Psychology,* 1927, *39,* 106–124.

Cannon, W. B., & Washburn, A. L. An explanation of hunger. *American Journal of Physiology,* 1912, *29,* 441–454.

Cerulli, M. A., Nikoomanesh, P., & Schuster, M. M. Progress in biofeedback conditioning for fecal incontinence. *Gastroenterology,* 1979, *76,* 742–746.

Clemens, W. J. *Heart beat discrimination and the learning and transfer of voluntary heart rate control.* Paper presented at the Southeastern Psychological Association meeting, New Orleans, March 1976.

Clemens, W. J., & MacDonald, D. F. Relationship between heart beat discrimination and heart rate control. *Psychophysiology,* 1976, *13,* 176.

Diagnostic and Statistical Manual of Mental Disorders (2nd edition). Washington, D.C.: American Psychiatric Association, 1968.

Dale, A., & Anderson, D. Information variables in voluntary control and classical conditioning of heart rate: Field dependence and heart-rate perception. *Perceptual and Motor Skills,* 1978, *47,* 79–85.
Deutsch, J. A., Young, W. G., & Kalogeris, T. J. The stomach signals satiety. *Science,* 1978, *201,* 165–167.
Garcia, J., Hankins, W. G., & Rusiniak, K. W. Behavioral regulation of the milieu interne in man and rat. *Science,* 1974, *185,* 824–831.
Goligher, J. C., & Hughes, E. S. R. Sensibility of the rectum and colon: Its role in the mechanism of anal continence. *Lancet,* 1951, *1,* 543–548.
Graham, D. T., Lundy, R. M., Benjamin, L. S., Kabler, J. D., Lewis, W. C., Kunsih, N. D., & Graham, F. K. Specific attitudes in initial interviews with patients having different "psychosomatic diseases." *Psychosomatic Medicine,* 1962, *24,* 257–266.
Griggs, R. C., & Stunkard, A. The interpretation of gastric motility. II. Sensitivity and bias in the perception of gastric motility. *Archives of General Psychiatry,* 1964, *11,* 82–89.
Grossman, M. I., Cummins, G. M., & Ivy, A. C. The effect of insulin on food intake after vagotomy and sympathectomy. *American Journal of Physiology,* 1947, *149,* 100–102.
Hefferline, A. F., Keenan, B., & Hartford, R. A. Escape and avoidance conditioning in human subjects without their observation of the response. *Science,* 1956, *130,* 1338–1339.
Hertz, A. F. *The sensibility of the alimentary canal.* London: Oxford University Press, 1911.
Hohmann, G. W. Some effects of spinal cord lesions on experienced emotional feelings. *Psychophysiology,* 1966, *3,* 143–156.
Holman, G. L. Intragastric reinforcement effect. *Journal of Comparative and Physiological Psychology,* 1968, *69,* 432–441.
Iggo, A. Gastric mucosal chemoreceptors with vagal afferent fibers in the cat. *Quarterly Journal of Experimental Physiology,* 1957, *42,* 398–409.
James, W. *The principles of psychology.* New York: Henry Holt, 1890.
James, W. What is emotion? *Mind,* 1884, *19,* 188–205.
Lange, C. The emotions (I. A. Haupt, Trans.). In K. Dunlap (Ed.), *The emotions.* Baltimore: Williams & Wilkins, 1922.
Leek, B. F. Abdominal visceral receptors. In E. Neil (Ed.), *Enteroceptors: Handbook of sensory physiology* (Vol. 3., No. 1.). New York: Springer-Verlag, 1972.
MacDonald, R. M., Inglefinger, F. J., & Belding, H. W. Late effects of total gastrectomy in man. *New England Journal of Medicine,* 1947, *237,* 887–896.
McFarland, R. A. Heart rate perception and heart rate control. *Psychophysiology,* 1975, *12,* 402–405.
McHugh, P. R. Aspects of the control of feeding: Application of quantitation in psychobiology. *Johns Hopkins Medical Journal,* 1979, *144,* 147–155.
Melzak, J., & Porter, N. H. Studies of the reflex activity of the external sphincter ani in spinal man. *Paraplegia,* 1964, *1,* 277–296.
Miller, N. E. Effect of learning on gastrointestinal functions. *Clinics in Gastroenterology,* 1977, *6,* 533–546.
Ritchie, J. Pain from distension of the pelvic colon by inflating a balloon in the irritable colon syndrome. *Gut,* 1973, *14,* 125–132.
Rodriquez, A. A., & Awad, E. Detrusor muscle and sphincteric response to anorectal stimulation in spinal cord injury. *Archives of Physical Medicine and Rehabilitation,* 1979, *60,* 269–272.
Ross, A., & Brener, J. Two procedures for training cardiac discrimination: A comparison of solution strategies and their relationship to heart rate control. *Psychophysiology,* 1981, *18,* 62–70.
Schachter, A., & Singer, J. E. Cognitive, social, and psychological determinants of emotional state. *Psychological Review,* 1962, *69,* 379–399.
Slucki, H., Ádám, G., & Porter, R. W. Operant discrimination of an interoceptive stimulus in rhesus monkeys. *Journal of the Experimental Analysis of Behavior,* 1965, *8,* 405–414.

Slucki, H., McCoy, F. B., & Porter, R. W. Interoceptive S^D of the large intestine established by mechanical stimulation. *Psychological Reports,* 1969, *24,* 35–42.

Stunkard, A. J., & Fox, S. The relationship of gastric motility and hunger: A summary of the evidence. *Psychosomatic Medicine,* 1971, *33,* 123–134.

Stunkard, A. J., & Koch, C. The interpretation of gastric motility. I. Apparent bias in the reports of hunger by obese persons. *Archives of General Psychiatry,* 1964, *11,* 74–82.

Swets, J. A. The relative operating characteristic in psychology. *Science,* 1973, *182,* 990–1000.

Tanner, W. R., Jr., & Swets, J. A. A decision-making theory of visual detection. *Psychological Review,* 1954, *61,* 401–409.

Weiss, T., & Engel, B. T. Operant conditioning of heart rate in patients with premature ventricular contractions. *Psychosomatic Medicine,* 1971, *33,* 301–321.

Whitehead, W. E., & Drescher, V. M. Perception of gastric contractions and self-control of gastric motility. *Psychophysiology,* 1980, *17,* 552–558.

Whitehead, W. E., Drescher, V. M., Heiman, P., & Blackwell, B. Relation of heart rate control to heart beat perception. *Biofeedback and Self-Regulation,* 1977, *2,* 371–392.

Whitehead, W. E., Engel, B. T., & Schuster, M. M. Irritable bowel syndrome: Physiological and psychological differences between diarrhea-predominant and constipation predominant patients. *Digestive Diseases and Sciences,* 1980, *25,* 404–413.

Whitehead, W. E., Engel, B. T., & Schuster, M. M. Perception of rectal distension is necessary to prevent fecal incontinence. In G. Ádám, I. Meszaros, & E. I. Banyai,(Eds.), *Advances in Physiological Sciences* (Vol. 17). *Brain and Behavior.* Budapest, Hungary: Akademiai Kiado, 1981.

Whitehead, W. E., Fedoravicius, A. S., Blackwell, B., & Wooley S. Psychosomatic symptoms as learned responses. In J. R. McNamara (Ed.), *Behavioral approaches in medicine: Application and analysis.* New York: Plenum Press, 1979.

Whitehead, W. E., Orr, W. C., Engel, B. T., & Schuster, M. M. External anal sphincter response to rectal distension: Learned response or reflex. *Psychophysiology,* 1981, *19,* 57–62.

Whitehead, W. E., Winget, C., Fedoravicius, A. S., Wooley, S., & Blackwell, B. Learned illness behavior in patients with irritable bowel syndrome and peptic ulcer. *Digestive Diseases and Sciences,* 1982, *27,* 202–208.

18

INTESTINAL AFFERENT INFLUENCE ON BEHAVIOR
GYÖRGY ÁDÁM

1. Introduction

Gastroenterology, as the scientific field separated recently from normal and pathological physiology, deals mainly with functions taking place in the alimentary tract itself. Thus, its general principle is inevitably organocentric. In other words, this branch of medicine pays relatively little attention to processes happening outside the main system, especially to such "distant" events as higher nervous or mental phenomena. The merit of contemporary psychophysiology consists in filling the gap between classical physiology of the gastrointestinal tract and experimental psychology.

The importance of the present book lies in its creating the necessary links between these two divisions of knowledge. Without accomplishing these essential contacts, it is impossible either for gastrointestinal physiology or for psychology to progress further.

The pursuit of gastroenterology for a synthesis with psychophysiology has a long and venerable tradition in the history of European medicine: The Heidenhainian and Pavlovian traditions are splendid examples of this respected past. Nevertheless—as with other branches of physiology—organocentric views still prevail. No wonder that mainly homeostatic activities of the visceral afferent pathways are considered, especially if the sensory functions of the vagus or of the splanchnic nerves are surveyed in the context of gastric or intestinal processes.

GYÖRGY ÁDÁM • Department of Comparative Physiology, Eötvös University of Budapest, Budapest, Hungary.

This statement leads us directly to the topic of the present chapter—the *extrahomeostatic function* of the visceral afferent system. As we all know from our basic physiological knowledge, the main function of the visceral afferent nerves reaching the central nervous system at the level of the spinal cord, the medulla, and the midbrain is the protection of homeostasis (in other words, the maintenance of the constancy of the internal environment). This does not, however, exclude the possibility of the role of these viscerosensory paths in processes far beyond the regulation of the viscera strictly considered. This extrahomeostatic role was not self-evident and was not regarded as a recognized function in major handbooks or surveys even 15–20 years ago. The gap between visceral (e.g., gastrointestinal) and behavioral physiology mentioned previously has not so far been surmounted in our field of visceroceptive physiology. That is why, despite our earlier and recent data, the alarming and rather controversial question still arises whether the visceral afferent system can be regarded as a sense organ (similar to the somatosensory system of the skin, etc.) carrying information to higher centers, and thus influencing the behavior of the organism in addition to the effect on internal homeostasis, or whether this extrahomeostatic function is merely a rudimentary activity of a diffuse, sparsely spread peripheral system.

I am not a gastroenterologist. My special field of research consists in comparative studies of animal and human psychological physiology concerning the visceral influence on behavior. I will present some data which seem to prove the existence of a well-organized viscerosensory system.

2. Research Strategies

Two main research strategies were applied in our several experimental studies carried out on humans and on chronically-operated animals. The aim of the investigations was to determine the role of visceral input in modifying:

1. The innate behavior, for example, signal detection of the brain using electrical recordings as indicators, sleep–wakefulness cycle research, motivational studies, etc.
2. The learned behavior, for example, classical and instrumental conditional reflexes, using visceral stimuli as CS or $S^{D-\Delta}$ stimuli.

The visceral afferent system was regarded by us as a more or less homogeneous apparatus obeying common, general rules as far as its influence on behavior is concerned. From a practical point of view, we select three main visceral sites of stimulation (Ádám, 1967), which could be reached relatively easily by using invasive methods: (1) The renal system was historically the first object of our interest. We stimulated both the renal pelvis and the ureter on specially operated dogs with ureteral fistulae; (2) The receptors of the cardiovascular system were studied by the stimulation or the extirpation of the carotid sinus on dogs and rats; (3) Finally, several loci of the gastrointestinal system—the stomach, the jejunum, and the ileum—were chosen for visceroceptive stimulation on rats, cats, dogs, monkeys, and, in special balloon experiments, on humans. Instead of stimulating the mucosa of these hollow viscera, the direct stimulation of the splanchnic or the vagus nerves was applied in some series by means of chronically-implanted, Teflon-coated bipolar electrodes.

The invasive approach of stimulation was carried out in two different modalities: Either mechanical excitation was applied in the form of distension of the walls of the hollow organ by means of a balloon, or electrical stimulation of the mucosa or of the nerves was undertaken. Both interventions could be quantified, but the later proved to be more reliable in this respect in animals. Our effort toward quantification of the visceroceptive stimuli excluded the use of spontaneous motility or other physiological visceral changes from the wide variety of possibilities to be used as internal stimuli.

We preferred to work on the gastrointestinal tract for both practical and theoretical reasons. Practical advantages of doing visceroceptive studies on the gastrointestinal system are obvious: The Haidenhainian and Pavlovian experimental surgical techniques facilitate invasive experiments on chronic preparations. For example, the completely innervated and vascularized U-shaped, isolated Thiry–Vella intestinal loop proved to be an adequate and advantageous preparation. The monkeys, dogs, cats, and even rats (Figure 1) tolerated this chronic fistula well for months and years, practically for their whole lifetime. Similarly to numerous well-known observations of the Pavlovian laboratories on dogs with chronic fistulae, it was easy to simultaneously observe extrahomeostatic and homeostatic regulatory effects in such preparations.

These empirical advantages cannot be disregarded. Nevertheless, some theoretical peculiarities of the gastrointestinal tract rendered this system even more remarkable for our visceroceptive studies. The gastrointestinal apparatus is probably the only functional system of the human organism which stands—from the point of view of the psychology of perception—on the boundary between extero- and visceroception; in other words, it is a perceptual field from which both conscious and nonconscious sensory input to the brain can be demonstrated. From this standpoint, the mucosal areas not far from the oral and anal orifices can be regarded as transitional perceptual territories between conscious extero- and nonconscious visceroception (Figure 2). Low intensity, nonpainful stimulation of the oral cavity or of the pharynx evokes marked subjective sensations, whereas the weak stimulation of the middle or lower segment of the esophagus does not elicit any sensations. The same circumstance is valid for the rectal and sigmoid cavity. The "transition line" between gastrointestinal areas with marked perceptual experience and nonconscious input is unknown so far. The centimeter by centimeter exploration of such a perceptive phenomenon in normal, awake humans encounters extreme technical difficulties. That is why only

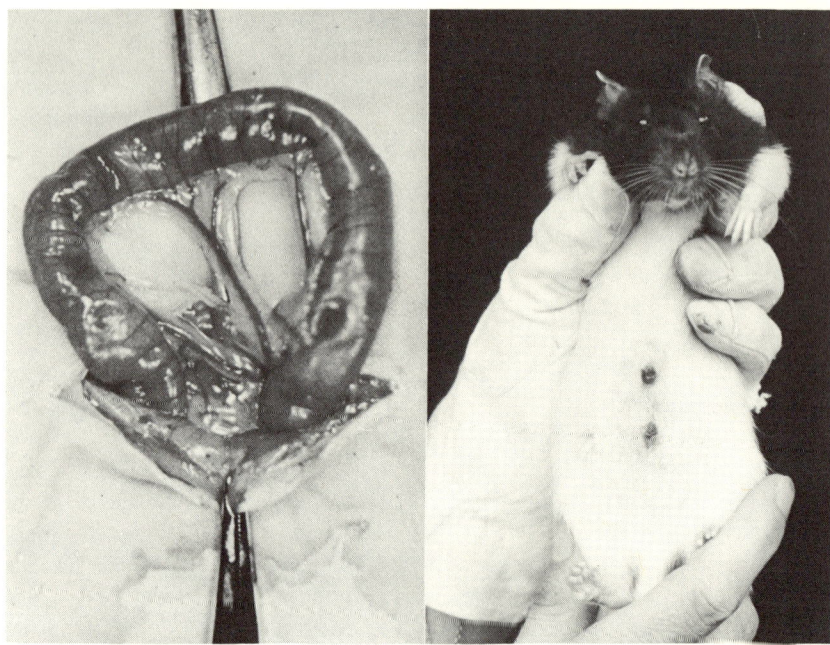

Figure 1. Isolated intestinal loop in rats. The modified Thiry-Vella loop was elaborated in our laboratory (Bárdos & Ádám, 1978). Left, the fully vascularized and innervated loop before the completion of surgery; right, the operated rat two months after surgery.

sporadic, mainly indirect data in the literature point to the sliding, movable character of such a boundary.

From the evolutionary viewpoint, the gastrointestinal system can be regarded as an "invaginated" external environment since it represents a tube open on both ends. This is explicitly true in lower invertebrates; in vertebrates it is true in a more hidden way.

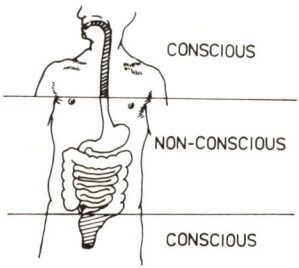

Figure 2. Simplified scheme of the gastrointestinal tract as a transitory system between extero- and interoception. Striated areas—borderline sites between conscious and nonconscious events.

The insufficiency of the Sherringtonian definition of "interoception" or "visceroception" becomes self-evident in this very case of a transitional system between real exteroception (e.g., the dermal organs of sense) and "true" visceroception (e.g., the receptors of the cardiovascular system). The deficiency turns into a "virtue" when gastrointestinal psychophysiology comes up: Both nonconscious and conscious sensory input could be demonstrated coming from the alimentary tract. We could also demonstrate the learned character of the latter.

Since the modest purpose of the present paper is merely the brief survey of our partly published data, I will emphasize the description of some experiments on humans which were preceded and/or succeeded by detailed studies on chronic animal preparations (Ádám, 1967, 1978).

3. Subjective Detection of Gastrointestinal Stimuli

In some early experiments on humans, it was demonstrated that the painless distension of the duodenal wall almost invariably caused EEG desynchronization proving that intestinal impulses may elicit electrical arousal reaching the ascending reticular activating system (Ádám, Preisich, Kukorelli, & Kelemen, 1965). It was noteworthy that in about 70% of the subjects the reticular activation was not accompanied by subjective sensations (e.g., by feeling of pressure, discomfort, etc.). Subsequently, by using verbal feedback it was possible to teach the experimental subjects to detect or to bring into consciousness, intestinal impulses which prior to conditioning had been unconscious (Ádám, 1967). These results indicate that intestinal signals can be detected by higher brain centers, the nonconscious range of this signal detection mechanism being represented by EEG arousals which were analyzed by us in detail in animal experiments (Ádám, Mészáros, Lehotzky, Nagy, & Rajk, 1960). The data prove, furthermore, that this extrahomeostatic intestinal input—usually nonconscious—can be converted into conscious sensation by means of feedback conditioning.

Extrahomeostatic visceroceptive signal detection was investigated by us using three different approaches. In addition to (1) the observation of EEG arousal mentioned previously, we analyzed (2) the morphology and the circumstances of appearance of visceroceptive evoked potentials (Ádám, 1967). Finally, gastrointestinal afferent influence on the brain was studied by us in its different aspects by using this sensory input as a (3) conditional stimulus (CS) in classical conditioning and as a discriminatory stimulus (S^D) or in instrumental conditioning experiments (Ádám, 1967). All these data verify that visceroceptive input starting from the gastrointestinal tract may have a marked influence on the activity of higher brain centers, and moreover, it can modify learned behavior.

4. Effects of Stimulus Intensity and Site of Stimulation

Our conditioning studies also prove that the brain can discriminate between visceral stimuli of several intensities or stimuli coming from different sites of excitation. Topical discrimination of intestinal impulses was studied by us in dogs (Figure 3) and even in humans by applying the habituation–discrimination test elaborated by us. The results of these habituation experiments have shown that the human brain can discriminate intestinal stimuli situated 15–20 cm apart.

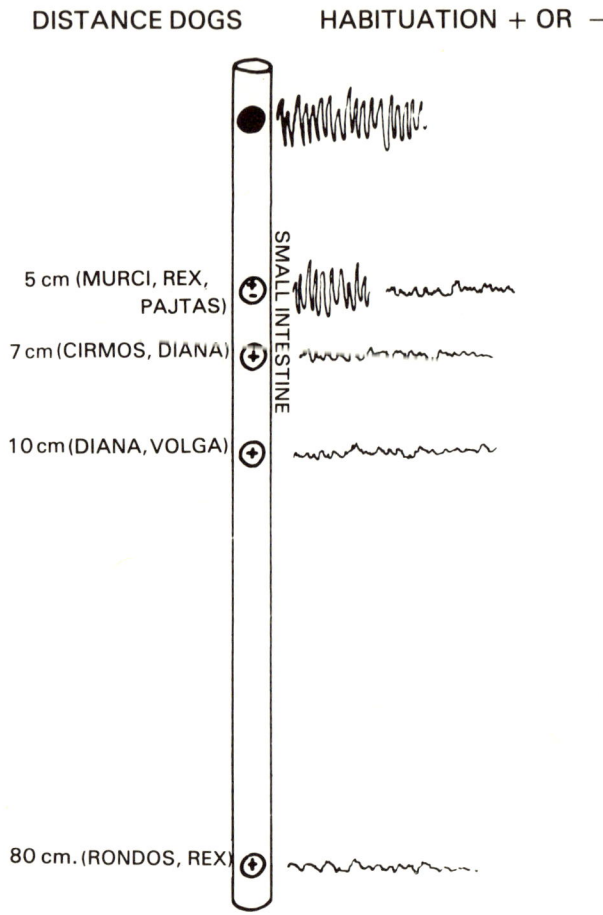

Figure 3. Schematic representation of the habituation–discrimination test of intestinal stimuli carried out with double-balloon stimulation. The distance between the sites of inflation was 5, 7, 10, and 80 cm in the 7 dogs taking part in this series. After habituation to stimulation at balloon A, desynchronization of the EEG invariably occurred upon stimulation of adjacent segments whenever the distance to A was more than 5 cm. (From Ádám, 1967.)

INTESTINAL AFFERENT INFLUENCE ON BEHAVIOR 357

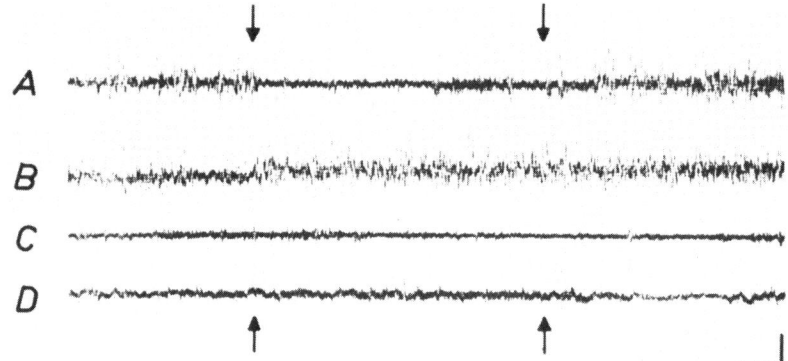

Figure 4. Desynchronization and synchronization triggered by stimulation of the splanchnic nerve with different intensities in the cat with chronically implanted cortical and splanchnic electrodes. Between arrows, stimulation with shocks of 0.10 msec duration and 3 cps at different voltages. A, cortical desynchronization at 2.6 V in drowsiness; B, synchronization at 2.4 V in drowsy state. The same intensity of stimulation had no effect in wakefulness (C) or in paradoxical sleep (D). Calibration, 10 sec and 100 μV. (From Kukorelli & Juhász, 1976.)

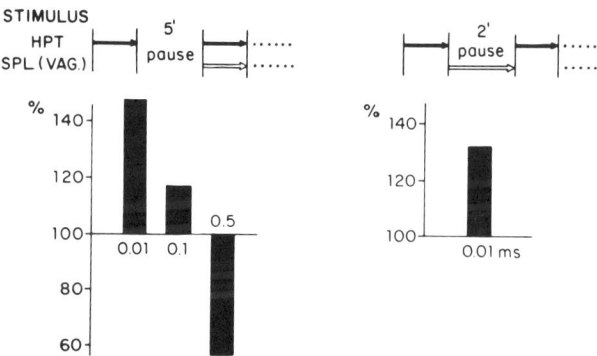

Figure 5. Latency modification of the aggressive behavior of the cat following simultaneous hypothalamic and visceral afferent nerve (splanchnic or vagal) stimulation. Left top, schedule of the experiment. Isolated hypothalamic stimulation for 1 sec resulted in a typical attack phenomenon with a latency of about 15 sec. After a pause of 5 sec simultaneous hypothalamic and visceral stimuli were applied. The procedure was repeated several times. Left bottom, average results of 6 cats showing an increase in the latency of aggressive reaction after weak visceral stimulation (square pulses of 0.01–0.10 msec duration). Right top, schedule of the experiment, when visceral stimulus was administered during the 2-sec pause between two hypothalamic stimulations. Right bottom, an increase in the latency of aggressiveness appeared in the 6 cats after weak pulses of 0.01 msec visceral stimulation. Ordinate, percentage of the latency of the hypothalamic attack reaction when 100% is the control value of hypothalamic aggressiveness. (From Juhász, Kukorelli, & Détári, 1980.)

This differentiation remains, however, outside the range of consciousness (Ádám, 1967).

In most of the previously mentioned studies we tried to avoid painful stimuli and such interventions in the gastrointestinal tract which could evoke overt startle reactions or orienting responses of the humans or animals, but otherwise in our earlier work we did not pay special attention to intensity or threshold aspects. In recent years, however, it became more and more evident that, similarly to exteroceptive input, visceroceptive impulses evoke different responses in the brain depending on the intensity of the stimulus applied. For example, different intensities of electrical stimulation of the splanchnic or vagal nerves may elicit desynchronizing or synchronizing effects (Figure 4).

This dual, and at the same time opposite function, called our attention to the threshold aspects of visceroception. In electrophysiological experiments on chronically operated cats, we started to judge stimuli "weak" or "strong" according to their relation to the "viscerosomatic" or "visceroabdominal" threshold (Kukorelli & Juhász, 1976, 1977). In behavioral studies on rats, the

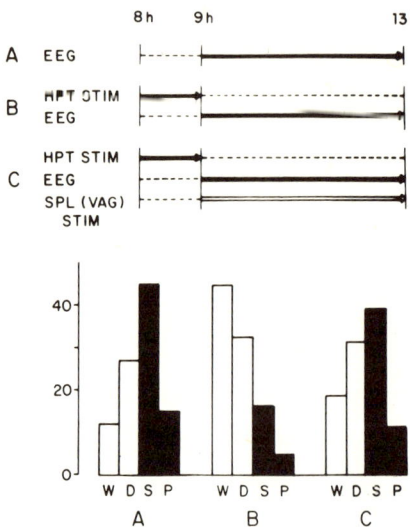

Figure 6. Modification of the sleep–wakefulness cycle in the cat following hypothalamic versus simultaneous hypothalamic and visceral stimulation. Top, schedule of the experiment. After feeding the cat was situated in the sound-attenuated box at 8:00 in the morning. EEG recording was carried out during 4 hr from 9:00 to 12:00. A, control EEG recording; B, EEG following random hypothalamic stimulation during one hour from 8:00 to 9:00; C, simultaneous random hypothalamic and weak visceral stimulation (pulses of 0.01 msec). Bottom, percentage of the different stages of the sleep–wakefulness cycle (W, wakefulness; D, drowsiness; S, slow-wave sleep; P, paradoxical sleep) calculated from the tape recordings of the EEG curves by the use of a special computer program. A, control; B, after hypothalamic stimulation; C, after simultaneous hypothalamic and visceral stimulation. Ordinate, percentage of the cycle. (From Juhász, Kukorelli, & Détári, 1980.)

Table 1
Intensity Continuum of Extrahomeostatic Effects of Visceral Afferent Input

Nociceptive intensity

Evoking arousal (desynchronized EEG)	Negative *motivation* enlarging reactivity to stress, aggressiveness	Natural signal detection and $S^D - S^\Delta$ discrimination	Conscious *in humans* natural visceral perception

Thresholds

Viscero-somatic—evoking slow wave sleep synchronized EEG	Modifying innate behavior—positive motovation reducing reactivity to stress, aggressiveness	Conditioned stimulus—signal detection and $S^D - S^\Delta$ discrimination only by learning	Verbal report—nonconscious *in humans* perception only by learning

Aspects

Electrophysiological	Behavioral	Learning	Consciousness

Zero intensity

threshold criterion was chosen according to the ability of the intestinal stimulus to modify the spontaneous, innate behavior of the animal (Bárdos, Nagy, & Ádám, 1980).

It turned out that gastrointestinal input below the viscerosomatic threshold will reduce hypothalamically induced aggressiveness in cats, and will induce synchronization of the EEG and enhance slow-wave sleep. On the contrary, stimuli above this threshold will augment aggressive reactions and will evoke arousal (Figures 5 and 6).

Thus, visceroceptive stimuli act along an intensity continuum in the middle of which a given "threshold" can be quantitatively determined (Table 1). This Janus-faced nature of the extrahomeostatic visceroception is remarkable, since it represents a common denominator with the other sense organs (visual, auditory, tactile functions, etc.). The most exciting face of this double-faced mechanism is the low-intensity, hidden level of visceral input, which can induce positively motivated behavior, and which may reduce reactivity to aggressiveness and evoke slow-wave sleep.

Interestingly enough, in accordance with our data on the gastrointestinal visceroceptive system, some authors emphasize the same calming, stress-reducing effect of weak viscerosensory impulses. Koch (1932), shortly after the discovery of the reflexogenix carotid area by Hering, described the taming effect of the stimulation of this region in dogs. Dell (1952) induced synchronization of the EEG by means of the stimulation of the sinus nerve in cats. Dworkin, Filewich, Miller, Craigmyle, and Pickering (1979) demonstrated that baroreceptor stimulation reduces reactivity to noxious stimuli in rats.

Our studies on humans, as well as our animal experiments, indicate that conscious signal detection and discrimination of weak, subthreshold stimuli may be possible but only following some kind of training procedure (classical conditioning or feedback training, etc.).

The intensity continuum hypothesis outlined above means that we can regard the receptive machinery of the gastrointestinal tract as a global, generalized apparatus, its actual level and intensity of activity influencing in different ways the behavior of the organism. Our mosaiclike results and the sporadic data in the literature, however, do not yet allow an integrated and well-balanced general theory on the role of intestinal afferent influence on behavior.

5. References

Ádám, G. *Interoception and behavior.* Budapest: Akadémiai Kiadó, 1967.
Ádám, G. Visceroception, awareness, and behavior. In G. E. Schwartz & D. Shapiro (Eds.), *Consciousness and self-regulation: Advances in research and theory* (Vol. 2). New York: Plenum Press, 1978.
Ádám, G., Mészáros, I., Lehotzky, K., Nagy, A., & Rajk, A. On the role of the brain stem activation system in the conditioning to visceral stimulation. *Acta Physiologica Academiae Scientiarum Hungaricae*, 1960, *18*, 143-148.
Ádám, G., Preisich, P., Kukorelli, T., & Kelemen, V. Changes in human cerebral electrical activity in response to mechanical stimulation of the duodenum. *Electroencephalography and Clinical Neurophysiology*, 1965, *18*, 409-415.
Bárdos, G., Nagy, J., & Ádám, G. Thresholds of behavioral reactions evoked by intestinal and skin stimulation in rats. *Physiology and Behavior* 1980, *24*, 661-665.
Dell, P. Corrélations entre le système nerveux végétatif et le système de la vie de relation. Mesencéphale, Diencéphale et cortex cérébrale. *Journal de Physiologie* 1952, *44*, 471-490.
Dworkin, B. R., Filewich, R. J., Miller, N. E., Craigmyle, N., & Pickering, T. G. Baroreceptor activation reduces reactivity to noxions stimulation: Implications for hypertension. *Science*, 1979, *205*, 1299-1301.
Juhász, G., Kukorelli, T., & Détári, L. Relationships between aggressive behavior, visceral afferentation and sleep in cats. *Proceedings of the International Union of Physiological Sciences*, 1980, *14*, 497.
Koch, E. B. Die Irradiation der pressoreceptorischen Kreislaufreflexe. *Klinische Wochenschrift*, 1932, *11*, 225.
Kukorelli, T., & Juhász, G. Electroencephalographic synchronization induced by stimulation of small intestine and splanchnic nerve in cats. *Electroencephalography and Clinical Neurophysiology*, 1976, *41*, 491-500.
Kukorelli, T., & Juhász, G. Sleep induced by intestinal stimulation in cats. *Physiology and Behavior*, 1977, *19*, 355-358.

INDEX

Behavioral analysis
  defined, 302–304
  in irritable bowel syndrome, 284–285
  of peptic ulcer, 225
Bernstein test of acid sensitivity in esophagus, 12
Biofeedback
  for aerophagia, 6
  fecal incontinence, 326–328
  gastric acid secretion, 168–169, 226–228
  ruminative vomiting, 6
Borborygmi (bowel sounds), 71

Compliance of colon and rectum, 245–247

Diabetes
  fecal incontinence in, 318–319
Diffuse esophegeal spasm
  chest pain, 5–6, 34
  motility, 11
  psychosomatic etiology, 23
Diverticular disease
  colon motility in, 271
  defined, 235
  etiology, 301
  fiber treatment, 296
  myoelectric abnormalities in, 258
Drugs
  aspirin and gastric ulceration, 213
  carbenoxolene in gastric ulcer treatment, 221
  cimetidine in peptic ulcer treatment, 221–222

Drugs (Cont.)
  corticosteroids and gastric ulceration, 213
  metaclopramide in peptic ulcer treatment, 221
  neostigimine induced colon motility, 268–270

Eating
  EEG effects, 189, 194
  gastric contractions induced by, 193
Emotion
  Cannon WB fight or flight reaction, 213–214
  colostomy observations of physiological correlates, 266–267
  effect on gastrointestinal functions, 263–264
  gastric motility and secretion, 69, 161, 196–199
  James–Lange theory of, 331, 341–342
  opposite effects of weak and strong visceral stimuli, 357–359
  psychosomatic etiology, 213–214
Esophageal manometry
  atlas of wave types, 5–6
  definition of wave types, 21–22
  diffuse esophegeal spasm, 11
  normal values, 9
  scleroderma, 10, 36
  sleep, 28–29
"Executive monkey" experiment, 200–201, 203–204, 217–218
Extinction of ruminative vomiting, 57–58

INDEX

Fecal incontinence
  habit treating for encopresis, 310
  prevalence, 299

Gastric contractions
  problems with pressure measurements, 72–73
  sleep effects on, 189–191
  typology of Code, 74–75
  See also Emotion, Hunger, Visceral perception
Gastrocolic reflex
  colon motility, 270–271
  definition, 241
  depressed patient with absence of, 267
  habit training for encopresis, 310
  hormone mediators of, 291–292
  irritable bowel syndrome abnormalities in, 269–270, 291, 293
General adaption syndrome of Hans Selye, 213
Globus hystericus, 23, 34
Gracilis muscle transfer
  surgery for incontinence, 320

Hertz AF(AF Hurst), 331, 334–335
Hirschsprung's disease, 321
Hormones
  gastrocolic reflex, 291–292
  motility response to, 242, 271–273
  esophegeal motility disorders in pregnancy, 22, 37
Hunger
  afferent pathways for satiety, 211
  Cannon WB theory, 331
  conditioned taste preferences, 341
  gastric contractions in, 69–70, 71, 75, 185–187

Individual response specificity and psychosomatic etiology, 214–215
Irritable bowel syndrome
  gastrocoloc reflex abnormal, 269–270, 291, 293
  myoelectric activity in, 258–259, 272–275, 290
  pain from distension, 281–282
  perception of colon contractions, 345–346
  prevalence, 235
  psychological symptoms, 236, 278–280

Learned helplessness, 203, 218

Morbidity of all gastrointestinal disorders, 209
Mother–infant bonding in psychogenic vomiting, 47
Motility index, 79–80
Myoelectric activity
  colon serosal recording, 251
  diverticular disease, 258
  electrical response activity (ERA) of the stomach, 78–79
  esophagus, 21–22
  irritable bowel syndrome, 258–259, 272–275, 290
  migrating myoelectric complex, 191
  relaxation oscillator theory, 77, 255, 323–326
  spikes and gastric contractions, 77–78, 80
  skin surface recording, 252
  See also Spectral analysis

Overcorrection treatment for ruminative vomiting, 58

Pavlovian conditioning
  cephalic phase of gastric secretion, 210
  conditioned taste preferences, 341
  of gastric acid secretion, 187, 263
  of lower esophageal sphincter in reflux esophagitis, 40–41
  psychogenic vomiting, 46–47
  reflex inhibition of acid secretion, 216
  of salivation, 263
Peptic ulcers
  animal models, 66
  aspirin in, 213
  behavioral analysis of ulcer pain, 225
  biofeedback for, 226–227
  carbenoxolene in, 221
  cimetidine for, 221–222
  corticosteroids in, 213
  "executive monkey" study, 200–204, 217–218
  learned helplessness, 218
  metaclopramide for, 221
  mucus in etiology of, 213
  prevalence, 65
  psychotherapy, 223
  Zollinger–Ellison syndrome in, 213

Pneumostatic dilation for achlasia, 35–36
Positive reinforcement treatment for ruminative vomiting, 57
Pregnancy
  esophageal motor disorders in, 22, 37
Presbyesophagus, 22, 34
Prevalence of gastrointestinal disorders
  all, 209
  diverticular disease, 235–236
  fecal incontinence, 299
  irritable bowel syndrome, 235
  peptic ulcers, 65
  presbyesophagus, 22, 34
Punishment
  ethics of taste aversion treatment, 56
  ethics of shock treatment, 54
  treatment of vomiting, 52–53

Radio-opaque marker study of bowel transit, 248
Reflux esophagitis
  acid clearance during sleep, 14–18
  Bernstein test of acid sensitivity, 12
  Pavlovian conditioning in, 40–41
  pH monitoring in, 12–14

Scleroderma
  esophageal motility in, 10, 36
Sleep
  acid clearance from the esophagus, 14–18
  esophageal motility, 28–29
  gastric motility and secretion, 189–191
  pulmonary aspiration in, 20
Smoking
  and gastric ulcers, 213
  and lower esophegeal sphincter, 37
Spectral analysis
  computer software for, 135, 140
  Fourier transforms defined, 97–98
  interpretive problems, 100–103, 107
  sampling rate theory, 138
  window transformations, 138–139
  See also Myoelectric activity
Spina bifida
  biofeedback for incontinence, 327–328
  external anal sphincter in, 315

Spina bifida *(Cont.)*
  fecal incontinence in, 299, 305, 307

Telemetry, 71–72, 165, 173–174
Thiry-Vella loop, 353–354

Ulcerative colitis
  colon motility in, 240, 247, 268–270
  psychological characteristics, 279

Visceral perception
  afferent nerves, 333
  alpha EEG blocking test of, 355
  animal models of, 337, 352–353
  awareness defined, 333–334
  awareness of gastrointestinal activity, 334–335, 353–354
  and behavioral self-regulation, 216, 341, 347
  of colon contractions, 345–346
  conditioned taste preferences, 341
  cultural differences in, 183–185
  discrimination without awareness, 334
  forced-choice test, 319
  habituation–discrimination test, 356
  of heart beats, 337
  Hertz, 331, 334–335
  Lacey intake–rejection theory, 215–216
  pain from colon distension, 281–282
  of rectal distension, 338
  stomach contractions, 334, 336–339, 344
  symptom perception questionnaire, 182–185
  Thiry-Vella loop preparation, 353–354
Vomiting (psychogenic)
  biofeedback treatment of, 6
  extinction for, 57–58
  mother–infant bonding, 47
  overcorrection for, 58
  Pavlovian conditioning, 46–47
  positive reinforcement, 57
  punishment, 52–54
  taste aversion punishment of, 56

Zollinger–Ellison syndrome
  gastric ulcers in, 213